Oxford American Handbook of

Urology

About the Oxford American Handbooks in Medicine

The Oxford American Handbooks are pocket clinical books, providing practical guidance in quick reference, note form. Titles cover major medical specialties or cross-specialty topics and are aimed at students, residents, internists, family physicians, and practicing physicians within specific disciplines.

Their reputation is built on including the best clinical information, complemented by hints, tips, and advice from the authors. Each one is carefully reviewed by senior subject experts, residents, and students to ensure that content reflects the reality of day-to-day medical practice.

Key series features

- Written in short chunks, each topic is covered in a two-page spread to enable readers to find information quickly. They are also perfect for test preparation and gaining a quick overview of a subject without scanning through unnecessary pages.
- Content is evidence based and complemented by the expertise and judgment of experienced authors.
- The Handbooks provide a humanistic approach to medicine – it's more than just treatment by numbers.
- A "friend in your pocket," the Handbooks offer honest, reliable guidance about the difficulties of practicing medicine and provide coverage of both the practice and art of medicine.
- For quick reference, useful "everyday" information is included on the inside covers.

Published and Forthcoming Oxford American Handbooks

Oxford American Handbook of Clinical Medicine
Oxford American Handbook of Anesthesiology
Oxford American Handbook of Cardiology
Oxford American Handbook of Clinical Dentistry
Oxford American Handbook of Clinical Diagnosis
Oxford American Handbook of Clinical Pharmacy
Oxford American Handbook of Critical Care
Oxford American Handbook of Emergency Medicine
Oxford American Handbook of Geriatric Medicine
Oxford American Handbook of Nephrology and Hypertension
Oxford American Handbook of Neurology
Oxford American Handbook of Obstetrics and Gynecology
Oxford American Handbook of Oncology
Oxford American Handbook of Otolaryngology
Oxford American Handbook of Pediatrics
Oxford American Handbook of Physical Medicine and Rehabilitation
Oxford American Handbook of Psychiatry
Oxford American Handbook of Pulmonary Medicine
Oxford American Handbook of Rheumatology
Oxford American Handbook of Sports Medicine
Oxford American Handbook of Surgery
Oxford American Handbook of Urology

Oxford American Handbook of **Urology**

Edited by

David M. Albala
Professor of Urology
Director of Minimally Invasive Urologic Surgery
Duke University Medical Center
Durham, North Carolina

Allen F. Morey
Chief, Urology Service
Parkland Memorial Hospital and Paul C. Peters Chair
Professor, Department of Urology
University of Texas Southwestern Medical Center
Dallas, Texas

Leonard G. Gomella
The Bernard W. Godwin Jr. Professor of Prostate Cancer
Chairman, Department of Urology
Thomas Jefferson University
Philadelphia, Pennsylvania

John P. Stein
Professor of Urology
Norris Comprehensive Cancer Center
University of Southern California Keck School of Medicine
Los Angeles, California

with

John Reynard
Simon Brewster
Suzanne Biers

OXFORD
UNIVERSITY PRESS

OXFORD
UNIVERSITY PRESS

Oxford University Press, Inc. publishes works that further
Oxford University's objective of excellence
in research, scholarship and education.

Oxford New York

Auckland Cape Town Dar es Salaam Hong Kong Karachi
Kuala Lumpur Madrid Melbourne Mexico City Nairobi
New Delhi Shanghai Taipei Toronto

With offices in

Argentina Austria Brazil Chile Czech Republic France Greece
Guatemala Hungary Italy Japan Poland Portugal
Singapore South Korea Switzerland Thailand Turkey Ukraine Vietnam

Published by Oxford University Press Inc.
198 Madison Avenue, New York, New York 10016

www.oup.com

Oxford is a registered trademark of Oxford University Press

First published 2011

Library of Congress Cataloging-in-Publication Data

Oxford American handbook of urology / edited by David M. Albala ... [et al.] ; with
John Reynard, Simon Brewster, Suzanne Biers.
p. ; cm.—Other title: Handbook of urology
Includes bibliographical references and index.
ISBN 978-0-19-537139-0

1. Urology—Handbooks, manuals, etc. 2. Urinary organs—Diseases—Handbooks,
manuals, etc. I. Albala, David M. II. Title: Handbook of urology.
[DNLM: 1. Urologic Diseases—Handbooks. 2. Female Urogenital Diseases—
Handbooks. 3. Male Urogenital Diseases—Handbooks. WJ 39 O973 2011]
RC872.9.O94 2011
616.6—dc22   2010003464

9 8 7 6 5 4 3 2 1

Printed in China
on acid-free paper

Preface

The goal of the *Oxford American Handbook of Urology* is to create a concise source of clinical information for medical students and physicians in training. This Handbook primarily presents the nonsurgical aspects of urology—the information needed for making a rapid diagnosis and determining the proper initial treatment course amid the confines of a busy clinical practice. It is meant to be a practical pocket reference, not an exhaustive treatise on urology.

As we witness the rapid pace of advancement in urological surgery, it becomes ever more difficult for any urologist to stay current in all areas of our specialty. The Handbook aims to provide the reader with an efficient information source that will be helpful in guiding effective management of our growing population of urological patients.

The book is written for our patients, with appreciation for the many mentors from whom we have learned, and for the many students and residents we have been fortunate to train. It is adapted for the American practice of urology from the *Oxford Handbook of Urology*, published in the UK, and we thank John Reynard, Simon Brewster, and Suzanne Biers for their fine book and the opportunity to "Americanize" it.

We dedicate this book to our colleague and friend, John P. Stein, M.D., whose untimely death has left a large void in our specialty. He was an accomplished clinician, researcher, and teacher who will be sorely missed.

David M. Albala, M.D.
Allen F. Morey, M.D.
Leonard G. Gomella, M.D.

Contents

Detailed contents *xi*
Symbols and Abbreviations *xxi*

1 Significance and preliminary investigation
of urological symptoms and signs | 1
2 Urological investigations | 35
3 Bladder outlet obstruction | 63
4 Incontinence | 109
5 Infections and inflammatory conditions | 133
6 Urological neoplasia | 185
7 Miscellaneous urological disease of the kidney | 331
8 Stone disease | 355
9 Upper tract obstruction, flank pain,
hydronephrosis | 405
10 Trauma to the urinary tract and other
urological emergencies | 419
11 Infertility | 465
12 Disorders of erectile function, ejaculation
and seminal vesicles | 483
13 Neuropathic bladder | 499
14 Urological problems in pregnancy | 531
15 Pediatric urology | 537
16 Urological surgery and equipment | 571
17 Basic science of relevance to urological practice | 659
18 Urological eponyms | 669

Index *673*

Detailed contents

1   Significance and preliminary investigation of urological symptoms and signs   1

Hematuria I: definition and types *2*
Hematuria II: causes and investigation *4*
Hematospermia *8*
Lower urinary tract symptoms (LUTS) *10*
Nocturia and nocturnal polyuria *14*
Flank pain *16*
Urinary incontinence in adults *20*
Genital symptoms *22*
Abdominal examination in urological disease *24*
Digital rectal examination (DRE) *28*
Lumps in the groin *30*
Lumps in the scrotum *32*

2   Urological investigations   35

Urine examination *36*
Urine cytology *38*
Prostatic specific antigen (PSA) *39*
Radiological imaging of the urinary tract *40*
Uses of plain abdominal radiography (KUB X-ray—kidneys, ureters, bladder) *42*
Intravenous pyelography (IVP) *44*
Other urological contrast studies *48*
Computed tomography (CT) and magnetic resonance imaging (MRI) *50*
Radioisotope imaging *52*
Uroflowmetry *54*
Post-void residual urine volume measurement *58*
Cystometry, pressure-flow studies, and videocystometry *60*

3   Bladder outlet obstruction   63

Regulation of prostate growth and development of benign prostatic hyperplasia (BPH) *64*
Pathophysiology and causes of bladder outlet obstruction (BOO) and BPH *66*
Benign prostatic obstruction (BPO): symptoms and signs *68*

Diagnostic tests in men with LUTS thought to be due to BPH *70*

Why do men seek treatment for their symptoms? *72*

Watchful waiting for uncomplicated BPH *74*

Medical management of BPH: α-blockers *76*

Medical management of BPH: 5α-reductase inhibitors *78*

Medical management of BPH: combination therapy *80*

Medical management of BPH: alternative drug therapy *82*

Minimally invasive management of BPH: surgical alternatives to TURP *84*

Invasive surgical alternatives to TURP *86*

TURP and open prostatectomy *88*

Acute urinary retention: definition, pathophysiology, and causes *90*

Acute urinary retention: initial and definitive management *94*

Indications for and technique of urethral catheterization *96*

Indications for and technique of suprapubic catheterization *98*

Management of nocturia and nocturnal polyuria *100*

High-pressure chronic retention (HPCR) *102*

Bladder outlet obstruction and retention in women *104*

Urethral stricture disease *106*

4   **Incontinence**   **109**

Classification *110*

Causes and pathophysiology *112*

Evaluation *114*

Treatment of sphincter weakness incontinence: injection therapy *116*

Treatment of sphincter weakness incontinence: retropubic suspension *117*

Treatment of sphincter weakness incontinence: pubovaginal slings *118*

Treatment of sphincter weakness incontinence: the artificial urinary sphincter *120*

Overactive bladder: conventional treatment *122*

Overactive bladder: options for failed conventional therapy *124*

"Mixed" incontinence *126*

Post-prostatectomy incontinence *128*

Vesicovaginal fistula (VVF) *130*

Incontinence in the elderly patient *132*

5   Infections and inflammatory conditions   133

Urinary tract infection: definitions, incidence, and
   investigations 134
Urinary tract infection: microbiology 138
Lower urinary tract infection 140
Recurrent urinary tract infection 142
Urinary tract infection: treatment 146
Acute pyelonephritis 148
Pyonephrosis and perinephric abscess 150
Other forms of pyelonephritis 152
Chronic pyelonephritis 154
Septicemia and urosepsis 156
Fournier gangrene 160
Epididymitis and orchitis 162
Periurethral abscess 164
Prostatitis: epidemiology and classification 166
Prostatitis: presentation, evaluation, and treatment 168
Other prostate infections 170
Interstitial cystitis 172
Tuberculosis 176
Parasitic infections 178
HIV in urological surgery 180
Inflammatory and other disorders of the penis 182

6   Urological neoplasia   185

Pathology and molecular biology 188
Prostate cancer: epidemiology and etiology 190
Prostate cancer: incidence, prevalence, and mortality 192
Prostate cancer pathology: premalignant lesions 193
Prostatic-specific antigen (PSA) and prostate cancer
   screening 194
Counseling before prostate cancer screening 195
Prostate cancer: clinical presentation 196
PSA and prostate cancer 198
PSA derivatives: free-to-total ratio, density, and velocity 200
Prostate cancer: transrectal ultrasonography and
   biopsies 202
Prostate cancer staging 206
Prostate cancer grading 212

Risk stratification in management of prostate cancer *214*

General principles of management of localized prostate cancer *215*

Management of localized prostate cancer: watchful waiting and active surveillance *216*

Management of localized prostate cancer: radical prostatectomy *218*

Postoperative course after radical prostatectomy *222*

Prostate cancer control with radical prostatectomy *224*

Management of localized prostate cancer: radical external beam radiotherapy (EBRT) *226*

Management of localized prostate cancer: brachytherapy (BT) *228*

Management of localized and radiorecurrent prostate cancer: cryotherapy and HIFU *230*

Management of locally advanced nonmetastatic prostate cancer (T3–4 N0M0) *232*

Management of advanced prostate cancer: hormone therapy I *233*

Management of advanced prostate cancer: hormone therapy II *234*

Management of advanced prostate cancer: hormone therapy III *238*

Management of advanced prostate cancer: androgen-independent/ castration-resistant disease *240*

Palliative management of prostate cancer *242*

Prostate cancer: prevention; complementary and alternative therapies *244*

Bladder cancer: epidemiology and etiology *246*

Bladder cancer: pathology and staging *248*

Bladder cancer: presentation *252*

Bladder cancer: diagnosis and staging *254*

Management of superficial UC: transurethral resection of bladder tumor (TURBT) *256*

Management of superficial UC: adjuvant intravesical chemotherapy and BCG *258*

Muscle-invasive bladder cancer: surgical management of localized (pT2/3a) disease *260*

Muscle-invasive bladder cancer: radical and palliative radiotherapy *263*

Muscle-invasive bladder cancer: management of locally advanced and metastatic disease *264*

Bladder cancer: urinary diversion after cystectomy *266*

Transitional cell carcinoma (UC) of the renal pelvis and ureter 270

Radiological assessment of renal masses 274

Benign renal masses 276

Renal cell carcinoma: epidemiology and etiology 278

Renal cell carcinoma: pathology, staging, and prognosis 280

Renal cell carcinoma: presentation and investigations 284

Renal cell carcinoma: active surveillance 286

Renal cell carcinoma: surgical treatment I 288

Renal cell carcinoma: surgical treatment II 290

Renal cell carcinoma: management of metastatic disease 292

Testicular cancer: epidemiology and etiology 294

Testicular cancer: clinical presentation 296

Testicular cancer: serum markers 299

Testicular cancer: pathology and staging 300

Testicular cancer: prognostic staging system for metastatic germ cell cancer 303

Testicular cancer: management of non-seminomatous germ cell tumors (NSGCT) 304

Testicular cancer: management of seminoma, IGCN, and lymphoma 308

Penile neoplasia: benign, viral-related, and premalignant lesions 310

Penile cancer: epidemiology, risk factors, and pathology 314

Squamous cell carcinoma of the penis: clinical management 318

Carcinoma of the scrotum 320

Tumors of the testicular adnexa 321

Urethral cancer 322

Retroperitoneal fibrosis 326

Wilms tumor and neuroblastoma 328

7   Miscellaneous urological diseases of the kidney   331

Cystic renal disease: simple cysts 332

Cystic renal disease: calyceal diverticulum 334

Cystic renal disease: medullary sponge kidney (MSK) 336

Acquired renal cystic disease (ARCD) 338

Autosomal dominant (adult) polycystic kidney disease (ADPKD) 340

Vesicoureteric reflux (VUR) in adults 342

Ureteropelvic junction (UPJ) obstruction in adults 346
Anomalies of renal ascent and fusion: horseshoe kidney,
    pelvic kidney, malrotation 348
Renal duplications 352

8   **Stone disease**   355

Kidney stones: epidemiology 356
Kidney stones: types and predisposing factors 358
Kidney stones: mechanisms of formation 360
Factors predisposing to specific stone types 362
Evaluation of the stone former 366
Kidney stones: presentation and diagnosis 368
Kidney stone treatment options: watchful waiting 370
Stone fragmentation techniques: extracorporeal lithotripsy
    (ESWL) 372
Intracorporeal techniques of stone fragmentation
    (fragmentation within the body) 374
Kidney stone treatment: flexible ureteroscopy and laser
    treatment 378
Kidney stone treatment: percutaneous nephrolithotomy
    (PCNL) 380
Kidney stones: open stone surgery 383
Kidney stones: medical therapy (dissolution therapy) 384
Ureteric stones: presentation 386
Ureteric stones: diagnostic radiological imaging 388
Ureteric stones: acute management 390
Ureteric stones: indications for intervention to relieve
    obstruction and/or remove the stone 392
Ureteric stone treatment 394
Treatment options for ureteric stones 396
Prevention of calcium oxalate stone formation 398
Bladder stones 400
Management of ureteric stones in pregnancy 402

9   **Upper tract obstruction, flank pain, hydronephrosis 405**

Hydronephrosis 406
Management of ureteric strictures (other than UPJ
    obstruction) 410
Pathophysiology of urinary tract obstruction 414
Physiology of urine flow from kidneys to bladder 416
Ureter innervation 417

10   Trauma to the urinary tract and other urological emergencies   **419**

Renal trauma: classification and grading *420*

Renal trauma: clinical and radiological assessment *422*

Renal trauma: treatment *426*

Ureteral injuries: mechanisms and diagnosis *432*

Ureteral injuries: management *434*

Bladder and urethral injuries associated with pelvic fractures *440*

Bladder injuries *444*

Posterior urethral injuries in males and urethral injuries in females *448*

Anterior urethral injuries *452*

Testicular injuries *454*

Penile injuries *456*

Torsion of the testis and testicular appendages *460*

Paraphimosis *462*

Malignant ureteral obstruction *463*

Spinal cord and cauda equina compression *464*

11   Infertility   **465**

Male reproductive physiology *466*

Etiology and evaluation of male infertility *470*

Lab investigation of male infertility *472*

Oligospermia and azoospermia *476*

Varicocele *478*

Treatment options for male factor infertility *480*

12   Disorders of erectile function, ejaculation, and seminal vesicles   **483**

Physiology of erection and ejaculation *484*

Impotence: evaluation *488*

Impotence: treatment *490*

Retrograde ejaculation *492*

Peyronie's disease *494*

Priapism *496*

13   Neuropathic bladder   **499**

Innervation of the lower urinary tract (LUT) *500*

Physiology of urine storage and micturition *504*

Bladder and sphincter behavior in the patient with
neurological disease 506

The neuropathic lower urinary tract: clinical consequences
of storage and emptying problems 508

Bladder management techniques for the neuropathic
patient 510

Catheters and sheaths and the neuropathic patient 516

Management of incontinence in the neuropathic
patient 518

Management of recurrent urinary tract infections (UTIs)
in the neuropathic patient 520

Management of hydronephrosis in the neuropathic
patient 522

Management of autonomic dysreflexia in the neuropathic
patient 523

Bladder dysfunction in multiple sclerosis, in Parkinson
disease, after stroke, and in other neurological
disease 524

Neuromodulation in lower urinary tract dysfunction 528

14   Urological problems in pregnancy   531

Physiological and anatomical changes in the urinary
tract 532

Urinary tract infection (UTI) 534

Hydronephrosis 536

15   Pediatric urology   537

Embryology: urinary tract 538

Undescended testes 540

Urinary tract infection (UTI) 542

Vesicoureteric reflux (VUR) 544

Ectopic ureter 546

Ureterocele 548

Ureteropelvic junction (UPJ) obstruction 549

Hypospadias 550

Normal sexual differentiation 552

Abnormal sexual differentiation 554

Cystic kidney disease 558

Exstrophy 560

Epispadias 562

Posterior urethral valves 564

Non-neurogenic voiding dysfunction *566*
Nocturnal enuresis *568*

16   **Urological surgery and equipment**   **571**

Preparation of the patient for urological surgery *572*
Antibiotic prophylaxis in urological surgery *574*
Complications of surgery in general: DVT and PE *576*
Fluid balance and management of shock in the surgical
    patient *580*
Patient safety in the operating room *582*
Transurethral resection (TUR) syndrome *583*
Catheters and drains in urological surgery *584*
Guide wires *590*
Irrigating fluids and techniques of bladder washout *592*
JJ stents *594*
Lasers in urological surgery *598*
Diathermy *600*
Sterilization of urological equipment *604*
Telescopes and light sources in urological endoscopy *606*
Consent: general principles *608*
Cystoscopy *610*
Transurethral resection of the prostate (TURP) *612*
Transurethral resection of bladder tumor (TURBT) *614*
Optical urethrotomy *616*
Circumcision *618*
Hydrocele and epididymal cyst removal *620*
Nesbit procedure *622*
Vasectomy and vasovasostomy *624*
Orchiectomy *626*
Urological incisions *628*
JJ stent insertion *630*
Nephrectomy and nephroureterectomy *632*
Radical prostatectomy *634*
Radical cystectomy *636*
Ileal conduit *640*
Percutaneous nephrolithotomy (PCNL) *642*
Ureteroscopes and ureteroscopy *646*
Pyeloplasty *650*
Laparoscopic surgery *652*

Endoscopic cystolitholapaxy and (open) cystolithotomy 654
Scrotal exploration for torsion and orchiopexy 656

17   Basic science of relevance to urological practice   659

Physiology of bladder and urethra 660
Renal anatomy: renal blood flow and renal function 661
Renal physiology: regulation of water balance 664
Renal physiology: regulation of sodium and potassium
    excretion 665
Renal physiology: acid–base balance 666

18   Urological eponyms   669

Index 673

Symbols and Abbreviations

↓	decreased
↑	increased
AAA	abdominal aortic aneurysm
AAOS	American Academy of Orthopedic Surgeons
ABC	airway, breathing, circulation
ABG	arterial blood gas
ABP	acute bacterial prostatitis
ACE	angiotensin-converting enzyme
ACTH	adrenocorticotrophic hormone
AD	autonomic dysreflexia
ADA	adenosine deaminase
ADH	antidiuretic hormone
ADPKD	autosomal dominant polycystic kidney disease
AFP	A-fetoprotein
AID	artificial insemination using donor
AK-TEDS	above-knee thromboembolic stocking
ALT	alanine aminotransferase
AML	angiomyolipoma
ANP	atrial natriuretic peptide
AP	anteroposterior
AR	adrenoreceptor
5-AR	5A-reductase
ARC	AIDS-related complex
ARCD	acquired renal cystic disease
ARF	acute renal failure
ART	assisted reproductive technique
ASAP	atypical small acinar proliferation
AST	aspartate aminotransferase
ASTRO	American Society of Therapeutic Radiation Oncologists
AUA	American Urological Association
AUS	artificial urinary sphincter
AV	arteriovenous
BCG	bacillus Calmette–Guérin
BCR	bulbocavernosus reflex
BEP	bleomycin, etoposide, cisplatin
bFGF	basic fibroblast growth factor
bid	twice daily

BMI	body mass index
BNI	bladder neck incision
BOO	bladder outlet obstruction
BP	blood pressure
BPE	benign prostatic enlargement
BPH	benign prostatic hyperplasia
BPO	benign prostatic obstruction
BSA	body surface area
BT	brachytherapy
BTX-A	botulinum toxin A
BUN	blood urea nitrogen
BUO	bilateral ureter obstruction
BXO	balanitis xerotica obliterans
CAH	congenital adrenal hyperplasia
CAR	cancer-associated retinopathy
CAVD	congenital absence of vas deferens
CBC	complete blood count
CBP	chronic bacterial prostatitis
CIS	carcinoma in situ
CISC	clean, intermittent self-catheterization
CMV	cisplatin, methotrexate, vinblastin or cytogmegalovirus
CNS	central nervous system
CPPS	chronic pelvic pain syndrome
Cr	creatinine
CRPC	castration-resistant prostatic cancer
CT	computerized tomography
CTPA	CT pulmonary angiogram
CTU	CT urogram
CXR	chest X-ray
DH	detrusor hyperreflexia
DHT	dihydrotestosterone
DI	diabetes insipidus
DIC	disseminated intravascular coagulation
DLPP	detrusor leak point pressure
DO	detrusor overactivity
DRE	digital rectal exam
DSD	detrusor sphincter dyssynergia; disorders of sexual development
DVT	deep venous thromboembolism
EAU	European Association of Urology
EBRT	external beam radiotherapy
EBV	Epstein–Barr virus

EC	etoposide, carboplatin (lung cancer) *or* epirubicin, cyclophosphamide (breast cancer)
ECG	electrocardiogram
ECF	extracellular fluid
EGF	epidermal growth factor
EHL	electrohydraulic lithotripsy
EMG	electromyogram
EMU	early morning urine
EORTC	European Organization for Research and Treatment of Cancer
EPS	expressed prostatic secretion
ERSPC	European Randomized Study of Screening for Prostate Cancer
ESR	erythrocyte sedimentation rate
ESWL	extracorporeal shock wave lithotripsy
FBC	full blood count
FDA	(U.S.) Food and Drug Administration
FEV_1	forced expiratory volume in 1 second
FISH	fluorescent in situ hybridization
FNA	fine needle aspiration
FSH	follicle-stimulating hormone
F:T	free-to-total (PSA ratio)
5-FU	5-fluorouracil
FVC	forced vital capacity
GAG	glycosaminoglycan
GCT	germ cell tumor
GFR	glomerular filtration rate
GH	growth hormone
GI	gastrointestinal
GIFT	gamete intrafallopian transfer
GnRH	gonadotrophin-releasing hormone
GU	genitourinary; gonococcal urethritis
Gy	Gray(s)
HA	hemagglutinin
hCG	human chorionic gonadotrophin
HDR	high-dose radiation
HGPIN	high-grade prostatic intraepithelial neoplasia
HIFU	high-intensity focused ultrasound
HIV	human immunodeficiency virus
HIVAN	HIV-associated nephropathy
HLA	human leukocyte antigen
HNPCC	hereditary nonpolyposis colorectal cancer
HoLEP	holium laser enucleation of the prostate

HoLRP	holium laser resection of the prostate
HPF	high-powered field
HPRC	high-pressure chronic retention
HPRCC	hereditary papillary renal cell carcinoma
HPV	human papillomavirus
HSV	herpes simplex virus
IC	intermittent catheterization; interstitial cystitis
ICF	intracellular fluid
ICS	International Continence Society
ICSI	intracytoplasmic sperm injection
IDC	indwelling catheterization
IFN	interferon (IFN-α, IFN-β, etc.)
IGCN	intratubular germ cell neoplasia
IGF	insulin-like growth factor
IL	interleukin (IL-1, IL-4, etc.)
ILP	interstitial laser prostatectomy
IM	intramuscular
INR	international normalized ratio
IORT	intraoperative radiotherapy
IPC	intermittent pneumatic calf compression
IPSS	International Prostate Symptom Score
ISC	intermittent self-catheterization
ISD	intrinsic sphincter deficiency
IUI	intrauterine insemination
IV	intravenous
IVC	inferior vena cava
IVF	in vitro fertilization
IVP	intravenous pyelography
IVU	intravenous urography
JVP	jugular venous pressure
KGF	keratinocyte growth factor
KUB	kidneys, ureters, bladder
LDH	lactate dehydrogenase
LDUH	low-dose unfractionated heparin
LFT	liver function test
LH	luteinizing hormone
LHRH	luteinizing hormone–releasing hormone
LMWH	low molecular-weight heparin
LUTS	lower urinary tract symptoms
MAB	maximal androgen blockade
MAR	mixed agglutination reaction (test)

MCUG	micturating cystourethrography
MESA	microsurgical epididymal sperm aspiration
MI	myocardial infarction
MMC	mitomycin C
MRI	magnetic resonance imaging
MRU	magnetic resonance urography
MRSA	methicillin-resistant *Staphylococcus aureas*
MS	multiple sclerosis
MSA	multiple system atrophy
MSK	medullary sponge kidney
MSU	mid-stream specimen of urine
MTX	methotrexate
MUCP	maximal urethral closure pressure
MVAC	methotrexate, vinblastine, doxorubicin, cisplatin
MVP	methotrexate, vinblastine, cisplatin
NCCN	National Comprehensive Cancer Network
NCI	National Cancer Institute
NDO	neurogenic detrusor overactivity
NGU	nongonococcal urethritis
NIDDK	National Institute of Diabetes, Digestive and Kidney Disease
NIH	National Institutes of Health
NO	nitrous oxide
NP	nocturnal polyuria
NSAID	nonsteroidal anti-inflammatory drug
OAB	overactive bladder
OP	open prostatectomy
PAG	periaqueductal gray matter
PC	prostate cancer
PCNL	percutaneous nephrolithotomy
PCPT	Prostate Cancer Prevention Trial
PD	Parkinson's disease
PDE5	phosphodiesterase type 5
PE	pulmonary embolism
PESA	percutaneous epididymal sperm aspiration
PFS	pressure-flow study
PGE	prostaglandin E
PLCO	Prostate, Lung, Colorectal, and Ovarian (study)
PMC	pontine micturition center
PO	orally, by mouth
PR	pulse rate
PSA	prostatic-specific antigen

PSADT	PSA doubling time
PTC	percutaneous transhepatic cholangiopancreatography
PTH	parathyroid hormone
PTTI	parenchymal transit time index
PUJO	pelviureteric junction obstruction
PUV	posterior urethral valve
PVR	post-void residual urine
qid	four times a day
RALP	robotically assisted laparoscopic prostatectomy
RBF	renal blood flow
RCC	renal cell carcinoma
RFA	radiofrequency ablation
RP	radical prostatectomy
RPF	retroperitoneal fibrosis; renal plasma flow
RPLND	retroperitoneal lymph node dissection
RR	respiratory rate
RT	radiation therapy
RTA	renal tubular acidosis
RTOG	Radiation Therapy Oncology Group
SBRT	stereotactic body radiotherapy
SC	subcutaneous
SCC	squamous cell carcinoma
SCI	spinal cord injury
SHBT	sex hormone–binding globulin
SIRS	systemic inflammatory response syndrome
SLE	systemic lupus erythematosus
SNM	sacral nerve modulation
SNS	sacral nerve stimulation
STD	sexually transmitted disease
SUI	stress urinary incontinence
SV	seminal vesicle
SWOG	Southwest Oncology Group
TB	tuberculosis
TBW	total body water
TC	testicular cancer
TCC	transitional cell carcinoma
TENS	transcutaneous electrical nerve stimulation
TESA	transcutaneous epididymal sperm aspiration
TGF	transforming growth factor
TIA	transient ischemic attack
tid	three times a day

TMP-SMZ	trimethoprim-sulfamethoxazole
TNF	tumor necrosis factor (TNF-α)
TNM	tumor–node–metastasis (staging system for cancer)
TRUS	transrectal ultrasound
TSE	testicular self-examination
TULIP	transurethral ultrasound-guided laser induced prostatectomy
TUMT	transurethral microwave thermotherapy
TUNA	transurethral radiofrequency needle aspiration
TUR	transurethral resection
TURBT	transurethral resection of bladder tumor
TURP	transurethral resection of the prostate
TUVP	transurethral electrovaporization of the prostate
TWOC	trial without catheter
UC	urothelial carcinoma
UFH	unfractionated heparin
UI	urinary incontinence
UPJO	ureteropelvic junction obstruction
US	ultrasound
UTI	urinary tract infection
UUI	urge urinary incontinence
UUO	unilateral obstruction of the ureter
VAD	vincristine, Adriamycin, dexamethasone
VAPEC-B	vincristine, doxorubicin, prednisolone, etoposide, cyclophosphamide, bleomycin
VAC	vacuum-assisted closure
VCUG	videocystourethrography
VEGF	vascular endothelial growth factor
VHL	von Hippel–Lindau (syndrome)
VLAP	visual laser ablation of the prostate
VLPP	Valsalva leak point pressure
VTE	venous thromboembolism
VUR	vesicoureteric reflux
VVF	vesicovaginal fistula
WAGR	Wilms tumor (associated with) aniridia, genitourinary abnormalities, mental retardation
WBC	white blood cell
WHO	World Health Organization
ZIFT	zygote intrafallopian transfer

Significance and preliminary investigation of urological symptoms and signs

Hematuria I: definition and types *2*
Hematuria II: causes and investigation *4*
Hematospermia *8*
Lower urinary tract symptoms (LUTS) *10*
Nocturia and nocturnal polyuria *14*
Flank pain *16*
Urinary incontinence in adults *20*
Genital symptoms *22*
Abdominal examination in urological disease *24*
Digital rectal examination (DRE) *28*
Lumps in the groin *30*
Lumps in the scrotum *32*

Hematuria I: definition and types

Definition

Hematuria is the presence of blood in the urine.

Macroscopic (gross) hematuria is visible to the naked eye.

Microscopic or dipstick hematuria is when blood is identified by urine microscopy or dipstick testing, either in association with other urological symptoms (*symptomatic* microscopic hematuria) or during a routine medical examination (*asymptomatic* microscopic hematuria).

Microscopic hematuria is generally defined as 3 or more red blood cells (RBCs) per high-power field on a centrifuged specimen confirmed on 2 of 3 properly collected specimens.[1,2]

Urine dipsticks test for heme test for hemoglobin and myoglobin in the urine. The peroxidase-like activity of heme is used to catalyze reactions that produce colored compounds ranging from orange to green and dark blue. Dipsticks have a sensitivity of 90%, detecting 5 RBC/microliter. Confirm the presence of RBCs on a dipstick with microscopic exam to rule out a false positive.

- *False positive urine dipstick:* menstrual or dysfunctional uterine bleeding contamination, or the presence of myoglobinuria, free hemoglobin (e.g., transfusion reaction), bacterial peroxidases, povidone, hypochlorite
- *False negative urine dipstick (rare):* in the presence of reducing agents (e.g., ascorbic acid prevents the reagent strip oxidation reaction)

Is microscopic or dipstick hematuria abnormal?

A few RBCs can be found in the urine of normal people. The upper limit of normal for RBC excretion is 1 million/24 hours (as seen in healthy medical students). In healthy male soldiers undergoing yearly urine examination over a 12-year period, 40% had microscopic hematuria on at least 1 occasion and 15% on 2 or more occasions. Transient microscopic hematuria may occur following rigorous exercise or sexual intercourse.

A catheterized urinary specimen may be needed if a voided specimen cannot be reliably obtained (e.g., vaginal contamination, obesity, men with nonretractile foreskin [phimosis]).

Because the presence of RBCs in the urine is normal, a substantial proportion of patients with microscopic and dipstick hematuria and even macroscopic hematuria will have normal hematuria investigations (i.e., no abnormality is found). No abnormality is found in approximately 50% of subjects with gross hematuria and 70% with microscopic hematuria, despite full conventional urological investigation (urine cytology, cystoscopy, upper tract imaging).[2]

1 Grossfeld GD, Litwin MS, Wolf JS, et al. (2001). Evaluation of asymptomatic microscopic hematuria in adults: the American Urological Association best practice policy—part I: definition, detection, prevalence, and etiology. *Urology* 57:599–603.
2 Khadra MH, Pickard RS, Charlton M, et al. (2000). A prospective analysis of 1930 patients with hematuria to evaluate current diagnostic practice. *J Urol* 163:524–527.

Hematuria II: causes and investigation

Any degree of confirmed hematuria should be evaluated, as it may be a sign of serious renal or urological disease, including malignancy (up to 20%). Gross hematuria is 5 times more likely to indicate a serious urological problem than is microscopic hematuria.

Common causes of hematuria

Although there is considerable overlap, hematuria in the clinical setting can be most broadly classified into surgical (urological) and medical causes, to help facilitate evaluation and management. Presence of white blood cells (WBCs) or bacteria, protein, red cell casts, or elevated serum creatine (Cr) and age of the patient may also be used to determine the cause.

Surgical (urological)

- Cancer: urothelial carcinoma or squamous cell carcinoma of the urethra, bladder, ureter, or renal pelvis; renal cell carcinoma; prostate cancer; other less common tumor types (sarcoma, adenocarcinoma)
- Stones (urolithiasis): kidney, renal pelvis, ureter, bladder
- Infection: pyelonephritis, cystitis, prostatitis, urethritis caused by agents such as bacterial, mycobacterial (TB), parasitic (schistosomiasis), fungal (Candida)
- Inflammation: cyclophosphamide cystitis, interstitial cystitis, radiation cystitis
- Trauma (blunt and penetrating): kidney, bladder, urethra (e.g., traumatic catheterization), pelvic fracture with urethral disruption
- Renal cystic disease: e.g., medullary sponge kidney
- Congenital abnormalities: vesicoureteral reflux, posterior urethral valves, ureteropelvic junction obstruction

Other urological causes include benign prostatic hyperpasia (BPH) (the large, vascular prostate), urethral stricture, fistula, urethral diverticulum, cystocele, recent surgical intervention, flank pain hematuria syndrome, and vascular malformations.

Medical (nephrological)

Medical causes of hematuria are more likely in children and young adults and if it is associated with proteinuria, elevated creatinine, or dysmorphic red cells/RBC casts. Glomerulonephritis is responsible for 30% of all cases of pediatric hematuria.

Renal parenchymal disease occurs with IgA nephropathy (Berger disease), postinfectious glomerulonephritis, and, less commonly, membrano-proliferative glomerulonephritis, Henoch–Schönlein purpura, vasculitis, Alport syndrome, thin basement membrane disease, and Fabry disease.

Other medical causes include coagulation disorders (congenital, such as hemophilia) or anticoagulation therapy; sickle cell trait or disease; renal papillary necrosis; hypercalcuria; and vascular disease (e.g., emboli to the kidney with infarction and hematuria).

Urological investigation of hematuria

In patients without evidence suggestive of medical renal disease, conventional urological investigation involves urine culture (if symptoms suggest urinary infection), urine cytology, cystoscopy, and upper tract imaging. Anticoagulation or aspirin use should never be automatically assumed to be the cause of hematuria. In these patients, malignancy can be seen in up to 24% and any hematuria should be evaluated.[1]

Patients with documented urinary tract infection (UTI) should be treated appropriately, and the urinalysis repeated approximately 4–6 weeks after treatment. If the hematuria resolves with treatment, no further evaluation is usually needed.[2]

In low-risk patients (<40 years without gross hematuria, no smoking history, no chemical exposure [i.e., benzenes or aromatic amines], no previous cyclophosphamide treatment, no irritative voiding complaints, no pelvic radiation, or no urological disease history), initial upper tract imaging is indicated, with further evaluation based on clinical findings.

In patients with high risk factors (high risk for urothelial carcinoma anywhere in the urinary tract), compete evaluation is indicated given the greater risk of malignancy.

Diagnostic cystoscopy

Typically this is carried out using a flexible, fiber-optic cystoscope in the outpatient setting with intraurethral lidocaine anesthesia.
- If radiological investigation demonstrates a lesion suggesting a urothelial carcinoma such as a bladder cancer, one may consider foregoing the flexible cystoscopy and proceed immediately to rigid cystoscopy and biopsy under anesthesia (transurethral resection of bladder tumor [TURBT]).
- Upper tract filling (renal pelvis, ureter) defects may also represent urothelial carcinoma or stones. Further intraoperative evaluation with retrograde pyelograms and ureteroscopy can be both diagnostic and therapeutic. However, the bladder must still be evaluated carefully with cystoscopy.

Should cystoscopy be performed in patients with asymptomatic microscopic hematuria?

The American Urological Association's (AUA's) *Best Practice Policy on Asymptomatic Microscopic Hematuria* recommends cystoscopy in all high-risk patients with microscopic hematuria (see risk factors on previous page).[3] In asymptomatic, low-risk patients <40 years of age, it states that "it may be appropriate to defer cystoscopy," but if this is done, urine should be sent for cytology.

1 Avidor Y, Nadu A, Matzkin H (2000). Clinical significance of gross hematuria and its evaluation in patients receiving anticoagulant and aspirin treatment. *Urology* 55(1):22–24.
2 Mariani AJ (1998). The evaluation of adult hematuria: a clinical update. In *AUA Update Series* 1998; Vol. XVII, lesson 24, pp. 185–192. Houston: AUA Office of Education.
3 Grossfeld GD (2001). Evaluation of asymptomatic microscopic hematuria in adults: the American Urological Association Best Practise Policy-Part II: patient evaluation, cytology, voided markers, imaging, cystoscopy, nephrology evaluation and follow-up. *Urology* 57:604–610.

However, the AUA also states that "the decision as to when to proceed with cystoscopy in low-risk patients with persistent microscopic hematuria must be made on an individual basis after a careful discussion between the patient and physician." Some clinicians believe that patients should be allowed to make a decision as to whether or not to proceed with cystoscopy, based on their interpretation of low risk.

What is the best upper tract imaging study for the evaluation of hematuria?

Intravenous pyelography (IVP), ultrasonography (US), and computed tomography (CT) are used in the workup of hematuria. Currently, there are no evidence-based imaging guidelines.

IVP is the traditional modality for urinary tract imaging. IVP alone can miss small renal masses and is unable to discriminate cystic from solid lesions and is therefore often combined with ultrasonography.

Ultrasonography can detect masses, stones, or obstruction. However, for the detection of urothelial carcinoma of the renal pelvis kidney or ureter, IVP or CT urogram is superior to US.

CT is considered the best modality for the evaluation of urinary stones, renal masses, and renal infections.

Contrast is not necessary to screen for urolithiasis and renal neoplasm. Contrast-enhanced CT urography results in visualization of the collecting system, comparable to that of IVP. At many centers, CT urography has completely replaced the IVP, as it combines visualization of the parenchyma and collecting system.[4]

Magnetic resonance imaging (MRI) is limited in the initial evaluation of hematuria.

Retrograde pyelography (RPG) is also considered an acceptable technique for upper tract collecting system evaluation. Because RPG is more invasive, it is generally reserved as a second-line study to further evaluate abnormalities detected initially on CT or IVP.

If no cause for hematuria is found (microscopic or macroscopic) is further investigation necessary?

Some say yes, quoting studies that show serious disease can be identified in a small number of patients in whom retrograde pyelography, endoscopic examination of the ureters and renal pelvis (ureteroscopy), contrast CT, and renal angiography were also done. Others say no, citing the absence of development of overt urological cancer during 2- to 4-year follow-up in patients originally presenting with microscopic or macroscopic hematuria (though without further investigations).[5]

When urine cytology, cystoscopy, renal US, and IVP are all normal, we perform CT scanning of the kidneys and ureters and retrograde pyelography in the following situations:

4 Stacul F, Rossi A, Cova MA (2008). CT urography: the end of IVU? *Radiol Med* 113(5):658–669.
5 Khadra MH (2000) A prospective analysis of 1930 patients with hematuria to evaluate current diagnostic practice. *J Urol* 163:524–527.

- Patients at high risk for transitional cell cancer (TCC). Risk factors for development of TCC of the urothelium (bladder, kidneys, renal pelvis, ureters) include positive smoking history, occupational exposure to chemicals or dyes, analgesic abuse (phenacetin), and history of pelvic irradiation.[6]
- Microscopic or dipstick hematuria persists at 3 months.
- Macroscopic hematuria persists.

At a minimum, follow-up routine urinalysis in patients with an initial negative workup is reasonable.

6 Patel JV, Chambers CV, Gomella LG (2008). Hematuria: etiology and evaluation for the primary care physician. *Can J Urol.* Suppl 1:54–61; discussion 62. Review.

Hematospermia

Sometimes spelled "hemospermia," *hematospermia* is the presence of blood in the semen. It can be bright red, coffee-colored, rusty, or darkened in appearance and may change as blood ages. Usually hematospermia is intermittent, benign, or self-limiting and has no cause identified.

Causes
- *Iatrogenic:* following prostate biopsy, cystoscopy or prostate intervention (resection, hyperthermia), prostate brachytherapy or radiation; usually clears in weeks to months
- *Age <40 years:* usually inflammatory (e.g., prostatitis, epididymo-orchitis, urethritis, urethral condylomata) or idiopathic (this cause likely reflects the limited investigation usually carried out in this age group). Rarely there is testicular tumor, or perineal or testicular trauma.
- *Age >40 years:* as for men aged <40, prostate cancer; bladder cancer; BPH with dilated veins in the prostatic urethra; prostatic or seminal vesicle (SV) calculi; hypertension; carcinoma of the seminal vesicles
- *Rare causes at any age:* bleeding diathesis; utricular cysts; Müllerian cysts; TB; schistosomiasis; amyloid of prostate or seminal vesicles; following therapeutic injection of hemorrhoids

Examination

Examine the testes, epididymis, prostate, and seminal vesicles. On digital rectal exam (DRE) evaluate for nodularity, tenderness, masses, midline and cystic structures. SV fullness can be associated with schistosomiasis (egg burden). Measure blood pressure.

Investigation

Send urine for culture. If the hematospermia resolves, an argument can be made for doing nothing else. If it recurs or persists, arrange a transrectal ultrasound (TRUS), flexible cystoscopy, and renal ultrasound. If hematuria coexists, investigate with an upper tract imaging study and cystoscopy (as described in Chapter 2). In general, evaluation in men >40 years of age should be more extensive.

Treatment
- Directed at the underlying abnormality, if found
- Watchful waiting in most men if no cause identified
- Empiric antibiotics (doxycycline or flouroqinolones) sometimes considered

Further reading
Ahmad I, Krishna NS (2007). Hemospermia. *J Urol* 177:1613–1618.
Kumar P, Kapoor S, Nargund V (2006). Haematospermia—a systemic review. *Ann R Coll Surg Engl* 88:339–342.
Leocadio DE, Stein BS (2009). Hematospermia: etiological and management considerations. *Int Urol Nephrol* 41(1):77–83.

Lower urinary tract symptoms (LUTS)

Many terms have been coined to describe the symptom complex traditionally associated with prostatic obstruction due to BPH. The classic
prostatic symptoms of hesitancy, poor flow, frequency, urgency, nocturia,
and terminal dribbling have in the past been termed *prostatism* or simply
BPH symptoms. One sometimes hears these symptoms being described
as due to BPO (benign prostatic obstruction) or BPE (benign prostatic
enlargement) or, more recently, LUTS/BPH.

However, these "classic" symptoms of prostatic disease bear little
relationship to prostate size, urinary flow rate, residual urine volume, or
urodynamic evidence of bladder outlet obstruction (BOO).[1] Furthermore,
age-matched men and women have similar "prostate" symptom scores;[2]
women obviously have no prostate.

Therefore, these terms are no longer used to describe the symptom
complex of hesitancy, poor flow, etc. Instead, the preferred term today
is *lower urinary tract symptoms (LUTS)*, which is purely a descriptive term
avoiding any implication about the possible underlying cause of these
symptoms.[3]

The new terminology of LUTS is useful because it reminds the urologist to consider possible alternative causes of symptoms, which may have
absolutely nothing to do with prostatic obstruction. It also reminds us to
avoid operating on an organ, such as the prostate, when the cause of the
symptoms may lie elsewhere.

Overactive bladder is a newly defined symptom complex during which
patients experience urgency with or without urge incontinence, usually
accompanied by frequency and/or nocturia.[4]

Baseline symptoms can be measured using a validated symptom index.
The most widely used in men is the International Prostate Symptom Score
(IPSS), a modified version of the AUA Symptom Index[5] (Fig. 1.1). It is
useful for the initial evaluation and for determining the effectiveness of
therapeutic intervention.

Other causes of LUTS

In broad terms, LUTS can be due to pathology in the prostate, the bladder,
the urethra, or other pelvic organs (uterus, rectum) or to neurological
disease affecting the nerves that innervate the bladder. These pathologic
processes can include benign enlargement of the prostate causing bladder
outflow obstruction (BPE causing BOO) and infective, inflammatory, and

1 Reynard JM, Yang Q, Donovan JL, et al. (1998) The ICS-'BPH' study: uroflowmetry, lower urinary tract symptoms and bladder outlet obstruction. *Br J Urol* 82:619–623.
2 Lepor H, Machi G (1993) Comparison of AUA symptom index in unselected males and females between fifty-five and seventy-nine years of age. *Urology* 42:36–41.
3 Abrams P (1994). New words for old—lower urinary tracy symptoms for 'prostatism'. *Br Med J* 308:929–930.
4 Voelzke BB (2007). Overactive bladder; prevalence, pathophysiology, and pharmacotherapy. *Urol Rep* 1:16–22.
5 Barry MJ, Fowler FJ Jr, O'Leary MP, et al. (1992) The American Urological Association Symptom Index for benign prostatic hyperplasia. *J Urol* 148:1549–1557.

	Not at all	Less than 1 time in 5	Less than half the time	About half the time	More than half the time	Almost always	Score
Incomplete emptying. Over the last month, how often have you had a sensation of not emptying your bladder completely after you finish urinating?	0	1	2	3	4	5	
Frequency. Over the last month, how often have you had to urinate again less than 2 hours after you finished urinating?	0	1	2	3	4	5	
Intermittency. Over the past month, how often have you found you stopped and started again several times when you urinated?	0	1	2	3	4	5	
Urgency. Over the past month, how often have you found it difficult to postpone urination?	0	1	2	3	4	5	
Weak stream. Over the past month, how often have you had a weak urinary stream?	0	1	2	3	4	5	
Straining. Over the past month, how often have you had to push or strain to begin urination?	0	1	2	3	4	5	
Nocturia. Over the past month, how many times did you most typically get up to urinate from the time you went to bed at night until the time you got up in the morning?	0	1	2	3	4	5	
Total IPSS score							

Quality of life due to symptoms	Delighted	Pleased	Mostly satisfied	Mixed—about equally satisfied and dissatisfied	Mostly dissatisfied	Unhappy	Terrible
If you were to spend the rest of your life with your urinary condition just the way it is now, how would you feel about that?	0	1	2	3	4	5	6

Figure 1.1 The International Prostate Symptom Score (IPSS). This figure was published in Barry MJ, Fowler FJ Jr, O'Leary MP, et al. (1992). The American Urological Association symptom index for benign prostatic hyperplasia. *J Urol* 148(5):1549–1557. Copyright Elsevier 1992.

neoplastic conditions of the bladder, prostate, or urethra. While LUTS are, in general, relatively nonspecific for a particular disease, the associated symptoms can indicate their cause.

For example, LUTS in association with hematuria suggests a possibility of bladder cancer. This is more likely if irritative symptoms (urinary frequency, urgency), and bladder (suprapubic) pain are prominent. Carcinoma in situ of the bladder, a superficial, noninvasive, and potentially very aggressive form of bladder cancer, which very often progresses to muscle invasive or metastatic cancer, classically presents in this way.

Recent onset of bed wetting in an elderly man is often due to high-pressure chronic retention. Visual inspection of the abdomen may show marked distension due to a grossly enlarged bladder. The diagnosis of chronic retention is confirmed by palpating the enlarged, tense bladder, which is dull to percussion; ultrasound measurement; and drainage of a large volume following catheterization.

Rarely, LUTS can be due to neurological disease.

Multiple sclerosis can cause urgency and urge incontinence.

Parkinson disease is associated with urinary symptoms and incontinence. Many patients also have detrusor overactivity and impaired contractility.

Spinal cord or cauda equina compression due to pelvic or sacral tumors can cause urinary symptoms. Associated symptoms include back pain, sciatica, ejaculatory disturbances, and sensory disturbances in the legs, feet, and perineum. In these rare cases, loss of pericoccygeal or perineal sensation (sacral nerve roots 2–4) indicates an interruption to the sensory innervation of the bladder, and an MRI scan often confirms the clinical suspicion that there is a neurological problem.

Further reading

Abrams P, et al. (2002). Lower urinary tract function. *Neurourol Urodyn* 21:167–178.

Gravas S, Melekos MD (2009). Male lower urinary tract symptoms: how do symptoms guide our choice of treatment? *Curr Opin Urol.* 19(1):49–54.

Vishwajit S, Anderson KE (2009). Terminology of lower urinary tract symptoms. Helpful or confusing? *Sci World J* 18;9:17–22.

Nocturia and nocturnal polyuria

Nocturia is the frequent need to get up and urinate at night. It is differentiated from enuresis (bed wetting) in that the person does not wake and the bladder empties.

Nocturnal polyuria (NP) refers to a condition in which the rate of urine output is excessive only at night and total 24-hour output is within normal limits.

Nocturia ≥2 is fairly common and is a bothersome cause of sleep disturbance.

Prevalence of nocturia ≥2: men—40% age 60–70 years, 55% age >70 years; women—10% age 20–40 years, 50% age >80 years.[1,2] Nocturia ≥2 is associated with a 2-fold increased risk of falls and injury in the active elderly.

Men who void more than twice at night have a 2-fold increased risk of death, possibly due to the associations of nocturia with endocrine and cardiovascular disease.[3]

Diagnostic approach to the patient with nocturia

Nocturia can be due to urological disease, but more often than not it is nonurological in origin. Most awakenings from sleep attributed by patients pressured to urinate were instead a result of sleep disorders—even in those patients with well-known medical reasons for noctruria Therefore, "approach the lower urinary tract last" (Neil Resnick,[4] Professor of Gerontology, Pittsburgh).[5,6]

Causes of nocturia

- *Urological:* benign prostatic obstruction, overactive bladder, incomplete bladder emptying
- *Nonurological:* renal failure, idiopathic nocturnal polyuria, diabetes mellitus, central diabetes insipidus, nephrogenic diabetes insipidus, primary polydipsia, hypercalcemia, drugs, autonomic failure, obstructive sleep apnea

Assessment of the nocturic patient

Ask the patient to complete a voiding diary that records time and volume of each void over a 24-hour period for 7 days. This establishes
- If the patient is polyuric or nonpolyuric
- If polyuric, is the polyuria present throughout 24 hours or is it confined to nighttime (nocturnal polyuria)?

1 Coyne KS, et al. (2003). The prevalence of nocturia and its effect on health-related quality of life and sleep in a community sample in the USA. *Br J Urol Int* 92:948–954.
2 Jackson S (199). Lower urinary tract symptoms and nocturia in women: prevalence, aetiology and diagnosis. *Br J Urol Int* 84:5–8.
3 McKeigue P, Reynard J (2000). Relation of nocturnal polyuria of the elderly to essential hypertension. *Lancet* 355:486–488.
4 Resnick NM (2002). Geriatric incontinence and voiding dysfunction. In Walsh PC, Retik AB, Vaughan ED, Wein AJ (Eds.), *Campbell's Urology*, 8th ed. Philadelphia: W.B. Saunders.
5 Pressman MR, Figueroa WG, Kendrick-Mohamed J, et al. (1996). Nocturia. A rarely recognized symptom of sleep apnea and other occult sleep disorders. *Arch Intern Med* 156:545.
6 Fitzgerald MP, Litman HJ, Link CL; McKinlay JB, et al. (2007). The association of nocturia with cardiac disease, diabetes, body mass index, age and diuretic use: results from the BACH survey. *J Urol* 177:1385–1389.

Polyuria (24-hour polyuria) is defined as >3 L of urine output per 24 hours (standardization).

Nocturnal polyuria is defined as the production of more than one-third of 24-hour urine output between midnight and 8 a.m. (It is a normal physiological mechanism to reduce urine output at night. Urine output between midnight and 8 a.m.—one-third of the 24-hour clock—should certainly be no more than one-third of 24-hour total urine output and, in most people, will be considerably less than one-third.)

Polyuria (urine output of >3 L/24 hours) is due to either a solute diuresis or water diuresis.

Measure urine osmolality: <250 mosm/kg = water diuresis, >300 mosm/kg = solute diuresis.

Excess levels of various solutes in the urine, such as glucose in the poorly controlled diabetic, lead to a solute diuresis. A water diuresis occurs in patients with primary polydipsia (an appropriate physiological response to high water intake) and diabetes insipidus (DI) (antidiuretic hormone [ADH] deficiency or resistance). Patients on lithium have renal resistance to ADH (nephrogenic DI).

Further reading

Guite HF, et al. (1988). Hypothesis: posture is one of the determinants of the circadian rhythm of urine flow and electrolyte excretion in elderly female patients. *Age Ageing* 17:241–248.

Matthiesen TB, Rittig S, Norgaard JP, Pedersen EB, Djurhuus JC (1996). Nocturnal polyuria and natriuresis in male patients with nocturia and lower urinary tract symptoms. *J Urol* 156:1292–1299.

van Kerrebroeck P, Abrams P, Chaikin D, et al. (2002). The standardisation of terminology in nocturia: Report from the Standardisation Sub-committee of the International Continence Society. *Neurourol Urodyn* 21:179–183.

Flank pain

Sometimes referred to as loin pain, *flank pain* is pain or discomfort in the side of the abdomen between the last rib and the hip. It can present suddenly with the severity reaching a peak within minutes or hours (*acute flank pain*). Alternatively, it may have a slower course of onset (*chronic flank pain*), developing over weeks or months.

Traditionally, flank pain is presumed to be urological in origin, based on the anatomic position of the kidney and ureters. However, other structures in this region and pathology within these structures, and pain arising from extra-abdominal organs may radiate to the flank as a referred pain. While flank pain may be urological, other possibilities must be considered in the differential diagnosis.

The speed of onset of flank pain gives some, though not an absolute, indication of the cause of urological flank pain. Acute flank pain is more likely to be due to something obstructing the ureter, such as a stone. Flank pain of more chronic onset suggests disease within the kidney or renal pelvis.

Acute flank pain

The most common cause of sudden onset of severe pain in the flank is the passage of a stone formed in the kidney that is passing down through the ureter. Ureteric stone pain characteristically starts very suddenly (within minutes), is colicky in nature (waves of increasing severity are followed by a reduction in severity, though seldom going away completely), and radiates to the groin as the stone passes into the lower ureter.

The pain may change in location, from flank to groin, but its location does not provide a good indication of the position of the stone, except when the patient has pain or discomfort in the penis and a strong desire to void, which suggests that the stone has moved into the intramural part of the ureter (the segment within the bladder) or bladder. The patient cannot get comfortable and often changes position frequently without relief.

Half of patients with these classic symptoms of ureteric colic do not have a stone confirmed on subsequent imaging studies or have no documentation of passing a stone.[1,2] They have some other cause for their pain (see next page).

A ureteric stone is only very rarely life threatening, but many of the differential diagnoses may be life threatening. Acute flank pain is less likely to be due to a ureteric stone in women and in patients at the extremes of age. Urolithiasis tends to be a disease of men (less common in women) between the ages of ~20 and 60 years, though it can occur in younger and older individuals.

1 Smith RC (1996). Diagnosis of acute flank pain: value of unenhanced helical CT. *AJR Am J Roentgen* 166:97–100.
2 Thomson JM (2001). Computed tomography versus intravenous urography in diagnosis of acute flank pain from urolithiasis: a randomized study comparing imaging costs and radiation dose. *Australas Radiol* 45:291–297.

Acute flank pain—non-stone, urological causes

- *Clot or tumor colic:* a clot may form from a bleeding source within the kidney (e.g., renal cell carcinoma or transitional cell carcinoma [TCC] of the upper urinary tract). A ureteral TCC may cause ureteric obstruction and acute flank pain. Flank pain and hematuria are often assumed due to a stone, but it is important to approach investigation of patients from the perspective of hematuria and to rule out cancer.
- *Ureteropelvic junction obstruction (UPJO)*, also known as ureteropelvic junction obstruction (UPJO), may present acutely with flank pain severe enough to mimic a ureteric colic. A CT scan will demonstrate hydronephrosis, with a normal-caliber ureter below the PUJ and no stone. MAG3 renography usually confirms the diagnosis, demonstrating delayed emptying.
- *Infection:* e.g., acute pyelonephritis, pyonephrosis, emphysematous pyelonephritis, xanthogranulomatous pyelonephritis. These patients have a high fever (>38°C), whereas patients with a ureteric stone do not (unless there is associated infection) and are often systemically ill. Imaging studies may or may not show a stone, and there will be radiological evidence of infection within the kidney and perirenal tissues (such as edema or perinephric stranding on CT scan).
- *Other less common causes* include ptotic kidney, renal infarction or necrosis, renal vein thrombosis, calyceal diverticulum, renal cystic disease (medullary sponge kidney, hemorrhagic cysts), renal bleed (trauma or spontaneous from renal cell carcinoma or angiomyelolipoma), testicular torsion.

Acute flank pain—nonurological causes

Vascular
- Leaking or dissecting abdominal aortic aneurysm

Medical
- Pneumonia/pleurisy
- Myocardial infarction
- Malaria with bilateral flank pain and dark hematuria: "black water fever"
- Herpes zoster

Musculoskeletal
- Muscle spasm, sprain, flank hernia

Gynecological and obstetric
- Ovarian pathology (e.g., twisted ovarian cyst)
- Ectopic pregnancy
- Ovarian vein syndrome

Gastrointestinal
- Acute appendicitis
- Inflammatory bowel disease (Crohn's, ulcerative colitis)
- Diverticulitis
- Perforated peptic ulcer
- Bowel obstruction
- Pancreatitis

Neurological/spinal
- Vertebral or spinal cord/nerve root irritation (bulging or herniated intervertebral disk, sciatica, tumor
- Vertebral body fracture or collapse

Distinguishing urological from nonurological flank pain

History and examination are most important. Patients with ureteric colic often move around the bed in extreme pain and are unable to find a comfortable position. Those with peritonitis lie still. With pancreatitis the patient gets relief when leaning forward.

Palpate the abdomen for signs of peritonitis (abdominal tenderness and/ or guarding) and examine for abdominal masses (pulsatile and bruit suggests aneurysm). In ovarian vein syndrome, pain can worsen on lying down or between ovulation and menstruation.

Examine the patient's back, chest, and testicles. Costovertebral angle tenderness suggests a renal process or musculoskeletal process. In women, do a pregnancy test.

Urinalysis is critical as it suggests or excludes a urinary tract cause. However, up to 26% of patients with a documented stone on CT do not have hematuria.[3,4]

Chronic flank pain—urological causes

Renal or ureteric cancer
- Renal cell carcinoma
- Urothelial carcinoma of the renal pelvis or ureter

Renal stones
- Staghorn calculi
- Non-staghorn calculi, calyceal diverticular stone

Renal infection
- TB, fungal, malarial
- Chronic pyelonephritis, renal abscess
- Ureteropelvic junction obstruction

Testicular pathology (referred pain)
- Testicular neoplasms
- Testicular trauma
- Epidimo-orchitis

Ureteric pathology
- Ureteric reflux
- Ureteric stone (may drop into the ureter, causing severe pain which then subsides to a lower level of chronic pain)

3 Bove P, Kaplan D, Dalrymple N, et al. (1999). Reexamining the value of hematuria testing in patients with acute flank pain. *J Urol* 162:685–687.
4 Jindal G (2007). Acute flank pain secondary to urolithiasis: radiologic evaluation and alternate diagnoses. *Radiol Clin North Am* 45(3):395–410.

Chronic flank pain—nonurological causes

Gastrointestinal
- Bowel neoplasms
- Liver disease

Spinal disease
- Prolapsed intervertebral disc
- Degenerative disease
- Spinal metastases

Urinary incontinence in adults

Definitions

Urinary incontinence (UI): involuntary loss of urine that is objectively demonstrable and is of social and/or hygienic concern (international Continence Society definition).

Stress urinary incontinence (SUI): urine loss associated with increased intra-abdominal pressure such as exertion, coughing, or sneezing. A diagnosis of *urodynamic* SUI is made during filling cystometry when there is involuntary leakage of urine during a rise in abdominal pressure (induced by coughing), in the absence of a detrusor contraction.

Urge urinary incontinence (UUI): sudden uncontrollable urgency, leading to leakage of urine.

Overactive bladder (OAB): urinary urgency, with or without urge incontinence, usually with frequency and nocturia, in the absence of causative infection or pathological conditions.

Overflow incontinence: increased residual or chronic urinary retention leads to urinary leakage from bladder overdistension.

Total incontinence: the continuous leakage of urine.

Functional incontinence: loss of urine related to deficits of cognition and mobility.

Mixed urinary incontinence (MUI): a combination of SUI and UUI.

- Both UUI/OAB and MUI require a perception of urgency by the patient.
- 25% of women aged >20 years have UI, of whom 50% have SUI, 10–20% have pure UUI, and 30–40% have MUI.
- UI impacts psychological health, social functioning, and quality of life.

Significance of SUI and UUI

SUI occurs in women as a result of bladder neck/urethral hypermobility and/or neuromuscular defects causing intrinsic sphincter deficiency (sphincter weakness incontinence). As a consequence, urine leaks whenever urethral resistance is exceeded by an increased abdominal pressure occurring during exercise or coughing, for example.

In women, obesity, childbirth, and cystocele/uterine prolapse are common causes. In men, prostate surgery (radical prostatectomy, TURP) can result in incompetence or weakness of the external sphincter.

UUI may be due to bladder overactivity (formerly known as detrusor instability) or, less commonly, to a pathological process that irritates the bladder (infection [UTI, vaginitis, pelvic inflammatory disease], tumor [urological, gynecological], urolithiasis) or neuropathy (multiple sclerosis, CNS neoplasms, stroke). The correlation between urodynamic evidence of bladder overactivity and the sensation of urgency is poor, particularly in patients with MUI.

Symptoms resulting from involuntary detrusor contractions may be difficult to distinguish from those due to sphincter weakness. Furthermore, in some patients, detrusor contractions can be provoked by coughing, thus distinguishing leakage due to SUI from that due to bladder overactivity can be very difficult. For the diagnosis of OAB, no cause can be identified.

Other types of incontinence

While SUI and especially UUI do not specifically allow identification of the underlying cause, some types of incontinence may allow a specific diagnosis to be made.

- **Bed wetting** in an elderly man suggests high-pressure chronic retention.
- **Total incontinence** suggests a fistulous communication between the bladder (usually) and vagina (e.g., due to surgical injury at the time of hysterectomy or C-section) or, rarely, the presence of an ectopic ureter draining into the vagina (in which case the urine leak is usually low in volume, but lifelong). Total disruption of the internal and external sphincter in men and women can also cause total incontinence.

Diagnosis and management of incontinence

A basic history and physical exam along with urinalysis may identify the cause. In women, a pelvic exam must be performed (cystocele, urethral diverticulum).

Residual urine determination and urinary flow rates can be used to diagnose retention or outflow obstruction. Good flow rate with minimal postvoid residual suggests sphincteric incontinence.

- Urodynamic studies are useful where the history does not clearly indicate the cause.
- Cystometrogram measures bladder compliance, sensations, and detrusor responses to filling. It is particularly useful with urgency and urge incontinence. Documentation of detrusor hyperreflexia or detrusor instability has important therapeutic implications.
- Valsalva leak point pressure determines the intra-abdominal pressure at which urine leaks. A low leak point pressure implies intrinsic sphincter deficiency (ISD).
- Videourodynamic studies are advanced testing if basic evaluation not informative.

Further reading

Anger JT. Saigal CS. Stothers L. Thom DH. Rodriguez LV. Litwin MS (2006). Urologic Diseases of America Project. The prevalence of urinary incontinence among community dwelling men: results from the National Health and Nutrition Examination survey. *J Urol* 176(5):2103–2108.
Atiemo HO, Vasavada SP (2006). Evaluation and management of refractory overactive bladder. *Curr Urol Rep* 7:370–375.
Wein AJ, Rackley RR (2006). Overactive bladder: a better understanding of pathophysiology, diagnosis, and management. *J Urol* 175:S5–S10.

Genital symptoms

Scrotal pain

Pathology within the scrotum
- Epididymitis, orchitis, epididymo-orchitis
- Torsion of the testicles
- Torsion of testicular appendages
- Testicular tumor (usually painless)

Referred pain
- Ureteric colic
- Inguinal hernia
- Nerve root irritation or entrapment (ilioinguinal or genitofemoral)

Testicular torsion
Ischemic pain is severe and often accompanied by nausea and vomiting. Torsion presents with sudden onset of pain in the hemiscrotum, sometimes waking the patient from sleep. It may radiate to the groin and/or flank. There is sometimes a history of mild trauma to the testis in the hours before the acute onset of pain.

Similar episodes may have occurred in the past, with spontaneous resolution of the pain (suggesting torsion or spontaneous detorsion). The testis is very tender. It may be high-riding (lying at a higher than normal position in the testis) and may lie horizontally due to twisting of the cord.

Torsion of testicular appendage
Pain is usually not as severe as testicular torsion, and onset can be more gradual, not usually associated with nausea/vomiting.

Epididymitis, orchitis, epididymo-orchitis
These conditions have similar presenting symptoms to those of testicular torsion. Tenderness is most commonly localized to the epididymis. Isolated orchitis is rare today. Untreated epididymitis may involve the testicle secondarily with massive swelling and diffuse tenderness. See p. 33 for advice on attempting to distinguish torsion from epididymo-orchitis.

Testicular tumor
Only 20% of patients present with testicular pain, and most often after minor trauma.

Acute presentations of testicular tumors
- Testicular swelling may occur rapidly (over days or weeks). An associated (secondary) hydrocele is common. A hydrocele, especially in a young person, should always be investigated with an ultrasound to determine whether the underlying testis is normal.
- Rapid onset (days) of testicular swelling can occur. Very rarely, patients present with advanced metastatic disease (high-volume disease in the retroperitoneum, chest, and neck, causing chest, back, or abdominal pain or shortness of breath).

- Approximately 10–15% of testis tumors present with signs suggesting inflammation (i.e., signs suggesting a diagnosis of epididymo-orchitis—a tender, swollen testis, with redness in the overlying scrotal skin and a fever).

Priapism

Priapism is painful, persistent, prolonged erection of the penis not related to sexual stimulation (see causes in Chapter 12). It can be associated with pharmacological therapies (oral and intracavernosal) for erectile dysfunction. Recurrent or "stuttering" priapism episodes are recurrent but of limited duration. There are two broad categories—low flow (most common) and high flow.

Low-flow ("ischemic") priapism is due to hematological disease (hemoglobinopathies, sickle cell anemia, thalassemia) or infiltration of the corpora cavernosa with malignant disease, or it is medication related. The corpora cavernosa are very rigid and painful because the corpora are ischemic.

High-flow priapism is due to perineal trauma, which creates an arteriovenous fistula. There is less pain and rigidity.

Diagnosis is usually obvious from the history and examination. Characteristically, the corpora cavernosa are rigid and the glans is flaccid. In low-flow priapism of the erect penis is very tender. Examine the abdomen for evidence of malignant disease and perform a digital rectal examination to examine the prostate. If necessary, corporal blood gas can be used to sort ischemic priapism ($pO_2 < 30$ mmHg, $pCO_2 > 60$ mm Hg, pH < 7.25) from non-ischemic priapism ($pO_2 > 90$ mmHg, $pCO_2 < 40$ mmHg, pH > 7.4).

Abdominal examination in urological disease

Because of their retroperitoneal (kidneys, ureters) or pelvic location (bladder and prostate) normal urologic organs are relatively inaccessible to the examining hand when compared with, for example, the spleen or liver. For the same reason, for the kidneys and bladder to be palpable typically implies a fairly advanced disease state in the adult.

It is important that the urologist appreciates the characteristics of other intra-abdominal organs when involved with disease, so that they may be distinguished from urologic organs.

Characteristics and causes of an enlarged kidney

The mass lies in a paracolic gutter, it moves with respiration, is dull to percussion, and can be felt bimanually. It can also be balloted (i.e., bounced, like a ball [balla = "ball" in Italian]) between the hands, one placed on the anterior abdominal wall and one on the posterior abdominal wall.

Common causes of an enlarged kidney

Causes include tumors (renal carcinoma, angiomyolipoma, sarcoma, nephroblastoma), hydronephrosis, pyonephrosis, perinephric abscess, and polycystic disease.

Characteristics and causes of an enlarged liver

The mass descends from underneath the right costal margin; one cannot get above it. It moves with respiration, is dull to percussion, and has a sharp or rounded edge. The surface may be smooth or irregular.

Causes of an enlarged liver

These include infection, congestion (heart failure, hepatic vein obstruction—Budd–Chiari syndrome), cellular infiltration (amyloid), cellular proliferation, space-occupying lesion (polycystic disease, metastatic infiltration, primary hepatic cancer, hydatid cyst, abscess), and cirrhosis.

Characteristics and causes of an enlarged spleen

The mass appears from underneath the costal margin, enlarges toward the right iliac fossa, is firm and smooth, and may have a palpable notch. It is not possible to get above the spleen, it moves with respiration, is dull to percussion, and cannot be felt bimanually.

Causes of an enlarged spleen

These include infections (bacterial, viral infection, protozoal, spirochete); hematological disease; cellular proliferation (leukemias); congestion (portal hypertension due to cirrhosis, portal vein thrombosis, hepatic vein obstruction, congestive heart failure); cellular infiltration; and space-occupying lesions (cysts, lymphoma, polycystic disease).

Characteristics of an enlarged bladder

The bladder arises out of the pelvis and is dull to percussion. Pressure of the examining hand may cause a desire to void. In infants and young children it is easier to palpate.

Abdominal distension: causes and characteristics

- Fetus/gravid uterus—very smooth, firm mass, dull to percussion, arising out of the pelvis
- Flatus—hyperresonant (there may be visible peristalsis if the accumulation of flatus is due to bowel obstruction)
- Feces—palpable in the flanks and across the epigastrium, firm and may be identifiable, there may be multiple separate masses in the line of the colon
- Fat
- Fluid (ascites)—fluid thrill, shifting dullness
- Large abdominal masses (massive hepatomegaly or splenomegaly, fibroids, polycystic kidneys, retroperitoneal sarcoma)

The umbilicus and signs and symptoms of associated pathology

The umbilicus represents the location of four fetal structures—the umbilical vein, two umbilical arteries, and the urachus, which is a tube extending from the superior aspect of the bladder toward the umbilicus. The urachus represents the obliterated vesicourethral canal). The urachus may remain open at various points leading to the following abnormalities (Fig. 1.2):[1]

- **Completely patent urachus** communicates with the bladder and leaks urine through the umbilicus. This usually does not present until adulthood because strong contractions of bladder of a child close the mouth of the fistula.
- **Vesicourachal diverticulum** is a diverticulum in the dome of the bladder. This is usually asymptomatic.
- **Umbilical cyst or sinus** can become infected, forming an abscess or may chronically discharge infected material from the umbilicus. A cyst can present as an immobile, midline swelling between the umbilicus and bladder, deep to the rectus sheath. It may have a small communication with the bladder, thus its size can fluctuate as it can become swollen with urine.

Other causes of umbilical masses

These include metastatic deposit (from abdominal cancer, metastatic spread occurring via lymphatics in the edge of the falciform ligament, running alongside the obliterated umbilical vein) and endometriosis (becomes painful and discharges blood at the same time as menstruation).

1 Hinman F Jr (1993). Atlas of Urosurgical Anatomy. Philadelphia: W.B. Saunders.

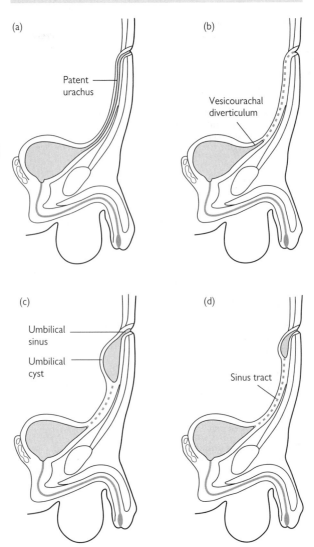

Figure 1.2 Urachal abnormalities. This figure was published in Hinman F Jr, *Atlas of Urosurgical Anatomy*. Copyright Elsevier 1993.

Digital rectal examination (DRE)

The immediate anterior relationship of the rectum in the male is the prostate. The DRE is the mainstay of examination of the prostate.

Explain to the patient the need for the examination. Ensure that the examination is done in privacy. The exam is usually performed with the patient leaning over the exam table, but may be done in the left lateral position with the patient lying on their left side and with the hips and knees flexed to 90° or more. This positioning may make it possible to examine the base of a large prostate or examine a more obese patient.

Examine the anal region for fistulae and fissures. Apply plenty of lubricating gel to the gloved finger. If in the lateral position, lift the buttock upward with your other hand to expose the anus. Apply gentle pressure with the lubricated index finger and slowly insert your finger into the anal canal and then into the rectum. Note the presence of any rectal masses or hemorrhoids. Rectal tone should also be noted.

Palpate anteriorly toward the pubis with the pulp of your finger, and feel the surface of the prostate. Note the consistency (normal, boggy, firm, rock hard), its surface (smooth or irregular), and symmetry and estimate its size. Describe any focal areas of firmness or frank nodularity.

A normal adult prostate is about 20 g and 3–4 cm long and wide. Normal prostate consistency is similar to that of the contracted thenar eminence of the thumb and is often described as rubbery.

It can be helpful to relate its size to common objects such as fruit or nuts: normal prostate (walnut or chestnut), moderately enlarged (tangerine), and markedly enlarged (apple or orange). A +1 to +4 system also gives a very rough idea of the prostate size. Estimating the gram size based on DRE is very unreliable and is best done by imaging such as transrectal ultrasound.

The normal bilobed prostate has a groove (the median sulcus) between the two lobes and in prostate cancer this groove may be obscured. The lateral sulci should be distinct. Obliteration can be seen after radiation therapy to the prostate or rectum or with locally advanced prostate cancer. Normal seminal vesicles should never be palpated and, if felt, suggest a pathological process, most often infiltration by prostate cancer.

Many men find DRE uncomfortable or even painful, and the inexperienced doctor may equate this normal discomfort with prostatic tenderness. Prostatic tenderness is best elicited by gentle pressure on the prostate with the examining finger. If the prostate is really involved by some acute, inflammatory condition, it will be very tender. However, it is best to avoid DRE with the possibility of abscess or acute bacterial prostatitis in the profoundly neutropenic patient (risk of septicemia).

Firmness or nodularity can be caused by BPH, prostate cancer or other malignancy such as urothelial carcinoma, lymphoma, sarcoma or other rare tumor, chronic prostatitis with calcifications, prior prostate surgery, ejaculatory duct cysts, and granulomatous prostatitis, among others.

Other features to elicit in the DRE

The integrity of the sacral nerves that innervate the bladder and of the sacral spinal cord can be established by eliciting the bulbocavernosus reflex (BCR) during a DRE. The sensory side of the reflex is elicited by squeezing the glans of the penis or the clitoris (or in catheterized patients, by gently pulling the balloon of the catheter onto the bladder neck).

The motor side of the reflex is tested by feeling for contraction of the anus during this sensory stimulus. Contraction of the anus represents a positive BCR and indicates that the afferent and efferent nerves of the sacral spinal cord (S2–S4) and the sacral cord are intact.

Lumps in the groin

Differential diagnosis

This includes inguinal hernia, femoral hernia, enlarged lymph nodes, saphena varix, hydrocele of the cord (or of the canal of Nück in women), vaginal hydrocele, undescended testis, lipoma of the cord, femoral aneurysm, and psoas abscess.

Determining the diagnosis

Hernia

A hernia (usually) has a cough impulse (i.e., it expands on coughing) and (usually) reduces with direct pressure or on lying down unless, uncommonly, it is incarcerated (i.e., the contents of the hernia are fixed in the hernia sac by their size and by adhesions). *Movement* of the lump is not the same as *expansion*. Many groin lumps have a transmitted impulse on coughing (i.e., they move) but do not expand on coughing.

Since inguinal and femoral hernias arise from within the abdomen and *descend* into the groin, it is not possible to get above them. For lumps that arise from within the scrotum, the superior edge can be palpated (i.e., it is possible to get above them).

Once a hernia has protruded through the abdominal wall, it can expand in any direction in the subcutaneous tissues. Therefore, the position of the unreduced hernia *cannot* be used to establish whether it is inguinal or femoral. The point of *reduction* of the hernia establishes whether it is an inguinal or femoral hernia.

- *Inguinal:* the hernia reduces through the abdominal wall at a point *above and medial* to the pubic tubercle. An indirect inguinal hernia often descends into the scrotum; a direct inguinal hernia rarely does.
- *Femoral:* the hernia reduces through the abdominal wall at a point *below and lateral* to the pubic tubercle.

Enlarged inguinal lymph nodes

These present as a firm, noncompressible, nodular lump in the groin. Look for pathology in the skin of the scrotum and penis, the perianal area and anus, and the skin and superficial tissues of the thigh and leg.

Penile cancer can spread to the inguinal nodes. Superficial infections of the leg and sexually transmitted disease (STD) such as chancroid, herpes, and lymphogranuloma venereum can cause tender inguinal lymphadenopathy.

Saphena varix

This is a dilatation of the proximal end of the saphenous vein. It can be confused with an inguinal or femoral hernia because it has an expansile cough impulse (i.e., expands on coughing) and disappears on lying down. It is easily compressible and has a fluid thrill when the distal saphenous vein is percussed.

Hydrocele of the cord (or of the canal of Nück in women)

A *hydrocele* is an abnormal quantity of peritoneal fluid between the parietal and visceral layers of the tunica vaginalis, the double layer of peritoneum surrounding the testis and which was the processus vaginalis in the fetus. Normally, the processus vaginalis becomes obliterated along its entire length, apart from where it surrounds the testis where a potential space remains between the parietal and visceral layers.

If the central part of the processus vaginalis remains patent, fluid secreted by the "trapped" peritoneum accumulates and forms a hydrocele of the cord (the equivalent in females is known as the canal of Nück). A hydrocele of the cord may therefore be present in the groin.

Undescended testis

The testis may be on the correct anatomical path, but may have failed to reach the scrotum (incompletely descended testis) or may have descended away from the normal anatomical path (ectopic testis). The "lump" is smooth, oval, tender to palpation, and noncompressible, and there is no testis in the scrotum.

Lipoma of the cord

A noncompressible lump is in the groin, with no cough impulse.

Femoral aneurysm

This usually occurs in the common femoral artery (rather than superficial or profunda femoris branches) and is therefore located just below the inguinal ligament. It is easily confused with a femoral hernia. Like all aneurysms, they are expansile (but unlike hernias they do not expand on coughing).

Psoas abscess

The scenario is one of a patient who is very ill with a fever, with a soft, fluctuant, compressible mass in the femoral triangle.

Lumps in the scrotum

Differential diagnosis

- *Testicle:* Testicular malignancy (germ cell tumor such as seminoma, embryonal, choriocarcinoma, yolk sac tumor), lymphoma, benign testicular tumor (adenomatoid tumor, Leydig or Sertoli cell tumor), torsion of testicle or appendix, trauma with testicular rupture, benign cysts, granulomatous orchitis, syphilitic gumma
- *Epididymis:* epididymitis/epididmo-orchitis, epididymal cyst, cystadenoma, adenomatoid tumor
- *Paratesticular masses:* hydrocele, spermatocele, varicocele, hematocele, hydrocele of the cord, cord lipoma, rhabdomyosarcoma of the cord
- *Others:* inguinal hernia, lesions of the scrotal wall (cysts, carcinoma)

Determining the diagnosis

Determination of the duration of the mass and whether it is painful can help establish the diagnosis. Painful masses include those from trauma, epididymitis, torsion, and hernia. Painless masses include tumors, hydrocele, spermatocele, varicocele, and epididymal masses.

Inguinal hernia

An indirect inguinal hernia often extends into the scrotum. It usually has a cough impulse (i.e., it expands on coughing) and usually reduces with direct pressure or on lying down. It is not possible to get above the lump.

Hydrocele

A *hydrocele* is an abnormal quantity of peritoneal fluid between the parietal and visceral layers of the tunica vaginalis, the double layer of peritoneum surrounding the testis and which was the processus vaginalis in the fetus. It is usually painless, unless the underlying testicular disease is painful.

A hydrocele has a smooth surface, and it is difficult or impossible to feel the testis, which is surrounded by the tense, fluid collection (unless, rarely, the hydrocele is very lax). The superior margin can be palpated (i.e., you can get above the lump). It is possible to transilluminate a hydrocele (i.e., the light from a flashlight applied on one side can be seen on the other side of the hydrocele). Ultrasound is most reliable to evaluate for underlying testicular pathology in this setting.

Hydroceles may be primary (idiopathic) or secondary. Primary hydroceles develop slowly (over the course of years, usually) and there is no precipitating event such as epididymo-orchitis or trauma, and the underlying testis appears normal on ultrasound (no testicular tumor). Secondary hydroceles (infection, tumor, trauma) represent an effusion between the layers of the tunica vaginalis (the visceral and parietal layers), analogous to a pleural or peritoneal effusion.

In filariasis (infection with the filarial worm *Wuchereria bancrofti*), obstruction of the lymphatics of the spermatic cord gives rise to the hydrocele.

Epididymal cyst

This is also known as a spermatocele if there are spermatozoa in the contained fluid. Cysts derive from the collecting tubules of the epididymis and contain clear fluid. They develop slowly over years, lie within the scrotum (you can get examining finders above them), and usually lie above and behind the testis. They are often multiple or multiloculated.

Orchitis

This occurs in the absence of involvement of the epididymitis and is due to a viral infection, e.g., mumps. Orchitis often occurs with enlargement of the salivary glands.

Epididymitis

This is often difficult to differentiate from testicular torsion. Typically, it is caused by an ascending infection. Common agents include coliform bacteria, *Pseudomonas, Chlamydia*, and gonorrhea.

Acute epididymitis can be accompanied by pain, frequency, and dysuria. Early the epididymis can be palpated and is very tender. Later the testicle can become involved secondarily.

Tuberculous epididymo-orchitis

Infection of the epididymis (principally) by tuberculosis (TB) spreads from the blood or urinary tract. The *absence* of pain and tenderness is noticeable. The epididymis is hard and has an irregular surface. The spermatic cord is thickened and the vas deferens also feels hard and irregular (a "string of beads").

Testicular tumor (seminoma, embryonal cell, yolk sac tumor, teratoma)

This is a solid mass on the testicle which, and if very large, may extend up into the spermatic cord. The typical malignant tumor in the testicle is painless and discovered incidentally, often after a minor trauma that probable calls attention to the area. Very rarely it can present with pain and tenderness in the testis and with fever.

The lump is usually firm or hard and may have a smooth or irregular surface. Examine the contralateral testicle and for abdominal and supraclavicular lymph nodes.

Gumma of the testis

This condition is rare. Syphilis of the testis results in a round, hard, insensitive mass involving the testis (a so-called billiard ball). It is difficult to distinguish from a tumor.

Varicocele

A *variocele* is dilatation of the pampiniform plexus—the collection of veins surrounding the testis and extending up into the spermatic cord (essentially varicose veins of the testis and spermatic cord). Small, symptomless varicoceles occur in approximately 20% of normal men and are more common on the left side.

They may cause a dragging sensation or ache in the scrotum; they are said to feel like a "bag of worms." The varicocele disappears when the patient lies down.

Sebaceous cyst
These are common in scrotal skin. They are fixed to the skin and have a smooth surface.

Carcinoma of scrotal skin
This appears as an ulcer on the scrotal skin, often with a purulent or bloody discharge.

Chapter 2

Urological investigations

Urine examination 36
Urine cytology 38
Prostatic specific antigen (PSA) 39
Radiological imaging of the urinary tract 40
Uses of plain abdominal radiography (KUB
    X-ray—kidneys, ureters, bladder) 42
Intravenous pyelography (IVP) 44
Other urological contrast studies 48
Computed tomography (CT) and magnetic
    resonance imaging (MRI) 50
Radioisotope imaging 52
Uroflowmetry 54
Post-void residual urine volume measurement 58
Cystometry, pressure-flow studies, and
    videocystometry 60

Urine examination

Dipstick testing

Analysis for pH, blood, protein, glucose, and white cells can be done with dipstick testing.

pH

Urinary pH varies between 4.5 and 8, averaging between 5.5 and 6.5.

Blood

Normal urine contains <3 RBCs per high-powered field (HPF) (~1000 erythrocytes/mL of urine; upper limit of 5000–8000 erythrocytes/mL). Positive dipstick for blood indicates the presence of hemoglobin in the urine.

Hemoglobin has a peroxidase-like activity and causes oxidation of a chromogen indicator, which changes color when oxidized. Sensitivity of urine dipsticks for identifying hematuria (>3 RBCs/HPF) is >90%; specificity is lower (i.e., a higher false-positive rate with the dipstick), due to contamination with menstrual blood or dehydration (concentrates what RBCs are normally present in urine).

Hematuria due to a urological cause does not elevate urinary protein. Hematuria of nephrological origin often occurs in association with casts, and there is almost always significant proteinuria.

Protein

Normal, healthy adults excrete about 80–150 mg of protein per day in their urine (normal protein concentration <20 mg/dL). Proteinuria suggests the presence of renal disease (glomerular, tubulointerstitial, renal vascular) or multiple myeloma, but it can occur following strenuous exercise. A dipstick test is based on a tetrabromophenol blue dye color change (green color develops in the presence of protein of >20 mg/dL).

White blood cells

Leukocyte esterase activity detects the presence of white blood cells (WBCS) in the urine. Leukocyte esterase is produced by neutrophils and causes a color change in a chromogen salt on the dipstick. Not all patients with bacteriuria have significant pyuria.

False negatives are due to concentrated urine, glycosuria, presence of urobilinogen, and consumption of large amounts of ascorbic acid. False positives are due to contamination.

Nitrite testing

Nitrites in the urine suggest the possibility of bacteriuria. They are not normally found in the urine. Many species of gram-negative bacteria can convert nitrates to nitrites, and these are detected in urine by a reaction with the reagents on the dipstick that form a red azo dye.

The specificity of the nitrite dipstick for detecting bacteriuria is >90% (false-positive nitrite testing is contamination). Sensitivity is 35–85% (i.e., lots of false negatives); it is less accurate in urine containing fewer than 10^5 organisms/mL.

Cloudy urine that is positive for WBCs and is nitrite positive is very likely to be infected.

Urine microscopy

Red blood cell morphology

This is determined by phase-contrast microscopy. RBCs derived from the glomerulus are dysmorphic (they have been distorted by their passage through the glomerulus). RBCs derived from tubular bleeding (tubulointerstitial disease) and those from lower down the urinary tract (i.e., urological bleeding from the renal pelvis, ureters, or bladder) have a normal shape. Glomerular bleeding is suggested by the presence of dysmorphic RBCs, RBC casts, and proteinuria.

Casts

A *cast* is a protein coagulum (principally, Tamm–Horsfall mucoprotein derived from tubular epithelial cells) formed in the renal tubule and "cast" in the shape of the tubule (i.e., long and thin). The protein matrix traps tubular luminal contents. If the cast contains only mucoproteins it is called a *hyaline cast*. It is seen after exercise, heat exposure, and in pyelonephritis or chronic renal disease.

RBC casts contain trapped erythrocytes and are diagnostic of glomerular bleeding, most often due to glomerulonephritis. WBC casts are seen in acute glomerulonephritis, acute pyelonephritis, and acute tubulointerstitial nephritis.

Crystals

Specific crystal types may be seen in urine and help diagnose underlying problems (e.g., cystine crystals establish the diagnosis of cystinuria). Calcium oxalate, uric acid, and cystine are precipitated in acidic urine. Crystals precipitated in alkaline urine include calcium phosphate and triple-phosphate (struvite).

Urine cytology

Urine collections for cytology

Exfoliated cells lying in urine that has been in the bladder for several hours (e.g., early morning specimens) or in a urine specimen that has been allowed to stand for several hours are degenerate. Such urine specimens are not suitable for cytological interpretation.

Cytological examination can be performed on bladder washings (using normal saline) obtained from the bladder at cystoscopy (or following catheterization) or from the ureter (via a ureteric catheter or ureteroscope). The urine is centrifuged, and the specimen obtained is fixed in alcohol and stained by the Papanicolaou technique.

Normal urothelial cells are shed into the urine. Under microscopy their nuclei appear regular and monomorphic (diffuse, fine chromatin pattern, single nucleolus).

Causes of a positive cytology report (i.e., abnormal urothelial cells seen—high nuclear–cytoplasmic ratio, hyperchromatic nuclei, prominent nucleoli) include the following:

- Urothelial malignancy (transitional cell carcinoma [TCC], squamous cell carcinoma, adenocarcinoma)
- Previous radiotherapy (especially if within the last 12 months)
- Previous cytotoxic drug treatment (especially if within the last 12 months; e.g., cyclophosphamide, busulphan, cysclosporin)
- Urinary tract stones

Renal adenocarcinoma (clear cell cancer of the kidney) usually does not exfoliate abnormal cells, though occasionally clusters of clear cells may be seen, suggesting the diagnosis.

High-grade urothelial cancer and carcinoma in situ exfoliate cells that look very abnormal, and usually the cytologist is able to indicate that there is a high likelihood of a malignancy. Low-grade bladder TCC exfoliates cells that look very much like normal urothelial cells. The difficulty arises where the cells look abnormal, but not that abnormal—here the likelihood that the cause of the abnormal cytology is a benign process is greater.

Sensitivity and specificity of positive urine cytology for detecting TCC of the bladder depend on the definition of positive—if only obviously malignant or highly suspicious samples are considered positive, then the specificity will be high. Urine cytology may be negative in as many as 20% of high-grade cancers.

If "atypical cells" are included in the definition of abnormal, the specificity of urine cytology for diagnosing urothelial cancer will be relatively poor (relatively high number of false positives) because many cases will have a benign cause (stones, inflammation).

Prostatic specific antigen (PSA)

PSA is a 34KD glycoprotein enzyme produced by the columnar acinar and ductal prostatic epithelial cells. It is a member of the human kallikrein family and its function is to liquefy the ejaculate, enabling fertilization. PSA is present in both benign and malignant cells, although the expression of PSA tends to be reduced in malignant cells and may be absent in poorly differentiated tumors. Large amounts are secreted into the semen, and small quantities are found in the urine and blood.

The function of serum PSA is unclear, although it is known to liberate the insulin-like growth factor type 1 (IGF-1) from one of its binding proteins. 75% of circulating PSA is bound to plasma proteins (complexed PSA) and metabolized in the liver, while 25% is free and excreted in the urine. Complexed PSA is stable, bound to α_1-antichymotrypsin and α_2- macroglobulin. Free PSA is unstable, recently found to consist of two isoforms: pro-PSA is a peripheral zone precursor, apparently elevated in the presence of prostate cancer, and BPSA is the transition zone precursor and associated with benign prostatic hyperplasia (BPH).

The half-life of serum PSA is 2.2 days. A prostate biopsy is often recommended for men with a PSA > 2.5 ng/mL, though this varies with age. Table 2.1 shows a published age-specific normal range (95th percentile).

In the absence of prostate cancer, serum PSA concentrations also vary physiologically, according to race and prostate volume.

Indications for checking serum PSA

- Patient request, following counseling
- Lower urinary tract symptoms
- Abnormal digital rectal examination
- Progressive bone pain, especially back pain
- Unexplained anemia, anorexia, or weight loss
- Spontaneous thromboembolism or unilateral leg swelling
- Monitoring of prostate cancer patients

Table 2.1 Age-adjusted normal range for PSA

Age range (years)	Normal PSA range (ng/mL)
40–49	<2.5
50–59	<3.5
60–69	<4.5
>70	<6.5

Radiological imaging of the urinary tract

Ultrasound

Ultrasound is a noninvasive method of urinary tract imaging. While it provides good images of the kidneys and bladder, anatomical detail of the ureter is poor and the mid-ureter cannot be imaged at all by ultrasound because of overlying bowel gas.

Uses of ultrasound

Renal

- Assessment of hematuria
- Determination of nature of renal masses—can differentiate simple cysts (smooth, well-demarcated wall, reflecting no echoes; benign) from solid masses (almost always malignant; cystic masses with solid components or multiple septae or calcification may be malignant) and from those casting an "acoustic shadow" (stones) (Fig. 2.1)
- Can determine the presence or absence of hydronephrosis (dilatation of the collecting system) in patients with abnormal renal function (Fig. 2.2)
- Allows ultrasound-guided nephrostomy insertion in patients with hydronephrosis and renal impairment or with infected, obstructed kidneys

Bladder

- Measurement of post-void residual urine volume
- Allows ultrasound-guided placement of a suprapubic catheter

Prostate: transrectal ultrasound (TRUS)

- Measurement of prostate size (where gross prostatic enlargement is suspected on the basis of a DRE, and surgery, in the form of open prostatectomy, is contemplated)
- To assist prostate biopsy (allows biopsy of hypoechoic or hyperechoic lesions)
- Investigation of azoospermia (can establish the presence of ejaculatory duct obstruction)

Urethra

- Can image the urethra and establish the depth and extent of spongiofibrosis in urethral stricture disease

Testes

- Assessment of the patient complaining of a lump in the testicle (or scrotum)—can differentiate benign lesions (hydrocele, epididymal cyst) from malignant testicular tumors (solid, echo poor or with abnormal echo pattern)
- When combined with power Doppler can establish the presence or absence of testicular blood flow in suspected torsion
- Assessment of testicular trauma (rupture is indicated by abnormal echo pattern, due to blood within the body of the testis; surrounding

hematoma may be seen—blood within the scrotal soft tissues that has escaped through a tear in the tunica albuginea and the visceral and parietal layers of the tunica vaginalis; hematocele—blood contained by an intact parietal layer of the tunica vaginalis)
- Investigation of infertility—varicoceles and testicular atrophy may be identified

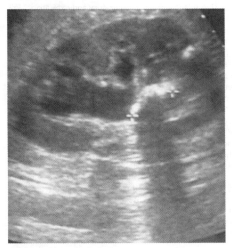

Figure 2.1 An acoustic shadow cast by a stone within the kidney.

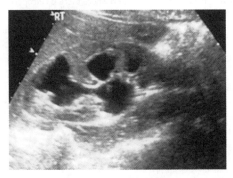

Figure 2.2 Hydronephrosis. Urine in dilated calyces appears black (hypoechoic).

Uses of plain abdominal radiography (KUB X-ray—kidneys, ureters, bladder)

Plain abdominal radiography is for detection of stones and determination of their size and (to an extent) their location within the kidneys, ureters, and bladder (Fig. 2.3).

For renal calculi, a calcification overlying the kidneys is intrarenal if it maintains its relationship to the kidney on inspiratory and expiratory films (i.e., if it moves with the kidney). If in doubt as to whether an opacity overlying the outline of the kidney is intrarenal or not, get an ultrasound (look for the characteristic acoustic shadow within the kidney), intravenous pyelography (IVP), or computed tomographic urography (CTU).

Sensitivity for *detection* of renal calculi is on the order of 50–70% (i.e., the false-negative rate is between 30% and 50%; it misses ureteric stones when these are present in 30–50% of cases). CTU or IVP, which relate the position of the opacity to the anatomical location of the ureters, are required to make a definitive diagnosis of a ureteric stone. However, once the presence of a ureteric stone has been confirmed by another imaging study (CTU or IVP), and as long as it is radio-opaque enough and large enough to be seen, plain radiography is a good way of following the patient to establish whether the stone is progressing distally, down the ureter.

Plain radiography is not useful for following ureteric stones that are radiolucent (e.g., uric acid) or small (generally a stone must be 3–4 mm to be visible on plain X-ray), or when the stones pass through the ureter as it lies over the sacrum. The ability of KUB X-ray to visualize stones is also dependent on the amount of overlying bowel gas.

Plain tomography (a plain X-ray taken of a fixed coronal plane through the kidneys) can be useful, but is rarely done with the availability of ultrasound and CT.

Opacities that may be confused with stones (renal, ureteric) on plain radiography include calcified lymph nodes and pelvic phleboliths (round, lucent center, usually below the ischial spines).

Look for the psoas shadow—this is obscured where there is retroperitoneal fluid (pus or blood) (Fig. 2.4).

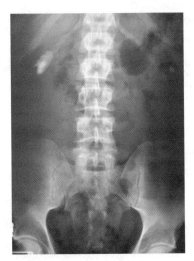

Figure 2.3 Small staghorn calculus on KUB X-ray.

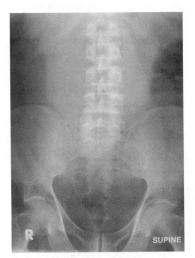

Figure 2.4 Leaking abdominal aortic aneurysm (AAA) on plain X-ray; the right psoas shadow cannot be seen because of retroperitoneal hemorrhage.

Intravenous pyelography (IVP)

IVP is also known as intravenous urography (IVU). A control film is obtained before contrast is given. Intravascular contrast is administered followed by a series of X-rays of the kidneys, ureters, and bladder over the following 30 minutes or so, to image their anatomy and pathology, and to give some indication of renal function.

- Radio-opacity of contrast agents depends on the presence of a tri-iodinated benzene ring in the molecule.
- Ionic monomers (sodium and meglumine salts) ionize, thereby producing high-osmolality solutions (e.g., iothalamate—Conray), diatrizoate—Hypaque, Urografin).
- Nonionic monomers have low osmolality (e.g., iopamidol—Niopam, iohexol—Omnipaque).
- At a concentration of 300 mg of iodine per mL, ionic monomers have an osmolality 5× higher than that of plasma, compared with nonionic monomers, which have an osmolality 2× that of plasma.
- Excreted from plasma by glomerular filtration.

Films and "phases" of IVP

Plain film

This is used to look for calcification overlying the region of the kidneys, ureters, and bladder.

Nephrogram phase

This is the first phase of IVP; film is taken immediately following intravenous administration of contrast (peak nephrogram density). The nephrogram is produced by filtered contrast within the lumen of the proximal convoluted tubule (it is a proximal tubular, rather than distal tubular, phenomenon).

Pyelogram phase

As the contrast passes along the renal tubule (into the distal tubule) it is concentrated (as water is absorbed, but the contrast agent is not). As a consequence, the contrast medium is concentrated in the pelvicalyceal system, thus this pyelogram phase (Fig. 2.5) is much denser than the nephrogram phase.

The pyelogram phase can be made denser by dehydrating the patient prior to contrast administration. Pelvic compression can be used to distend the pelvicalyceal system and demonstrate their anatomy more precisely. Compression is released and a film taken (20–30 min) (Fig. 2.6).

Side effects of administration of intravenous contrast media

These occur in 1% of patients given nonionic and 5% given ionic contrast media.

The most serious reactions represent an anaphylactic reaction—hypotension with flushing of the skin (marked peripheral vasodilatation), edema (face, neck, body, and limbs), bronchospasm, and urticaria. Rarely, cardiac arrest can occur. The death rate, as a consequence of these reactions, is ~1 in 40,000 to 1 in 70,000 with the ionic media, and ~1 in 200,000 with nonionic contrast agents.

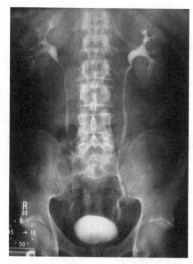

Figure 2.5 Normal IVP at 15 minutes.

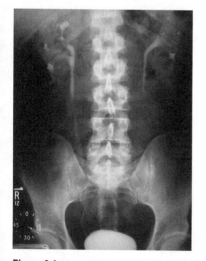

Figure 2.6 Normal IVP at 20 minutes. Lower abdominal compression has been released.

A contrast reaction is more likely to occur in patients with an iodine allergy, previous contrast reaction, asthma, multiple other allergies, and heart disease and is less likely with nonionic contrast media. Steroid premedication (prednisone 50 mg given at 13, 7, and 1 hour prior to the procedure) can reduce the risk of a contrast reaction.

Contrast media are also nephrotoxic; 10% of patients with a raised creatinine will develop an increase in creatinine after an IVP (more likely in diabetics, with dehydration, and with large contrast doses). The increase in creatinine usually resolves spontaneously.

Uses of IVP

- Investigation of hematuria—detection of renal masses, filling defects within the collecting system of the kidney and within the ureters (stones, TCCs)
- Localization of calcification overlying the urinary tract (i.e., is it a stone or not?)
- Investigation of patients with flank pain (e.g., suspected ureteric colic). IVP is increasingly being replaced with CTU, which has superior sensitivity and specificity.
- Very good for identification of congenital urinary tract abnormalities (e.g., ureteric anatomy in duplex systems) (Fig. 2.7); malrotation; horseshoe kidneys
- Used for follow-up postureteric surgery to identify strictures

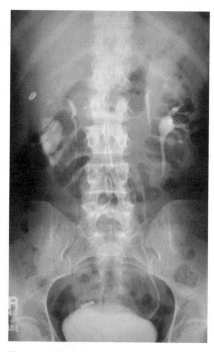

Figure 2.7 Bilateral duplex as seen on a tomogram from an IVP.

Other urological contrast studies

Voiding cystourethrography (VCUG) (Fig. 2.8)

VCUG is used to identify the presence of vesicoureteric reflux during filling and emptying of the bladder and presence and site of obstruction in the outlet of the bladder and within the urethra, particularly in patients with neuropathic bladder problems (e.g., spinal cord injury). This study is helpful for delineating the proximal extent of urethral strictures.

Cystography

This study consists of retrograde filling of the bladder, via a catheter, with contrast. It is used to identify vesicocolic and vesicovaginal fistulae and bladder rupture (extraperitoneal and intraperitoneal).

Urethrography (Fig. 2.9)

Retrograde filling of the urethra with contrast is used to identify the site and length of urethral strictures (Fig. 2.10) or presence, extent, and site of urethral injury (in pelvic fracture, for example).

Ileal loopogram

Retrograde filling of an ileal conduit with contrast is used to establish the presence of free reflux into the ureters (a normal finding; absence of free reflux suggests obstruction at the ureteroileal junction due to ischemic stenosis or recurrent TCC in the ureters at the ureteroileal junction) and the presence of TCCs in the ureters or renal pelvis (an occasional finding in patients who have had a cystectomy for bladder TCC with ileal conduit urinary diversion).

Retrograde pyelography

This study consists of retrograde instillation of contrast into the ureters by a ureteric catheter inserted into the ureter via a cystocope (rigid or flexible). It provides excellent definition of the ureter and renal pelvis for detection of ureteric and renal pelvic TCCs or radiolucent stones in patients with persistent hematuria in whom other tests have shown no abnormality.

Retrograde pyelography is also used to diagnose the presence and site of ureteric injury (obstruction, ureteric leak) in cases of ureteric injury (e.g., after hysterectomy or caesarean section).

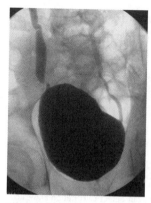

Figure 2.8 VCUG showing bilateral ureteric reflux.

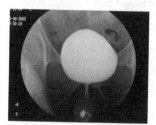

Figure 2.9 Normal urethrogram.

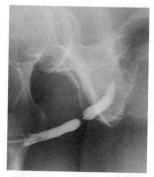

Figure 2.10 A urethrogram showing a bulbar urethral stricture.

Computed tomography (CT) and magnetic resonance imaging (MRI)

Computed tomography

CT is widely used for investigation of urological symptoms and disease. It can detect very small differences in X-ray absorption values of tissues, providing a very wide range of densities (and therefore differentiation between tissues) when compared with plain radiography.

The computer calculates the absorption value (attenuation) of each pixel and reconstructs this into an image. The attenuation values are expressed on a scale from -1000 to $+1000$ Hounsfield units (water = 0, air = -1000, bone = $+1000$).

More recently, advances in computing power have enabled the data to be reformatted so that images can be produced in sagittal and coronal planes as well as in the more familiar horizontal plane (Figs. 2.11 and 2.12).

"Plain" CT scans (without contrast) can detect calcification and calculi within the urinary tract. Administration of intravenous contrast is used to evaluate the nature of solid renal lesions and determine the nature of soft tissue masses (e.g., to differentiate bowel from lymph nodes in cancer staging CTs).

"Spiral" or "helical" CT is very rapid scanning while the table on which the patient is lying is moved though the scanner. A large volume of the body can be imaged in a single breath hold, thus eliminating movement artifact. This is particularly useful for identifying suspected ureteric stones in patients with acute flank pain.

Uses of CT

Renal
- Investigation of renal masses—characterizes solid from cystic lesions; differentiates benign (e.g., angiomyolipoma) from malignant solid masses (e.g., renal cell carcinoma)
- Staging of renal cancer (establishes local, nodal, and distant spread)
- Assessment of stone size and location (within the collecting system or within the parenchyma of the kidney)
- Detection and localization of site of intrarenal and perirenal collections of pus (pyonephrosis, perinephric abscess)
- Staging (grading) of renal trauma
- Determination of cause of hydronephrosis

Ureters
- Locates and measures size of ureteric stones

Bladder
- Bladder cancer staging (establishes local, nodal, and distant spread)

Uses of MRI

- Staging of pelvic cancer—bladder and prostate cancer staging (establishes local, nodal, and distant spread). As with CT, edema and fibrosis cannot be reliably distinguished from tumor within the bladder

wall, leading to overstaging of cancer. Again, as with CT, microscopic disease cannot be identified, leading to understaging of cancer.
- Localization of undescended testes
- Identification of ureteric stones, where ionizing radiation is best avoided (e.g., pregnant women with flank pain)

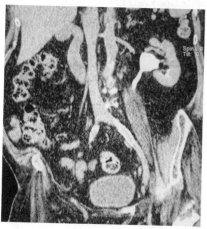

Figure 2.11 Coronal CT image of abdomen showing the left kidney, aorta, and IVC.

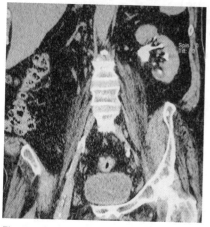

Figure 2.12 Coronal CT image of abdomen, showing the left kidney and paravertebral muscles.

Radioisotope imaging

A variety of organic compounds can be labeled with a radioactive isotope that emits gamma rays, allowing the radiation to penetrate through tissues and reach a gamma camera placed adjacent to the patient. The most commonly used radioisotope is technetium—^{99m}Tc (half-life 6 hours, gamma-ray emission energy 0.14 MeV). The excretion characteristics of the organic compound to which the ^{99m}Tc is bound determine the clinical use.

MAG3 renogram

^{99m}Tc is bound to mercapto-acetyl-triglycine. Over 90% of MAG3 becomes bound to plasma proteins following intravenous injection. It is excreted from the kidneys principally by tubular secretion (glomerular filtration is minimal).

Following intravenous injection, MAG3 is very rapidly excreted (appearing in the kidney within 15 seconds of the injection and starting to appear in the bladder within about 3 minutes). Approximately two-thirds of the injected dose of MAG3 is taken up by the kidneys with each passage of blood through the kidney. The radioactivity over each kidney thus increases rapidly.

The peak of radioactivity represents the point at which delivery of MAG3 to the kidney from the renal artery is equivalent to excretion of MAG3. The radioactivity starts to decline as excretion outstrips supply. Thus, a time–activity curve can be recorded for each kidney. This time–activity curve is known as a renogram.

Images are collected onto a film at 30-second intervals for the first 3 minutes and then at 5-minute intervals for the remainder of the study (usually a total of 30 minutes).

A normal renogram has 3 phases

- *First phase:* a steeply rising curve lasting 20–30 seconds
- *Second phase:* a more slowly rising curve, rising to a peak. If the curve does not reach a peak, the second phase is said to rise continually. A normal second phase ends with a sharp peak.
- *Third phase:* a curve that descends after the peak. There can be no third phase if there is no peak.

Description of the renogram

No comment is made about the first phase. The second phase is described as being absent, impaired, or normal. The third phase is described as being absent, impaired, or normal.

The time to the peak depends on urine flow and level of hydration and is a crude measure of the time it takes the tracer to travel through the parenchyma of the kidney and through the renal pelvis. The time to the peak of the renogram normally varies between 2 and 4.5 minutes.

If the renogram continues beyond the time at which the peak should normally occur, then there may be a distal obstruction (e.g., at the PUJ or lower down the ureter). In this situation, an injection of 40 mg of Lasix is given (at about 18 minutes) and if the curves start to fall rapidly, this is taken as proof that there is no obstruction. If it continues to rise, there is obstruction. If it remains flat (neither rising nor falling), this is described as an "equivocal" result.

Parenchymal transit time can also be measured (parenchymal transit time index [PTTI]). The normal range for PTTI is 40–140 seconds, and averages 70 seconds. PTTI is prolonged (to >156 seconds) in obstruction and in renal ischemia. A normal PTTI excludes obstruction.

Uses

- "Split" renal function (i.e., the % function contributed by each kidney)
- Determine presence of renal obstruction—based on shape of renogram curve and PTTI
- Determine presence of renal obstruction in response to IV Lasix injection

DMSA scanning

Dimercaptosuccinic acid (DMSA) is labeled with ^{99m}Tc. It is taken up by the proximal tubules and retained there, with very little being excreted in the urine. A "static" image of the kidneys is thus obtained (at about 3–4 hours after intravenous injection of radioisotope). It demonstrates whether a lesion contains functioning nephrons or not.

Uses

- "Split" renal function (i.e., the % function contributed by each kidney)
- Detection of scars in the kidney (these appear as defects in the cortical outline, representing areas in which the radioisotope is not taken up)

Radioisotope bone imaging

^{99m}Tc-labeled methylene-disphosphonate (MDP) is taken up by areas of bone where there is increased blood supply and increased osteoblastic activity. There are many causes of a focal increase in isotope uptake—bone metastases, site of fractures, osteomyelitis, TB, benign bone lesions (e.g., osteoma).

Metastases from urological cancers are characterized by their predilection for the spine and the fact that they are multiple (single foci of metastasis are rare). Prostate cancer classically metastasizes in this way.

Uroflowmetry

Uroflowmetry is the measurement of flow rate (Fig. 2.13). It provides a visual image of the "strength" of a patient's urinary stream. Urine flow rate is measured in mL/s and is determined using commercially available electronic flowmeters (Fig. 2.14).

These flowmeters are able to provide a printout recording the voided volume, maximum flow rate, and time taken to complete the void, together with a record of the flow pattern. Maximum flow rate, Q_{max}, is influenced by the volume of urine voided, by the contractility of the patient's bladder, and by the conductivity (resistance) of their urethra.

A number of nomograms are available that relate voided volume to flow rate (Fig. 2.15).

Interpretation and misinterpretation of urine flow rate

The "wag" artifact (see Fig. 2.13b) is seen as a sudden, rapid increase in flow rate on the uroflow tracing and is due to the urine flow suddenly being directed at the center of the flowmeter, producing a sudden artifactual surge in flow rate.

In men with prostatic symptoms, for the same voided volume, flow rate varies substantially on a given day (by as much as 5 mL/s if four flows are done[1]). Most guidelines recommend measuring at least two flow rates, and using the highest as representing the patient's best effort.

What does a low flow mean?

Uroflowmetry alone cannot tell you why the flow is abnormal. It cannot distinguish between low flow due to bladder outlet obstruction and that due to a poorly contractile bladder.

(a) 25ml/s flow rate

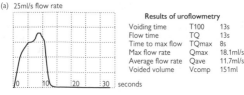

Results of uroflowmetry		
Voiding time	T100	13s
Flow time	TQ	13s
Time to max flow	TQmax	8s
Max flow rate	Qmax	18.1ml/s
Average flow rate	Qave	11.7ml/s
Voided volume	Vcomp	151ml

(b) 25ml/s flow rate

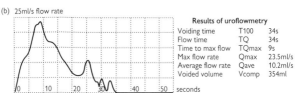

Results of uroflowmetry		
Voiding time	T100	34s
Flow time	TQ	34s
Time to max flow	TQmax	9s
Max flow rate	Qmax	23.5ml/s
Average flow rate	Qave	10.2ml/s
Voided volume	Vcomp	354ml

Figure 2.13 a) A uroflow trace; b) a uroflow trace with a "wag" artifact. The true Qmax is not 23.5mL/s as the readout suggests but is nearer 18 mL/s.

1 Reynard JM, Peters TJ, Lim C, Abrams P (1996). The value of multiple free-flow studies in men with lower urinary tract symptoms. *Br J Urol* 77:813–818.

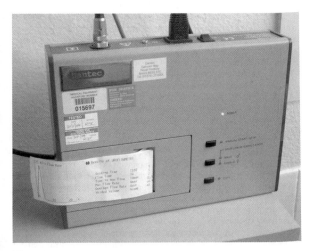

Figure 2.14 Dantec flowmeter.

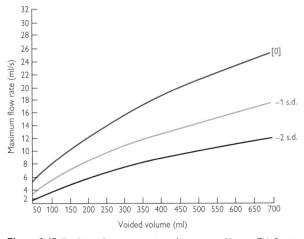

Figure 2.15 The Bristol flow rate nomogram for men over 50 years. This figure was published in Fitzpatrick J, Societe Internationale D'Urologie Reports. Non-surgical Treatment of BPH, p. 39. Copyright Elsevier 1992.

The principal use of urine flow rate measurement is in the assessment of elderly men with suspected prostatic obstruction (LUTS/BPH), although there is debate about its usefulness as a test for predicting outcome of various treatments.

Some studies suggest that men with poor outcomes are more likely to have had higher flows preoperatively compared with those with good outcomes, whereas other studies report equivalent improvements in symptoms regardless of whether the preoperative flow rate is high or low. A recent Veterans Administration trial comparing transurethral resection of the prostate (TURP) with watchful waiting in men with LUTS/BPH found that flow rate could not predict the likelihood of a good symptomatic outcome after TURP.[2]

As a consequence, different guidelines give different guidance with regard to performing uroflowmetry in men with LUTS/BPH. It is regarded as an optional test by the American Urological Association (AUA)[3] and is recommended by the Fourth International Consultation on BPH.[4] The European Association of Urology (EAU) BPH Guidelines state that it "is obligatory prior to undertaking surgical treatment."[5]

Generally speaking, urine flow rate measurement is regarded as having insufficient diagnostic accuracy for it to be useful in the assessment of female lower urinary tract dysfunction. Although urine flow measurement can be used to assess voiding function in men with urethral strictures, it has limited value in younger men because in this age group the bladder can compensate for a marked degree of obstruction by contracting more forcefully. Thus, a young man may have a normal flow rate despite having a significant urethral stricture.

2 Bruskewitz RC, Reda DJ, Wasson JH, et al. (1997). Testing to predict outcome after transurethral resection of the prostate. *J Urol* 157:1304–1308.
3 McConnell JD, Barry MJ, Bruskewitz RC, et al. (1994). Benign prostatic hyperplasia: diagnosis and treatment. Clinical practice guideline. Rockville, MD: Agency for Health Care Policy and Research.
4 Denis L (Ed.) (1997). *Fourth International Consultation on Benign Prostatic Hyperplasis (BPH)*, Paris 1997.
5 EAU guidelines for diagnosis of BPH (2001). *Eur Urol* 40:256–263.

Post-void residual urine volume measurement

Post-void residual urine (PVR) volume is the volume of urine remaining in the bladder at the end of micturition. In normal individuals there should be no urine remaining in the bladder at the end of micturition.

A PVR may be caused by detrusor underactivity (due to aging, as the older bladder is less able to sustain a contraction than the younger bladder, or neurological disease affecting bladder innervation), bladder outlet obstruction, or a combination of both.

In clinical practice, PVR volume is measured by ultrasound after the patient has attempted to empty their bladder. A commonly used formula for calculating bladder volume is

Bladder volume (mL) = bladder height (cm) × width (cm) × depth (cm) × 0.7

Interpretation and misinterpretation of PVR volume

PVR volume shows considerable day-to-day variability, with volumes recorded on different days over a 3-month period varying between 150 and 670 mL.[1]

Clinical usefulness of PVR volume measurement

PVR volume measurement cannot predict symptomatic outcome from TURP. For these reasons, residual urine volume measurement is regarded as an optional test in the AUA guidelines, but is recommended by the Fourth International Consultation on BPH.[2]

Residual urine volume measurement is useful (along with measurement of serum creatinine) as a safety measure. It indicates the likelihood of back pressure on the kidneys and thus it tells the urologist whether it is safe to offer watchful waiting rather than TURP.

In men with moderate LUTS it is safe not to operate when the PVR volume is <350 mL, and this probably holds true for those with higher PVR volumes (<700 mL).[3]

Does an elevated residual urine volume predispose to urinary infection?

Though intuition would suggest yes, what evidence there is relating residual volume to urine infection suggests that an elevated residual urine may not, at least in the neurologically normal adult, predispose to urine infection.[4,5]

---

1 Dunsmuir WD, Feneley M, Corry DA, et al. (1996). The day-to-day variation (test–retest reliability) of residual urine measurement. *Br J Urol* 77:192–193.
2 Denis L (Ed.) (1997). *Fourth International Consultation on Benign Prostatic Hyperplasia (BPH)*, Paris, 1997.
3 Bates TS, Sugiono M, James ED, et al. (2003). Is the conservative management of chronic retention in men ever justified? *Br J Urol Int* 92:581–583.
4 Riehmann M, Goetzmann B, Langer E, et al. (1994). Risk factor for bacteriuria in men. *Urology* 43:617–620.
5 Hampson SJ, Noble JG, Rickards D, Milroy EG (1992). Does residual urine predispose to urinary tract infection. *Br J Urol* 70:506–508.

Cystometry, pressure-flow studies, and videocystometry

- **Cystometry** is the recording of bladder pressure during bladder filling.
- **Pressure-flow study (PFS)** is the simultaneous recording of bladder pressure during voiding.
- **Videocystometry** is fluoroscopy (X-ray screening) combined with PFS during voiding (see Fig. 2.8).

These techniques provide the most precise measurements of bladder and urethral sphincter behavior during bladder filling and during voiding. Cystometry precedes the pressure-flow study.

Bladder pressure (P_{ves}, measured by a urethral or suprapubic catheter) and abdominal pressure (P_{abd}, measured by a pressure line inserted into the rectum) are recorded as the bladder fills (cystometric phase) and empties (voiding phase), and flow rate is simultaneously measured during the voiding phase.

The pressure developed by the detrusor (the bladder muscle), P_{det}, cannot be directly measured, but it can be derived by subtracting abdominal pressure from the pressure measured within the bladder (the intravesical pressure). This allows the effect of rises in intra-abdominal pressure caused by coughing or straining to be subtracted from the total (intravesical) pressure, so that a pure detrusor pressure is obtained.

All pressures are recorded in cm H_2O and flow rate is measured in mL/s. The pressure lines are small-bore, fluid-filled catheters attached to an external pressure transducer, or catheter-tip pressure transducers can be used.

A computerized printout of intravesical pressure (P_{ves}), intra-abdominal pressure (P_{abd}), and detrusor pressure (P_{det}) and flow rate (Q_{max}) is obtained (Fig. 2.16).

During bladder filling, the presence of overactive bladder contractions can be detected. During voiding, the key parameters are Q_{max} and the detrusor pressure at the point at which Q_{max} is reached, $P_{det} Q_{max}$. This pressure, relative to Q_{max}, can be used to define the presence of bladder outlet obstruction by using a variety of nomograms, of which the ICS nomogram is most widely used.

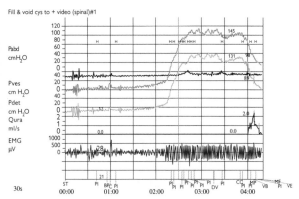

Figure 2.16 Computerized printout of intravesical pressure (Pves), intra-abdominal pressure (Pabd), subtracted detrusor pressure (Pdet), and flow rate (Qmax).

Bladder outlet obstruction

Regulation of prostate growth and development of benign
    prostatic hyperplasia (BPH) 64
Pathophysiology and causes of bladder outlet obstruction
    (BOO) and BPH 66
Benign prostatic obstruction (BPO): symptoms and
    signs 68
Diagnostic tests in men with LUTS thought to be
    due to BPH 70
Why do men seek treatment for their symptoms? 72
Watchful waiting for uncomplicated BPH 74
Medical management of BPH: α-blockers 76
Medical management of BPH: 5α-reductase inhibitors 78
Medical management of BPH: combination therapy 80
Medical management of BPH: alternative drug therapy 82
Minimally invasive management of BPH: surgical
    alternatives to TURP 84
Invasive surgical alternatives to TURP 86
TURP and open prostatectomy 88
Acute urinary retention: definition, pathophysiology,
    and causes 90
Acute urinary retention: initial and definitive
    management 94
Indications for and technique of urethral
    catheterization 96
Indications for and technique of suprapubic
    catheterization 98
Management of nocturia and nocturnal polyuria 100
High-pressure chronic retention (HPCR) 102
Bladder outlet obstruction and retention in women 104
Urethral stricture disease 106

Regulation of prostate growth and development of benign prostatic hyperplasia (BPH)

BPH is characterized by an increase in epithelial and stromal cell numbers (hyperplasia) in the periurethral area of the prostate. New epithelial gland formation is normally only seen during fetal development. The development of new glands in the adult prostate has given rise to the concept of 'reawakening' of the inductive effect of the prostatic stroma on the prostatic epithelium.

The increase in prostate cell number could reflect proliferation of epithelial and stromal cells, impairment of programmed cell death, or a combination of both. During the early phases of development of BPH, cell proliferation occurs rapidly. In established BPH, cell proliferation slows down and there is impairment of programmed cell death (androgens and estrogens actively inhibit cell death).

The role of androgens in BPH (Fig. 3.1)

Testosterone can bind directly to the androgen receptor, or may be converted to a more potent form, dihydrotestosterone (DHT), by the enzyme 5α-reductase (5AR).

There are two isoforms of 5AR: type I, or extraprostatic, 5AR (which is absent in prostatic tissue and present in, for example, skin and liver) and type II, or prostatic, 5AR (which is found exclusively on the nuclear membrane of stromal cells, but not within prostatic epithelial cells). Type I 5AR is not inhibited by finasteride, whereas type II 5AR is. Dutesteride will block both type I and type II 5AR isoforms.

Testosterone diffuses into prostate and stromal epithelial cells. Within *epithelial* cells it binds directly to the androgen receptor. In prostate *stromal* cells a small proportion binds directly to the androgen receptor, but the majority binds to 5AR (type II) on the nuclear membrane, is converted to DHT, and then binds (with greater affinity and therefore greater potency than testosterone) to the androgen receptor in the stromal cell.

Some of the DHT formed in the stromal cells diffuses out of these cells and into nearby epithelial cells (a paracrine action). The androgen receptor–testosterone or androgen receptor–DHT complex then binds to specific binding sites in the nucleus, thereby inducing transcription of androgen-dependent genes and subsequent protein synthesis.

It is thought that stromal–epithelial interactions may be mediated by soluble growth factors—small peptides that stimulate or inhibit cell division and differentiation. Growth stimulating factors include basic fibroblastic growth factor (bFGF), epidermal growth factor (EGF), keratinocyte growth factor (KGF), and insulin-like growth factor (IGF).

Transforming growth factors (e.g., TGF-β) normally inhibit epithelial cell proliferation, and it is possible that in BPH, TGF-β is down-regulated.

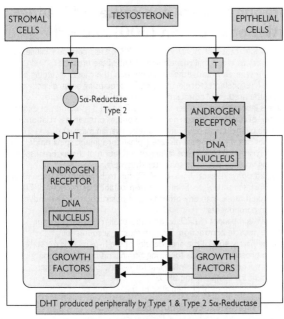

Figure 3.1 Testosterone (T) diffuses into the prostate epithelial and stromal cell (see text). This figure was published in Walsh PC, et al. Campbell's Urology, 8th edition, p. 1299. Copyright Elsevier 2002.

Pathophysiology and causes of bladder outlet obstruction (BOO) and BPH

The principle cause of BOO in men is BPH. Less common causes are urethral stricture and malignant enlargement of the prostate.

BOO in women is altogether less common, the causes including pelvic prolapse (cystocele, rectocele, uterine), the prolapsing organ directly compressing the urethra; urethral stricture; urethral diverticulum; post-surgery for stress incontinence; Fowler syndrome (impaired relaxation of external sphincter occurring in premenopausal women, often in association with polycystic ovaries); and pelvic masses (e.g., ovarian masses).

In either sex, neurological disease (spinal cord injury, spina bifida, multiple sclerosis [MS]) can cause failure of relaxation of the external sphincter during voiding (detrusor sphincter dyssynergia [DSD]).

The pathophysiological basis of BOO due to benign prostatic enlargement (BPE) secondary to BPH (benign prostatic obstruction, BPO) has been studied more than any other type of obstruction. BPO has dynamic and static components:

- *Dynamic component of BPO:* α_1-adrenoceptor-mediated prostatic smooth muscle contraction. Smooth muscle accounts for approximately 40% of the area density of the hyperplastic prostate and human prostate contracts following administration of α-adrenergic agonists. This effect is the rationale for α-adrenoceptor blocker treatment for symptomatic BPO.
- *Static component of BPO:* mediated by the volume effect of BPE.

Pathophysiological consequences of BOO

John Hunter (1786), who founded the Royal College of Surgeons of England, noted that "the disease of the bladder arising from obstruction alone is increased irritability and its consequences, by which it admits of little distension, becomes quick in its action and thick and strong in its coats."

BOO causes thickening of the wall of the bladder. Microscopically, smooth muscle cells enlarge and there is an increase in connective tissue (collagen and elastin) between the smooth muscle bundles. In some cases, this may lead to poor compliance, with development of high bladder and intrarenal pressures. Progressive hydronephrosis can develop, with impairment of renal function and even renal failure (high-pressure chronic urinary retention).

Experimentally created BOO causes development of bladder overactivity (unstable bladder contractions during bladder filling). This may be due to prolonged increased intravesical pressure during voiding causing ischemia and leading to ischemic damage to neurons within the bladder (i.e., denervation).

Symptomatically, many patients with BOO develop frequency, urgency, and urge incontinence.

Benign prostatic obstruction (BPO): symptoms and signs

Clinical practice guidelines

Such guidelines were developed to standardize the approach to diagnosis (and treatment) of men presenting with symptoms suggestive of BPH (see Box 3.1).[1] Every guideline agrees that a history should be taken, an examination performed, and the severity of urinary symptoms be formally assessed using the IPSS (the International Prostate Symptom Score). This includes a measure of the "problems" caused by the patient's symptoms (i.e., the degree to which the symptoms are troubling).

Urinary symptoms—what do they mean?

During the 1990s, the classic "prostatic" symptoms of frequency, urgency, nocturia, hesitancy, poor flow, an intermittent flow, and terminal dribbling—traditionally said to indicate the presence of BOO due to benign prostatic enlargement—were shown to bear little relationship to prostate size, flow rate, residual urine volume, or urodynamic evidence of BOO. Age-matched elderly men and women have similar symptom scores (IPSS), despite the fact that women have no prostate and rarely have BOO.

Prostatism vs. LUTS vs. LUTS/BPH

Prostatism has thus been replaced by the expression *lower urinary tract symptoms (LUTS)*, which avoids any implication about the cause of these symptoms. More recently, the expression *LUTS/BPH* has been used to describe the symptoms of BPH.

It doesn't really matter whether you use prostatism, LUTS, or LUTS/BPH as long as you remember that urinary symptoms may have nonprostatic causes. Try to avoid treating the prostate when the problem may lie elsewhere.

Ask specifically about the presence of the following:

- **Bed-wetting** suggests the presence of high-pressure chronic retention (look for distension of the abdomen due to a grossly enlarged bladder which is tense on palpation and dull to percussion).
- **Marked frequency and urgency**, particularly when also combined with bladder pain: look for carcinoma in situ of the bladder (urine cytology, flexible cystoscopy, and bladder biopsy).
- **Macroscopic hematuria** is sometimes due to a large vascular prostate, but exclude other causes (bladder and kidney cancer and stones) by flexible cystoscopy and upper tract imaging.
- **Back pain and neurological symptoms** (sciatica, lower limb weakness or tingling). Rarely, LUTS can be due to neurological disease.

---

1 Irani J, Brown CT, van der Meulen J, Emberton M (2003). A review of guidelines on benign prostatic hyperplasia and lower urinary tract symptoms: are all guidelines the same? *Br J Urol Int* 92:937–942.

Box 3.1 Websites for BPH clinical practice guidelines

- AUA guidelines: http://www.auanet.org/content/guidelines-and-quality-care/clinical-guidelines.cfm
- EAU guidelines: http://www.uroweb.org/files/uploaded_files/bph.pdf
- WHO (International Consensus Committee) guidelines: http://www.who.int/ina-ngo/ngo/ngo048.htm
- Australian guidelines: http://www.health.gov.au/nhmrc/publications/pdf/cp42.pdf
- German guidelines: http://dgu.springer.de/leit/pdf/3_99.pdf
- Singapore guidelines: http://www.urology-singapore.org.html/guidelines_bph.htm
- Malaysian guidelines: http://www.mohtrg.gov.my/guidelines/bph98.pdf
- UK guidelines: http://www.rcseng.ac.uk/publications/

Diagnostic tests in men with LUTS thought to be due to BPH

Clinical practice guidelines

Guidelines were developed as an attempt to standardize the approach to diagnosis and treatment of men presenting with symptoms suggestive of BPH[1] (see Box 3.1). All agree that a history should be taken and an examination performed, and all recommend assessment of symptom severity using the IPSS (International Prostate Symptom Score). This includes a measure of the problems caused by the patient's symptoms.

There is considerable variation among guidelines in terms of recommended diagnostic tests. High-quality guidelines (e.g., based on results of randomized trials) recommend few diagnostic tests[2]—urine analysis, completion of a voiding diary (frequency–volume chart) to detect the presence of polyuria and nocturnal polyuria (which may be the cause of a patient's increased frequency or nocturia), and measurement of serum creatinine. They regard flow rate measurement and assessment of residual urine volume as optional tests.

Digital rectal examination (DRE) and PSA

DRE and PSA testing are done to detect nodules that may indicate an underlying prostate cancer and to provide a rough indication of prostate size. Size alone is not an indication for treatment, but if surgical treatment is contemplated, marked prostatic enlargement can be confirmed by transrectal ultrasound (TRUS) scan (prostate volume in the order of 100 mL or more increases the likelihood of an open prostatectomy).

Discuss the pros and cons of PSA testing with the patient.

Serum creatinine

This is a baseline measure of renal function, used to detect renal failure secondary to high-pressure urinary retention.

Post-void residual urine volume (PVR)

PVR varies considerably (by as much as 600 mL between repeat measurements) on the same or on different days.[3] It cannot predict symptomatic outcome from transurethral resection of the prostate (TURP). Along with serum creatinine, it indicates whether watchful waiting is safe.

It is safe *not* to operate when the PVR volume is <350 mL,[4,5] since the majority of men show no worsening of creatinine, no increase in PVR, and no worsening of symptoms and do not require TURP or other bladder outlet procedure.

Flow rate measurement

This is variously regarded as *optional*, *recommended*, and *obligatory* prior to undertaking surgical treatment for BPH. Like PVR, measured flow rate varies substantially on a given day,[6] cannot distinguish between BOO and a poorly contractile bladder, and is not good at predicting the likelihood of a good symptomatic outcome after TURP.

Pressure-flow studies

Such studies are reasonably good at predicting symptomatic outcome after TURP. However, most patients without obstruction have a good outcome, and the time, cost, and invasiveness of pressure-flow studies are perceived by most urologists as not justifying their routine use.

Renal ultrasonography

This is used to detect hydronephrosis if serum creatinine is elevated. The percentage of patients having upper tract dilatation on ultrasound according to serum creatinine is as follows: creatinine <115 mmol/L (1.5 mg/dL), 0.8%; creatinine 115–130 mmol/L (1.5–1.7 mg/dL), 9%; and creatinine >130 mmol/L (1.7 mg/dL), 33%.[7]

Further reading

Roehrborn CG (2008). Currently available treatment guidelines for men with lower urinary tract symptoms. Br J Urol 102:18–23.

Wei JT, Calhoun E, Jacobsen SJ (2005). Urologic diseases in America project: benign prostatic hyperplasia. J Urol 173:1256–1261.

Emberton M, Andriole GL, de la Rosette J, Djavan B, Hoefner K, Nvarette R et al. (2003). Benign prostatic hyperplasia: a progressive disease of aging men. Urol 61:267–273.

1 Roehrborn CG, Bartsch G, Kirby R, et al. (2001) Guidelines for the diagnosis and treatment of benign prostatic hyperplasia: a comparative international overview. Urology 58:642–650.

2 Irani J, Brown CT, van der Meulen J, Emberton M (2003) A review of guidelines on benign prostatic hyperplasia and lower urinary tract symptoms: are all guidelines the same? Br J Urol Int 92:937–942.

3 Dunsmuir WD, Feneley M, Corry DA, et al. (1996) The day-to-day variation (test–retest reliability) of residual urine measurement. Br J Urol 77:192–193.

4 Bates TS, Sugiono M, James ED, et al. (2003) Is the conservative management of chronic retention in men ever justified? Br J Urol Int 92:581–583.

5 Wasson JH, Reda DJ, Bruskewitz RC, et al. (1995) A comparison of transurethral surgery with watchful waiting for moderate symptom of benign prostatic hyperplasia. The Veterans Administration Cooperative Study Group on Transurethral Resection of the Prostate. N Engll Med 332:75–79.

6 Reynard JM, Peters TJ, Lim C, Abrams P (1996) The value of multiple free-flow studies in men with lower urinary tract symptoms. Br J Urol 77:813–818.

7 Koch WF, Ezz el Din KE, De Wildt MJ, et al. (1996) The outcome of renal ultrasound in the assessment of 556 consecutive patients with benign prostatic hyperplasia. J Urol 155:186–189.

Why do men seek treatment for their symptoms?

Men seek treatment for their LUTS for several reasons:
• The symptoms may be bothersome.
• They may fear that the symptoms are a warning sign that acute urinary retention will develop.
• They may be concerned that their symptoms indicate that they have prostate cancer.

Establish what the patient wants from his consultation with you. Once reassured that the likelihood of urinary retention and prostate cancer is low, he may not want treatment for symptoms that on the surface may appear quite bad and he may be happy to adopt a policy of watchful waiting.

Bothersome symptoms

Bothersome symptoms do not necessarily equate with symptom severity as assessed by symptom scores. Thus, a man with a low symptom score may find his symptoms very bothersome and may want treatment, whereas another man with a high symptom score may not be bothered and may want no treatment.

If one symptom is particularly bad, but the other 6 symptoms in the 7-symptom score are minimal, overall symptom score will obviously be relatively low, but the patient may find that one symptom very bothersome (e.g., urgency and nocturia tend to be more bothersome than hesitancy or poor flow).

"Are my symptoms due to prostate cancer?"

No particular LUTS are specific for prostate cancer. Even if it turns out that the patient does have prostate cancer, a patient's symptoms might be due to coexistent BPH or some other LUT pathology. If he is concerned about the possibility of prostate cancer, counsel him with regard to PSA testing and prostate biopsy.

"Am I likely to develop retention of urine?"

Many patients are understandably concerned that their urinary symptoms may be a harbinger for the development of acute urinary retention. This may influence their decision to seek help for symptoms that they may perceive as indicating a risk of subsequent retention, and it may affect the type of treatment they choose.

Table 3.1 can help give the patient some idea of his risk of developing urinary retention.

Table 3.1 Yearly risk of retention according to age and symptom score (number of men experiencing an episode of retention every year)*

Age (years)	Mild symptoms (AUA symptom score ≤7)	Moderate or severe symptoms (AUA symptom score >7)
40–49	3 men in every 1000	3 men in every 1000
70–79	9 men in every 1000	34 men in every 1000

Adjusting for age and flow rate, those with an AUA symptom score of 8 or more had a 2.3-fold increased risk of going into urinary retention compared with those with an AUA score of 7 or less. Those men with a peak flow rate of <12 mL/s had a 4-fold increased risk of urinary retention compared with those with a flow rate of >12 mL/s. Prostate volume over 30 mL was associated with a 3-fold increased risk of urinary retention compared with those with prostate volumes <30 mL

This table is from Jacobsen et al.'s (1997) report,[1] a 4-year prospective study of a cohort of >2000 men. The presence of LUTS, a low flow rate, an enlarged prostate, and old age were associated with an increased risk of urinary retention.

1 Jacobsen SJ, Jacobson DJ, Girman CJ, et al. (1997) Natural history of prostatism: risk factors for acute urinary retention. *J Urol* 158:481–487.

Further reading

McConnell JD, Bruskewitz R, Walsh P, et al. (1998). The effect of finasteride on the risk of acute urinary retention and the need for surgical treatment among men with benign prostatic hyperplasia. Finasteride Long-Term Efficacy and Safety Study Group. *N Engl J Med* 338(9):557–563.

Watchful waiting for uncomplicated BPH

A number of studies have shown that in a substantial proportion of men, symptoms do not progress, even for those with severe symptoms.

Ball et al. study[1]

A total of 107 men were followed with watchful waiting over 5 years, and none developed an absolute indication for surgery. Half of the patients were obstructed on urodynamic testing. A third of the patients got better, just under a half stayed the same, a quarter got worse (of whom 8 underwent TURP), and 2% went into retention.

PLESS study[2]

In the Proscar long-term efficacy and safety study (PLESS), 1500 men with moderate to severe symptoms were randomized to placebo (and a similar number to active drug). Those on placebo had an average fall in symptom score of 1 point at 4 years.

Wasson study of watchful waiting vs. TURP[3]

For men with moderate symptoms, the risk of progression to retention, worsening symptoms, or need for TURP was relatively low in those who chose watchful waiting. Forty percent noticed an improvement in their symptoms, 30% got worse, and TURP was required in about a quarter.

Five centers' study[4]

In this study, 500 men referred by their family doctors for consideration for TURP were managed nonoperatively after viewing an educational program. Over the following 4-year period, a proportion of the men chose drug treatment or surgery. For men with mild, moderate, or severe symptoms, 10%, 24%, and 39%, respectively, had undergone surgery at the end of 4 years. For the same symptom categories, 63%, 45%, and 33% were still not receiving any treatment at the end of 4 years. Almost a quarter of men who initially presented with severe symptoms noted an improvement in their symptoms, to mild or moderate.

On the basis of all of these studies we can say that symptoms, even if severe, do not necessarily get worse even over fairly long periods of time. This forms the foundation of watchful waiting as an option for many patients, even if the symptoms at baseline are severe.

The International Prostate Symptom Score (IPSS) measures not only symptom severity but also, more importantly, the *bother* that the symptoms cause the patient. Thus, if a patient has a high symptom score (severe symptoms) but is not bothered by these symptoms, there is no indication for treatment.

By contrast, some patients have a low symptom score but may find even this degree of symptoms very bothersome. Treatment is indicated in such cases (usually starting with medical therapy such as an α-blocker or 5α-reductase inhibitor).

Further reading

Chapple CR (2004). Pharmacological therapy of benign prostatic hyperplasia/lower urinary tract symptoms: an overview for the practicing clinician. *Br J Urol Int* 94:738–744.

O'Leary MP (2003). Lower urinary tract symptoms/benign prostatic hyperplasia: maintaining symptom control and reducing complications. *Urol* 62:15–23.

1 Ball AJ, Feneley RC, Abrams PH (1981). Natural history of untreated 'prostatism'. *Br J Urol* 53:613–616.

2 McConnell JD, Bruskewitz R, Walsh PC, et al. (1998). The effect of finasteride on the risk of acute urinary retention and the need for surgical treatment among men with benign prostatic hyperplasia. Finasteride Long-Term Efficacy and Safety Study (PLESS) Group *N Engl J Med* 338:557–563.

3 Wasson JH, Reda DJ, Bruskewitz RC, et al. (1995). A comparison of transurethral surgery with watchful waiting for moderate symptoms of benign prostatic hyperplasia. The Veterans Affairs Cooperative Study Group on Transurethral Resection of the Prostate. *N Engl J Med* 332:75–79.

4 Barry MJ, Fowler FJJ, Bin L, et al. (1997). The natural history of patients with benign prostatic hyperplasia as diagnosed by North American urologists. *J Urol* 157:10–14.

Medical management of BPH: α-blockers

The rationale for α-blocker therapy in BPH

As described earlier, BPO is caused partly by α_1-adrenoceptor-mediated prostatic smooth muscle contraction, and this is the rationale for α-adrenoceptor blocker treatment for symptomatic BPO.

There are two broad subtypes of α-adrenoceptor (AR)—α_1 and α_2. Molecular cloning studies have identified three α_1-AR subtypes—α_{1a} (predominant in human stroma and therefore mediates prostate smooth muscle contraction), α_{1b} (predominant in human prostate epithelium), and α_{1L} (believed to be a conformational state of the α_{1a}-AR). The AR subtypes mediating efficacy and side effects of α-adrenoceptor blocking drugs are unknown.

α-Blocker classification

α-Blockers are categorized by their selectivity for the AR and by their elimination half-life.
- Nonselective: phenoxybenzamine or prazosin—effective symptom control, but high side-effect profile
- Long-acting α_1: terazosin, doxazosin
- Subtype selective: tamsulosin, alfuzosin, and silodosin—relatively selective for α_{1a}-AR subtype compared to the α_{1b} subtype

No study has directly compared one α-blocker with another in terms of efficacy or side effects.

Indications for treatment

These include bothersome lower urinary tract symptoms where watchful waiting has failed or the patient wishes to have treatment.

Efficacy

Percentage of patients who respond to α-blockers
If response is defined as >25% improvement in symptoms relative to placebo, most studies describe response rates of 30–40%.[1] The mean probability for improvement in symptom score after TURP is on the order of 80% (i.e., 8 out of 10 men will notice an improvement in their symptoms after TURP).

Improvements in symptom score in men who respond to α-blockers
The average improvement in symptom score after TURP is about 85%.[2] While some of this may represent a placebo response, this improvement is considerably better than that seen with the α-blockers, which result in a 10–30% improvement in symptom score relative to placebo.[3] This equates to a 4–5 point improvement in symptom score over placebo.

Side effects

A substantial proportion of men stop taking their medication because of either side effects (15–30% report some constellation of side effects) or a perceived lack of effectiveness.

Side effects include asthenia (weakness, in 5%), dizziness (6%), headache (2%) and postural hypotension (1%), and retrograde ejaculation (8%).

1 Lowe F (1999). Alpha-1-adrenoceptor blockade in the treatment of benign prostatic hyperplasia. *Prost Cancer Prost Dis* 2:110–119.

2 McConnell JD, Barry MD, Bruskewitz RC, et al. (1994). The BPH Guideline Panel. Benign prostatic hyperplasia: diagnosis and treatment. Clinical practice guideline. Agency for Health Care Policy and Research, publication No.94–0582, 1994, Rockville, MD: Public Health Service, U.S. Department of Health and Human Sciences.

3 Boyle P, Robertson C, Manski R, et al. (2001). Meta-analysis of randomized trials of terazosin in the treatment of benign prostatic hyperplasia. *Urology* 58:717–722.

Medical management of BPH: 5α-reductase inhibitors

5α-reductase inhibitors inhibit the conversion of testosterone to dihydro-testosterone (DHT), the more potent androgen in the prostate. This causes shrinkage of the prostatic epithelium and thus a reduction in prostate volume, thereby reducing the static component of benign prostatic enlargement. This takes some months to occur, so urinary symptoms will not improve initially.

Finasteride is a competitive inhibitor of the enzyme 5α-reductase (type II isoenzyme), which converts testosterone to DHT. Finasteride therefore lowers serum and intraprostatic DHT levels.

Dutasteride is a dual inhibitor (type I and II isoenzyme) of 5α-reductase. Whether it has any clinically significant advantages over finasteride in the treatment of BPH remains to be established.

Efficacy

A number of large studies have shown symptom improvement over placebo on the order of 2–3 points on the IPSS and improvements in flow rate on the order of 1–2 mL/s (SCARP[1] [Scandinavian BPH Study Group], PROSPECT[2] [Proscar Safety Plus Efficacy Canadian Two-year Study], PROWESS [Proscar Worldwide Efficacy and Safety Study] Group,[3] and, more recently, PLESS[4] [Proscar Long-term Efficacy and Safety Study]). The PLESS data also show a small reduction in the risk of urinary retention.

Side effects

Generally speaking, these are fairly mild. Principally they center on sexual problems (e.g., loss of libido, 5%; impotence, 5%; reduced volume of ejaculate in a few percent of patients).

5α-reductase inhibitors and risk of urinary retention

The PLESS data[4] have been widely publicized as showing a substantial reduction in the risk of urinary retention. In this 4-year follow-up study, 42 of 1471 men on finasteride went into urinary retention (3%), while 99 of 1404 on placebo experienced an episode of retention (7%). This represents an impressive 43% *relative* reduction in risk in those taking finasteride.

However, the *absolute* risk reduction over a 4-year period is a less impressive 4%. So, finasteride does reduce the risk of retention, but it is reducing the risk of an event that is actually quite rare, as suggested by the fact that 93% of men on placebo in this study did not experience retention over a 4-year period. Put another way, to prevent 1 episode of retention, 25 men would have to continue treatment with finasteride for 4 years.

5α-reductase inhibitors for hematuria due to BPH

Shrinking large vascular prostates probably helps reduce the frequency of hematuria in men with BPH.[5]

Further reading

Debruyne FM, Jardin A, Colloi D, et al. (1998). Sustained-release alfuzosin, finasteride and the combination of both in the treatment of benign prostatic hyperplasia. *Eur Urol* 34:169–175.

Kirby RS, Roerborn C, Boyle P, et al. (2003). Efficacy and tolerability of doxazosin and finasteride, alone or in combination, in treatment of symptomatic benign prostatic hyperplasia: the Prospective European Doxazosin and Combination Therapy (PREDICT) trial. *Urology* 61:119–126.

Lepor H, Williford WO, Barry MJ, et al. (1996). The efficacy of terazosin, finasteride, or both in benign prostatic hypertrophy. *N Engl J Med* 335:533–539.

McConnell JD, Roehrborn CG, Bautista OM, et al. (2003). The long-term effect of doxazosin, finasteride, and combination therapy on the clinical progression of benign prostatic hyperplasia. *New Engl J Med* 349:2387–2398.

1 Andersen JT, Ekman P, Wolf H, et al. (1995). Can finasteride reverse the progress of benign prostatic hyperplasia? A two-year placebo-controlled study. The Scandinavian BPH Study Group. *Urology* 46:631–637.

2 Nickel J, Fradet Y, Boake RC, et al. (1996). Efficacy and safety of finasteride therapy for benign prostatic hyperplasia: results of a 2-year randomised controlled trial (the PROSPECT study). PROscar Safety Plus Efficacy Canadian Two Year Study. *Can Med Assoc J* 155:1251–1259.

3 Marberger MJ (1998). Long-term effects of finasteride in patients with benign prostatic hyperplasia: a double-blind, placebo-controlled, multicenter study. PROWESS Study Group. *Urology* 51:677–686.

4 McConnell JD, Bruskewitz R, Walsh PC, et al. (1998). The effect of finasteride on the risk of acute urinary retention and the need for surgical treatment among men with benign prostatic hyperplasia. Finasteride Long-Term Efficacy and Safety Study (PLESS) Group. *N Engl J Med* 338:557–563.

5 Foley SJ, Soloman LZ, Wedderburn AW, et al. (2000). Finasteride for haematuria due to BPH. A prospective study of the natural history of hematuria associated with BPH and the effect of finasteride. *J Urol* 163:496–498.

Medical management of BPH: combination therapy

A combination of an α-blocker and a 5α-reductase inhibitor can be used to manage BPH. The relevant studies are as follows:

- **MTOPS study**[1] (Medical Therapy of Prostatic Symptoms): This combination prevented progression of BPH (progression being defined as a worsening of symptom score by 4 or more, or the development of complications such as UTI or acute urinary retention).
- **Veterans Affairs Combination Therapy Study**[2]: 1200 men were randomized to placebo, finasteride, terazosin, or a combination of terazosin and finasteride. At 1-year follow-up, relative to placebo, finasteride had reduced the symptom score by an average of 3 points, whereas terazosin alone or in combination with finasteride had reduced the symptom score by an average of 6 points.
- **PREDICT study**[3] (Prospective European Doxazosin and Combination Therapy): randomized over 1000 men to placebo, finasteride, doxazosin, or a combination of finasteride and doxazosin. The differences in symptom score at baseline and at 1-year follow-up were −5.7 and −6.6 for placebo and finasteride, and −8.3 and −8.5 for doxazosin and combination therapy.
- **ALFIN study**[4] (ALFuzosin, FINasteride, and combination in the treatment of BPH): 1000 men were randomized to alfuzosin, finasteride, or a combination. At 6 months, the improvement in the IPSS was not significantly different in the alfuzosin vs. the combination group.
- **CombAT study**[4,5] (tamsulosin, dutasteride, and combination in the treatment of BPH): 4844 men were randomized to tamsulosin, dutasteride, or a combination. At 24 months, the improvement in the IPSS was significantly different in the tamsulosin vs. the combination group. Combination therapy was better in patients with a large prostate than monotherapy with the α-blocker or 5α-reductase inhibitor alone.

Thus, in two large studies (CombAT and MTOPS), combination therapy was more useful than monotherapy with either an α-blocker or 5α-reductase inhibitor alone. Currently, dual therapy with an α-blocker and a 5α-reductase inhibitor is usually reserved for patients who are symptomatic with a large prostate (>40 g or a PSA >1.5 ng/mL).

In addition, 5α-reductase inhibitor therapy has been studied in patients with prostate cancer (Prostate Cancer Prevention Trial).[6] Over 18,000 men were randomized to finasteride or placebo over a 7-year period. Those in the finasteride group had a 25% lower prevalence of prostate cancer detected on prostate biopsy. However, higher-grade tumors, which are biologically more aggressive than low-grade cancers, were more common in the finasteride group. Further research in this area has suggested that prostate reduced in size by finasteride may have made higher-grade disease easier to biopsy and find.

The REDUCE trial enrolled over 8000 men to study the effect of dutasteride on prostate cancer prevention. This international 4-year study examined patients with intermediate risk for the development of prostate cancer. In order to enroll in the study, patients were required to have a 10 core prostate biopsy on entry and at years 2 and 4. Results showed a 23% reduction in the development of prostate cancer, and those that did develop cancer did not have higher-grade disease.[7]

1 McConnell JD, Roehrborn CG, Bautista OM, et al. (2003). The long-term effect of doxazosin, finasteride, and combination therapy on the clinical progression of benign prostatic hyperplasia. N Engl J Med 349:2387–2398.
2 Lepor H, Williford WO, Barry MJ, et al. (1996). The efficacy of terazosin, finasteride, or both in benign prostatic hypertrophy. N Engl J Med 335:533–539.
3 Kirby RS, Roerborn C, Boyle P, et al. (2003). Efficacy and tolerability of doxazosin and finasteride, alone or in combination, in treatment of symptomatic benign prostatic hyperplasia: the Prospective European Doxazosin and Combination Therapy (PREDICT) trial. Urology 61:119–126.
4 Debruyne FM, Jardin A, Colloi D, et al. (1998). Sustained-release alfuzosin, finasteride and the combination of both in the treatment of benign prostatic hyperplasia. Eur Urol 34:169–175.
5 Barkin J, Roehrborn CG, Siami P, et al. (2009). CombAT Study Group. Effect of dutasteride, tamsulosin and the combination on patient-reported quality of life and treatment satisfaction in men with moderate-to-severe benign prostatic hyperplasia: 2-year data from the CombAT trial. BJU Int 103(7):919–926.
6 Thompson IM, Goodman PJ, Tangen CM, et al. (2003). The influence of finasteride on the development of prostate cancer. N Engl J Med 349:215–224.
7 Andriole GL, Bostwick D, Brawley O, et al. (2010). The influence of dutasteride on the risk of biopsy-detectable prostate cancer: outcomes of the REduction by DUtasteride of Prostate Cancer Events (REDUCE) study. N Engl J Med 362:1192–1202.

Medical management of BPH: alternative drug therapy

Anticholinergics

For a man with frequency, urgency, and urge incontinence—symptoms suggestive of an overactive bladder—consider prescribing an anticholinergic (e.g., oxybutynin, tolterodine, trospium chloride, or flavoxate). There is the concern that these drugs could precipitate urinary retention in men with BOO (because they block parasympathetic/cholinergic mediated contraction of the detrusor), but the risk of this occurring is probably very low, even in men with urodynamically proven BOO.[1]

Phytotherapy

An alternative drug treatment for BPH symptoms, and one that is widely used in Europe and increasingly in North America, is phytotherapy. Half of all medications consumed for BPH symptoms are phytotherapeutic ones.[2] These agents are derived from plants and include the African plum (*Pygeum africanum*), purple coneflower (*Echinacea purpurea*), South African star grass (*Hipoxis rooperi*), and saw palmetto berry (*Seronoa Repens, Permixon*).

Saw palmetto contains an anti-inflammatory, antiproliferative, estrogenic drug with 5α-reductase inhibitory activity, derived from the American dwarf palm. It has been compared with finasteride in a large double-blind, randomized trial, and equivalent (40%) reductions in symptom score were found with both agents over a 6-month period. A meta-analysis of 18 randomized controlled trials of almost 3000 men has suggested that *Seronoa repens* produces similar improvements in symptoms and flow rates to those produced by finasteride.[3]

A recent *New England Journal of Medicine* study found saw palmetto no better than placebo in relieving BPH symptoms.[4]

South African star grass (*Hipoxis rooperi*, marketed as Harzol) contains β-sitosterol, which may induce apoptosis in prostate stromal cells by causing elevated levels of TGF-β_1. In a double-blind, randomized control trial, symptom improvement was 5 points over that with placebo.

For other agents (e.g., *Urtica dioica*—stinging nettle; the African plum) the studies have not been placebo controlled and lack sufficient statistical power to prove conclusively that they work.[2]

1 Reynard J (2004). Does anticholinergic medication have a role for men with lower urinary tract symptoms/benign prostatic hyperplasia either alone or in combination with other agents? *Curr Opin Urol* 14:13–16.
2 Lowe FC, Fagelman E (1999). Phytotherapy in the treatment of benign prostatic hyperplasia: an update. *Urology* 53:671–678.
3 Wilt JW, Ishani A, Stark G, et al. (1998). Saw palmetto extracts for treatment of benign prostatic hyperplasia: a systematic review. *JAMA* 280:1604–1608.
4 Bent S, et al. (2006) Saw palmetto extracts for treatment of benign prostatic hyperplasia. *N Engl J Med* 354:557–566.

Minimally invasive management of BPH: surgical alternatives to TURP

In 1989, Roos reported a seemingly higher mortality and reoperation rate after TURP than with open prostatectomy.[1] This result, combined with other studies suggesting that symptomatic outcome after TURP was poor in a substantial proportion of patients and that TURP was associated with substantial morbidity, prompted the search for less invasive treatments.

The two broad categories of alternative surgical techniques are minimally invasive and invasive. All are essentially heat treatments, delivered at variable temperature and power and producing variable degrees of coagulative necrosis of the prostate or vaporization of prostatic tissue.

Transurethral radiofrequency needle ablation (TUNA) of the prostate

Low-level radiofrequency is transmitted to the prostate via a transurethral needle delivery system, the needles that transmit the energy being deployed in the prostatic urethra once the instrument has been advanced into the prostatic urethra. It is done under local anesthetic, with or without intravenous sedation. The resultant heat causes localized necrosis of the prostate.

Improvements in symptom score and flow rate are modest. Side effects include bleeding (one-third of patients), UTI (10%), and urethral stricture (2%). No adverse effects on sexual function have been reported.[2]

The UK National Institute for Clinical Excellence[3] and the AUA Guidelines Committee[4] have endorsed TUNA as a minimally invasive treatment option for symptoms associated with prostatic enlargement. Concerns remain with regard to long-term effectiveness and retreatment rates.

Transurethral microwave thermotherapy (TUMT)

Microwave energy can be delivered to the prostate via an intraurethral catheter (high-energy system with a cooling system to prevent damage to the adjacent urethra or a low-energy system without a cooling mechanism), producing prostatic heating and coagulative necrosis. Subsequent shrinkage of the prostate and thermal damage to adrenergic neurons (i.e., heat-induced adrenergic nerve block) relieve obstruction and symptoms.

1 Roos NP, Wennberg J, Malenka DJ, et al. (1989). Mortality and reoperation after open and transurethral resection of the prostate for benign prostatic hyperplasia. *N Engl J Med* 320:1120–1124.
2 Fitzpatrick JM, Mebust WK (2002). Minimally invasive and endoscopic management of benign prostatic hyperplasia. In Walsh PC, Retik AB, Vaughan ED, Wein AJ (Eds.), *Campbell's Urology*, 8th ed. Philadelphia: Saunders.
3 Transurethral radiofrequency needle ablation of the prostate. National Institute for Clinical Excellence Interventional Procedure Guidance, October 2003.
4 AUA Clinical Guidelines: Management of BPH (2003; updated 2006). http://www.auanet.org/content/guidelines-and-quality-care/clinical-guidelines.cfm?sub=bph

Many reports of TUMT treatment are open studies, with *all* patients receiving treatment (no "sham" treatment group where the microwave catheter is inserted, but no microwave energy is given—this results in 10-point symptom improvement in approximately 75% of men). Compared with TURP, TUMT results in symptom improvement in 55% of men and TURP in 75%. Sexual side effects after TUMT (e.g., impotence, retrograde ejaculation) are less frequent than after TURP, but the catheterization period is longer, and UTI and irritative urinary symptoms are more common.[5]

The American Urological Association (AUA) and European Association of Urology (EUA) guidelines state that TUMT "should be reserved for patients who prefer to avoid surgery or who no longer respond favorably to medication."

High-intensity focused ultrasound (HIFU)

A focused ultrasound beam can be used to induce a rise in temperature in the prostate or, indeed, in any other tissue to which it is applied. For HIFU treatment of the prostate, a transrectal probe is used. A general anesthetic or heavy intravenous sedation is required during the treatment. It is regarded as an investigational therapy.

5 D'Ancona FCH, Francisca EAE, Witjes WPJ, et al. (1998). Transurethral resection of the prostate vs high-energy thermotherapy of the prostate in patients with benign prostatic hyperplasia: long-term results. *Br J Urol* 81:259–264.

Invasive surgical alternatives to TURP

Transurethral electrovaporization of the prostate (TUVP)
TUVP vaporizes and dessicates the prostate. TUVP seems to be as effective as TURP for symptom control and relief of BOO, with durable (5-year) results. Operating time and inpatient hospital stay are equivalent. Requirement for blood transfusion may be slightly less after TUVP.

TUVP does not provide tissue for histological examination, so prostate cancers cannot be detected. The AUA guidelines have endorsed TUVP as a surgical treatment option for prostatic symptoms.[1]

Laser prostatectomy
Several different techniques of laser prostatectomy evolved during the 1990s.

Transurethral ultrasound-guided laser-induced prostatectomy (TULIP)
This is performed using a probe consisting of a Nd:YAG laser adjacent to an ultrasound transducer. This is currently not used.

Visual laser ablation of the prostate (VLAP)
This side-firing system used a mirror to reflect or a prism to refract the laser energy at various angles (usually 90°) from a laser fiber located in the prostatic urethra onto the surface of the prostate. The principle tissue effect was one of coagulation with subsequent necrosis.

Contact laser prostatectomy
This technique produces a greater degree of vaporization than with VLAP, allowing the immediate removal of tissue.

Interstitial laser prostatectomy (ILP)
ILP is performed by transurethral placement of a laser fiber directly into the prostate, which produces a zone of coagulative necrosis some distance from the prostatic urethra.

TULIP, VLAP, contact laser prostatectomy, and ILP have been succeeded by holmium laser prostatectomy.

Holmium laser prostatectomy
The wavelength of the holmium:YAG laser is such that it is strongly absorbed by water within prostatic tissue. It produces vaporization at the tip of the laser fiber. Its depth of penetration is <0.5 mm, thus it can be used to produce precise incisions in tissue. When the beam is de-focused, it provides excellent hemostasis.

This method can be used with normal saline, thus avoiding the possibility of TURP syndrome.

Three techniques of Holmium laser prostatectomy have been developed in progression:
- Vaporization (holmium-only laser ablation of the prostate, HoLAP), which is time consuming and suitable only for small prostates
- Resection (holmium laser resection of the prostate, HoLRP), which has a similar symptomatic outcome to that of TURP.

- Enucleation (holmium laser enucleation of the prostate, HoLEP): lobes of the prostate are dissected off the capsule of the prostate and then pushed back into the bladder. A transurethral tissue morcellator is introduced into the bladder and used to slice the freed lobes into pieces that can then be removed. Improvement in symptom scores and flow rates are equivalent, and though the operation time with HoLEP is longer, catheter times and in-hospital stays are less with HoLEP.[2]

Greenlight Laser Prostatectomy

The KTP laser has been used for thermal ablation of prostatic tissue (Greenlight PV and HPS, American Medical Systems, Minnetonka, MN). When the Nd:YAG laser beam is passed through a KTP crystal, it doubles its frequency and halves its wavelength to 532nm. The laser emits a visible green light that is highly absorbed by hemoglobin but not water. Hence, the green laser light gets strongly absorbed within a very superficial layer of tissue by virtue of the fact that blood vessels and hemoglobin contained therein serve as primary absorbers. This photoselective vaporization of the prostate (PVP) leads to heat formation and vaporization of prostatic tissue. The prostate tissue is vaporized under direct vision using the laser fiber in a side-firing, near-contact sweeping technique. A TURP-like cavity is achieved with this procedure. The endpoint of a PVP procedure is noted by a significant reduction in the generation of vapor bubbles, indicating that the adenoma has been completely removed.

Advantages: Safe for patients taking anticoagulants, good results for larger prostates and those with a median lobe. Shorter stay or outpatient procedure requires local anesthesia ± sedation in the majority of patients.

Disadvantages: No tissue available for pathology, must handle with caution and need laser safety equipment.

Further reading

Bachmann, A, Schurch, L, Ruszat, R, et al. (2005). Photoselective Vaporization (PVP) versus Transurethral Resection of the Prostate (TURP): A Prospective Bi-Centre Study of Perioperative Morbidity and Early Functional Outcome. *European Urology.* 48(6):965–972.

Hammadeh MY, Madaan S, Hines J, Philp T (2000). Transurethral electrovaporization of the prostate after 5 years: is it effective and durable? *Br J Urol Int* 86:648–651.

McAllister WJ, Karim O, Plail RO, et al. (2003). Transurethral electrovaporization of the prostate: is it any better than conventional transurethral resection of the prostate? *Br J Urol Int* 91:211–214.

Sulser, T, Reich, O, Wyler, S, et al. (2004). Photoselective KTP Laser Vaporization of the Prostate: First Experiences with 65 Procedures. *Journal of Endourology* 18(10):976–981.

1 National Institute for Clinical Excellence Interventional Procedure Guidance 14, London, October 2003.

2 Gilling PJ, Kennett KM, Westenberg AM, et al. (2003). Holmium laser enucleation of the prostate (HoLEP) is superior to TURP for the relief of bladder outflow obstruction (BOO): a randomised trial with 2-year follow-up. *J Urol* 169:1465.

TURP and open prostatectomy

TURP

TURP involves removal of the obstructing tissue of BPH or obstructing prostate cancer from within the prostatic urethra, leaving the compressed outer zone intact (the "surgical capsule").

An electrically heated wire loop is used, through a resectoscope, to cut the tissue and diathermy bleeding vessels. The cut chips of prostate are pushed back into the bladder by the flow of irrigating fluid, and at the end of resection are evacuated using specially designed evacuators—a plastic or glass chamber attached to a rubber bulb that allows fluid to be flushed in and out of the bladder.

Indications for TURP

- Bothersome lower urinary tract symptoms that fail to respond to changes in life style or medical therapy
- Recurrent acute urinary retention
- Renal impairment due to BOO (high-pressure *chronic* urinary retention)
- Recurrent hematuria due to benign prostatic enlargement
- Bladder stones due to prostatic obstruction

Open prostatectomy

Indications

- Large prostate (>100 g)
- TURP not technically possible (e.g., limited hip abduction)
- Failed TURP (e.g., because of bleeding)
- Urethra too long for the resectoscope to gain access to the prostate
- Presence of bladder stones that are too large for endoscopic cystolitholapaxy, combined with marked enlargement of the prostate

Contraindications

- Small fibrous prostate
- Prior prostatectomy in which most of the gland has been resected or removed; this obliterates the tissue planes
- Carcinoma of the prostate

Techniques

Suprapubic (transvesical)

This is the preferred operation if enlargement of the prostate involves mainly the middle lobe. The bladder is opened, the mucosa around the protruding adenoma is incised, and the plane between the adenoma and capsule is developed to enucleate the adenoma. A 22 Fr urethral and a suprapubic catheter are left, together with a retropubic drain.

Remove the urethral catheter in 3 days and clamp the suprapubic Fr. at 6 days, removing it 24 hours later. The drain can be removed 24 hours after this (day 8).

Simple retropubic

Compared with the suprapubic (transvesical) approach, this procedure allows more precise anatomic exposure of the prostate. It allows better visualization of the prostatic cavity and more accurate removal of the adenoma. Better control of bleeding points and more accurate division of the urethra can be accomplished, reducing the risk of incontinence.

As well as the contraindications noted above, the retropubic approach should not be employed when the middle lobe is very large because it is difficult to get behind the middle lobe and to incise the mucosa (safely) distal to the ureters.

The prostate is exposed by a Pfannenstiel or lower midline incision. Hemostasis is achieved before enucleating the prostate, by ligating the dorsal vein complex with sutures placed deeply through the prostate.

The prostatic capsule and adenoma are incised transversely with the cautery just distal to the bladder neck. The plane between the capsule and adenoma is found with scissors and developed with a finger. Sutures are used for hemostasis. A wedge of bladder neck is resected.

A catheter is inserted and left for 5 days and the transverse capsular incision is closed. A large tube drain (30 Fr. Robinson's) is left for 1–2 days.

Complications

These include hemorrhage, urinary infection, and rectal perforation (close and cover with a colostomy).

Acute urinary retention: definition, pathophysiology, and causes

Definition

Acute urinary retention is the painful inability to void, with relief of pain following drainage of the bladder by catheterization.

The combination of reduced or absent urine output with lower abdominal pain is not in itself enough to make a diagnosis of acute retention. Many acute surgical conditions cause abdominal pain and fluid depletion, the latter leading to reduced urine output, and this reduced urine output can give the erroneous impression that the patient is in retention when, in fact, they are not.

Thus, central to the diagnosis is the presence of a *large* volume of urine, which when drained by catheterization leads to resolution of the pain. What represents "large" has not been strictly defined, but volumes of 500–800 mL are typical. Volumes <500 mL should lead one to question the diagnosis. Volumes >800 mL may be defined as acute or chronic retention.

Pathophysiology

Normal micturition requires the following:
- Afferent input to the brainstem and cerebral cortex
- Coordinated relaxation of the external sphincter
- Sustained detrusor contraction
- The absence of an anatomic obstruction in the outlet of the bladder

Four broad mechanisms can lead to urinary retention:
- Increased urethral *resistance* (i.e., BOO)
- Low bladder *pressure* (i.e., impaired bladder contractility)
- Interruption of sensory or motor innervation of bladder
- Central failure of coordination of bladder contraction with external sphincter relaxation

Causes in men

Causes include benign prostatic enlargement, malignant enlargement of the prostate, urethral stricture, and prostatic abscess (see also Box 3.2).

Urinary retention in men is either *spontaneous* or *precipitated* by an event. Precipitated retention is less likely to recur once the event causing it has been removed. Spontaneous retention is more likely to recur after a trial of catheter removal and more likely to require definitive treatment (e.g., TURP).

Precipitated retention can be caused by events such as anesthetic and other drugs (anticholinergics, sympathomimetic agents such as ephedrine in nasal decongestants), nonprostatic abdominal or perineal surgery, and immobility following surgical procedures.

Box 3.2 Causes of acute urinary retention in either sex

- Hematuria leading to clot retention
- Drugs (e.g., anticholinergics, sympathomimetic agents)
- Pain (adrenergic stimulation of the bladder neck)
- Postoperative retention (see below)
- Sacral cord (S2–4) injury
- Sacral (S2–4) nerve or compression or damage, resulting in detrusor areflexia—cauda equina compression (due to prolapsed L2–L3 disc or L3–L4 intervertebral disc pressing on sacral nerve roots of the cauda equina, trauma to vertebrae, or tumors [benign or metastatic])
- Suprasacral spinal cord injury (results in loss of coordination of external sphincter relaxation with detrusor contraction—detrusor-sphincter dyssynergia (DSD)—so external sphincter contracts when bladder contracts)
- Radical pelvic surgery damaging pelvic parasympathetic plexus (radical hysterectomy, abdominoperineal resection): unilateral injury to pelvic plexus (preganglionic parasympathetic and postganglionic sympathetic neurons) denervates motor innervation of detrusor muscle
- Pelvic fracture rupturing urethra (more likely in men than in women)
- Neurotropic viruses involving sensory dorsal root ganglia of S2–4 (herpes simplex or zoster)
- Multiple sclerosis (can affect any part of the CNS—Fig. 3.2); retention caused by detrusor areflexia or DSD
- Transverse myelitis
- Diabetic cystopathy (causes sensory and motor dysfunction)
- Damage to dorsal columns of spinal cord causing loss of bladder sensation (tabes dorsalis, pernicious anemia)

Causes in women

These include pelvic prolapse (cystocele, rectocele, uterine); urethral stricture; urethral diverticulum; post-surgery for stress incontinence; pelvic masses (e.g., ovarian masses); and Fowler syndrome.

Fowler syndrome

Increased electromyographic activity can be recorded in the external urethral sphincters of these women (which on ultrasound are of increased volume) and is hypothesized to cause impaired relaxation of the external sphincter.

Fowler syndrome occurs in premenopausal women, often in association with polycystic ovaries.

Risk factors for postoperative retention

Risk factors include instrumentation of the lower urinary tract; surgery to the perineum or anorectum; gynecological surgery; bladder overdistension; reduced sensation of bladder fullness; pre-existing prostatic obstruction; and epidural anesthesia. Postpartum retention is not uncommon, particularly with epidural anesthesia and instrumental delivery.

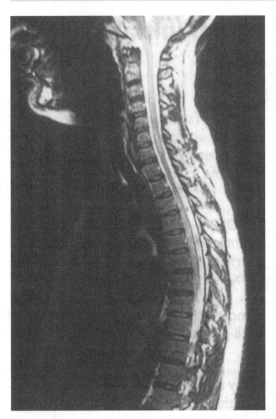

Figure 3.2 MRI of cervical and sacral cord in a young patient presenting with urinary retention. The patient had undiagnosed MS. Signal changes are seen in the cervical, thoracic, and lumbosacral cord.

Acute urinary retention: initial and definitive management

Initial management

Urethral catheterization is used to relieve pain (suprapubic catheterization if urethral route not possible). Record the volume drained—this confirms the diagnosis, determines subsequent management, and provides prognostic information on outcome from this treatment.

Definitive management in men

Discuss trial without catheter (TWOC) with the patient. Precipitated retention often does not recur; spontaneous retention often does. Half of patients with *spontaneous* retention will experience a second episode of retention within the next week or so, and 70% within the next year.

A maximum flow rate (Q_{max}) <5 mL/s and low voiding detrusor pressure predicts subsequent retention. Thus, while most patients will require definitive treatment (e.g., TURP), a substantial minority will not need surgery.

Options to avoid TURP

- Prostate-shrinking drugs followed by a voiding trial several months later (5α-reductase inhibitors in those with benign-feeling prostates, LHRH agonists in those with malignant-feeling prostates on DRE, confirmed by TRUS-guided prostate biopsy)
- Prostatic stents
- Long-term urethral or suprapubic catheter
- Clean, intermittent self-catheterization (CISC) is not a realistic option for most men, but some will be able and happy to do this.

Definitive management in women

Use CISC either until normal voiding function recovers or permanently if it does not. For Fowler syndrome use sacral neuromodulation (e.g., Medtronic InterStim).

Risks and outcomes of TURP for retention

Relative risks of TURP for retention vs. TURP for lower urinary tract symptoms (LUTS) are as follows: postoperative complications 26:1; blood transfusion 2.5:1; in-hospital death 3:1.[1]

High retention volume, greater age, and low maximum detrusor pressure are predictive for failure to void after TURP; 10% of those with acute retention of urine and 40% of those with chronic retention fail to void after initial post-turp. Overall, 1% of men will fail to void after subsequent voiding trial and will require long-term catheterization.[2]

---

1 Pickard R, Emberton M, Neal D (1998). The management of men with acute urinary retention. *Br J Urol* 81:712–720.

2 Reynard JM (1999). Failure to void after transurethral resection of the prostate and mode of presentation. *Urology* 53:336–339.

Indications for and technique of urethral catheterization

Indications

For relief of urinary retention and prevention of urinary retention, a period of postoperative catheterization is commonly employed after many operations where limited mobility makes normal voiding difficult.

Other indications for catheterization include monitoring of urine output (e.g., postoperatively); prevention of damage to the bladder during cesarean section; bladder drainage following surgery to the bladder, prostate, or urethra (e.g., TURP, TURBT, open bladder stone removal, radical prostatectomy); and bladder drainage following injuries to the bladder.

Technique

Explain the need for and method of catheterization to the patient. Use the smallest catheter—in practical terms, usually a 12 Fr., with a 10 mL balloon. For longer catheterization periods (weeks) use a silastic catheter to limit tissue reaction, thereby reducing the risk of a catheter-induced urethral stricture. If there is clot retention, use a three-way catheter (20 Fr. or greater) to allow evacuation of clots and bladder irrigation to prevent subsequent catheter blockage.

The technique is aseptic. One gloved hand is sterile; the other is "dirty." The dirty hand holds the penis or separates the labia to allow cleansing of urethral meatus; this hand should not touch the catheter. Use sterile water or sterile cleaning solution to prep skin around meatus.

Apply lubricant jelly to the urethra. Traditionally, this contains local anesthetic (e.g., 2% lidocaine), which takes 3–5 minutes to work. However, a randomized, placebo-controlled trial showed that 2% lidocaine was no more effective for pain relief than anesthetic-free lubricant,[1] suggesting that it is lubricant action that prevents urethral pain.

If using local anesthetic lubricant, warn the patient that it may STING. Local anesthetic lubricant is contraindicated in patients with allergies to local anesthetics and in those with urethral trauma, where there is a (theoretical) risk of complications arising from systemic absorption of lidocaine.

When instilling jelly, do so gently—a sudden, forceful depression of the plunger of the syringe can rupture the urethra! In males, milk the gel toward the posterior urethra, while squeezing the meatus to prevent it from coming back out of the meatus.

Insert the catheter using a sterile hand, until flow of urine confirms it is in the bladder. Failure of urine flow may indicate that the catheter balloon is in the urethra. Intraurethral inflation of the balloon can rupture the urethra. If no urine flows, attempt aspiration of urine using a 50 mL bladder syringe (lubricant gel can occlude eyeholes of the catheter).

Absence of urine flow indicates either that the catheter is not in the bladder or, if the indication for catheterization is retention, that the diagnosis is wrong (there will usually be a few mL of urine in the bladder even in cases where the absence of micturition is due to oliguria or anuria, so complete absence of urine flow usually indicates the catheter is not in the bladder). If the catheter will not pass into the bladder and you are sure that the patient is in retention, proceed with suprapubic catheterization.[1]

1 Birch BR (1994). Flexible cystoscopy in men: is topical anesthesia with lidocaine gel worthwhile? *Br J Urol* 73:155.

Indications for and technique of suprapubic catheterization

Indications

Suprapubic catheterization is indicated if there is failed urethral catheterization in urinary retention; it is the preferred site for long-term catheters.

Long-term *urethral* catheters commonly lead to acquired hypospadias in males (ventral splitting of glans penis) and patulous urethra in females (leading to frequent balloon expulsion and bypassing of urine around the catheter). Hence, a suprapubic site is preferred for long-term catheters.

Contraindications

Suprapubic catheterization is best avoided in the following:
- Patients with clot retention, the cause of which may be an underlying bladder cancer (the cancer could be spread along the catheter track to involve the skin)
- Patients with lower midline incisions (bowel may be stuck to the deep aspect of the scar, leading to the potential for bowel perforation)
- Pelvic fractures, where the catheter may inadvertently enter the large pelvic hematoma that always accompanies severe pelvic fracture. This can lead to infection of the hematoma, and the resulting sepsis can be fatal. Failure to pass a urethral catheter in a patient with a pelvic fracture usually indicates a urethral rupture (confirmed by urethrography) and is an indication for formal open, suprapubic cystotomy.

Technique

Prior to insertion of the trocar, be sure to confirm the diagnosis by
- Abdominal examination (palpate and percuss the lower abdomen to confirm bladder is distended),
- Ultrasound (in practice, usually not available), and
- Aspiration of urine (using a green needle).

Patients with lower abdominal scars may have bowel interposed between the abdominal wall and bladder and this can be perforated if the trocar is inserted near the scar and without prior aspiration of urine. In such cases, ultrasound-guided catheterization may be sensible.

Use a wide-bore trocar if you anticipate that the catheter will be in place for more than 24 hours (small-bore catheters will block within a few days). Aim to place the catheter about 2–3 fingerbreadths above the pubis symphysis. Placement too close to the symphysis will result in a difficult trocar insertion (the trocar will hit the symphysis).

Instill a few mL of local anesthetic into the skin of the intended puncture site and down to the rectus sheath. Confirm location of the bladder by drawing back on the needle to aspirate urine from the bladder. This helps guide the angle of trocar insertion.

Make a 1 cm incision with a sharp blade through the skin. Hold the trocar handle in your right hand, and steady the needle end with your left hand (this hand helps prevent insertion too deeply). Push the trocar in the same direction as that in which you previously aspirated urine.

As soon as urine passes from the trocar, withdraw the latter, holding the attached sheath in place. Push the catheter in as far as it will go. Inflate the balloon.

Peel away the side of the sheath and remove it.

Management of nocturia and nocturnal polyuria

Nocturia can be particularly resistant to treatment.

First, establish whether the patient is polyuric (>3 L of urine/24 hr) by having the patient complete a frequency–volume chart. If polyuric, this may account for the daytime and nighttime voiding frequency. Establish whether the patient has a solute or water diuresis and the causes thereof (see Box 3.3).

If nonpolyuric (<3 L urine output/24 hr), determine the *distribution* of urine output over the 24-hour period. If >1/3 of urine output is between the hours of midnight and 8 a.m., then the patient has nocturnal polyuria (NP).

Nonpolyuric nocturia
BPH medical therapy
The impact of α-blockers, 5α-reductase inhibitors, and anticholinergics on nocturia is modest.

TURP
Nocturia persists in 20–40% of men after TURP.

Medtronic InterStim therapy for nocturia
Patients preselected on the basis of a favorable symptomatic response to a test stimulation can experience a reduction in nocturia,[1] but not all patients respond to the test stimulation. The treatment is expensive and not yet widely available in all countries.

Treatment for nocturnal polyuria
The evidence base for NP treatments is limited (very few randomized, placebo-controlled trials).[2]

Fluid restriction
Many patients have reduced their afternoon and evening fluid intake in an attempt to reduce their nighttime diuresis.

Diuretics
Diuretics, taken several hours before bedtime, reduce nocturnal voiding frequency in some patients.[3]

DDAVP
DDAVP is a synthetic analogue of arginine vasopressin (endogenous ADH), which, if taken at night, can reduce urine flow by its antidiuretic action. It has been suggested that NP may be caused by a lack of endogenous production of ADH in elderly people.

However, adults both with and without NP have no rise in ADH at night (i.e., ADH secretion remains remarkably *constant* throughout the day in adults with and without NP). Furthermore, the diuresis in adults with NP is a *solute* diuresis due to a nocturnal natriuresis.[4]

Thus, lack of ADH secretion at night is *not* the cause of the diuresis in nocturnal polyuric adults, and thus from a theoretical perspective, there is no logical basis for using DDAVP in NP.[5] There is limited evidence that it reduces nighttime voiding frequency (at least in responder enrichment studies) and increases sleep duration in a proportion of patients with NP.[6]

Side effects include hyponatremia (Na <130 mmol/L) in 5% of patients. Measure serum Na 3 days after starting DDAVP and stop its use if hyponatremia develops.

Nocturia and sleep apnea

Obstructive sleep apnea (OSA) is highly prevalent in those over 65 years of age. It is often manifested by snoring. There is a strong association between OSA symptoms and nocturia.[7]

Large negative intrathoracic pressure swings may trigger a cardiac-mediated natriuresis and hence cause NP.

Box 3.3 Investigation of the polyuric patient (urine output of >3 L/24 hr)

Urine osmolality?
- >250mosm/kg = solute diuresis
- <250mosm/kg = water diuresis

Solute diuresis
- Poorly controlled diabetes mellitus; saline loading (e.g., postoperative diuresis); diuresis following relief of high-pressure chronic retention

Water diuresis
- Primary polydipsia; diabetes insipidus (nephrogenic—e.g., lithium therapy, central—ADH deficiency)

---

1 Spinelli M (2003). New sacral neuromodulation lead for percutaneous implantation using local anesthesia: description and first experience. *J Urol* 170:1905–1907.

2 Kujubu DA, Aboseif SR (2008). An overview of nocturia and the syndrome of nocturnal polyuria in the elderly. *Nat Clin Pract Nephrol* 4(8):426–435.

3 Reynard JM, Cannon A, Yang Q, Abrams P (1998). A novel therapy for nocturnal polyuria: a double-blind randomized trial of frusemide against placebo. *Br J Urol* 81:215–218.

4 Matthiesen TB, Rittig S, Norgaard JP, Pedersen EB, Djurhuus JD (1996). Nocturnal polyuria and natriuresis in male patients with nocturia and lower urinary tract symptoms. *J Urol* 81:215–218.

5 McKeigue P, Reynard J (2000). Relation of nocturnal polyuria of the elderly to essential hypertension. *Lancet* 355:486–488.

6 Mattiasson A (2002). Efficacy of desmopressin in the treatment of nocturia: a double-blind placebo-controlled study in men. *Br J Urol* 89:855–862.

7 Umlauf M (1999). Nocturia and sleep apnea symptoms in older patients: clinical interview. *Sleep* 22:S127.

High-pressure chronic retention (HPCR)

HPCR is maintenance of voiding, with a bladder volume of >800 mL and an intravesical pressure above 30 cmH_2O, accompanied by hydronephrosis.[1,2] Over time, this leads to renal failure. When the patient is suddenly unable to pass urine, acute-on-chronic high-pressure retention of urine has occurred.

A man with high-pressure retention who continues to void spontaneously may be unaware that there is anything wrong. He will often have no sensation of incomplete emptying and his bladder may be insensitive to the gross distension. Often the first presenting symptom is that of bedwetting. This is such an unpleasant and disruptive symptom that it will cause most people to visit their doctor.

Visual inspection of the patient's abdomen may show marked distension due to a grossly enlarged bladder. The diagnosis of chronic retention can be confirmed by palpation of the enlarged, tense bladder, which is dull to percussion.

Acute treatment

Catheterization relieves the pressure on the kidneys and allows normalization of renal function. A large volume of urine is drained from the bladder (often on the order of 1–2 L, and sometimes much greater).

The serum creatinine is elevated and an ultrasound will show hydronephrosis with a grossly distended bladder if the scan is done before relief of retention.

Anticipate a profound diuresis following drainage of the bladder. This is due to the following:

- Excretion of salt and water that has accumulated during the period of renal failure
- Loss of the corticomedullary concentration gradient, due to continued perfusion of the kidneys with diminished flow of urine through the nephron (this washes out the concentration gradient between the cortex and medulla)
- An osmotic diuresis caused by elevated serum urea concentration

A small percentage of patients have a postural drop in blood pressure. It is wise to admit patients with HPCR for a short period of observation, until the diuresis has settled.

A few patients will require intravenous fluid replacement if they experience a symptomatic fall in blood pressure when standing.

Definitive treatment

Treatment is with TURP or a long-term catheter. In those unable to void who have been catheterized, a trial without catheter is clearly not appropriate in cases where there is back-pressure on the kidneys.

Very rarely, a patient who wants to avoid a TURP and does not want an indwelling catheter will be able to empty their bladder by intermittent self-catheterization, but such cases are exceptional.

1 Mitchell JP (1984). Management of chronic urinary retention. *BMJ* 289:515–516.
2 Abrams P, Dunn M, George N (1978). Urodynamic findings in chronic retention of urine and their relevance to results of surgery. *BMJ* 2:1258–1260.

Bladder outlet obstruction and retention in women

In women this condition is relatively rare (~5% of women undergoing pressure-flow studies have BOO, compared with 60% of unselected men with LUTS).[1]

It may be symptom-free, present with LUTS or as acute urinary retention. In broad terms, the causes are related to obstruction of the urethra (e.g., urethral stricture, compression by a prolapsing pelvic organ such as the uterus, post-surgery for stress incontinence) or have a neurological basis (e.g., injury to sacral cord or parasympathetic plexus, degenerative neurological disease, e.g., MS, diabetic cystopathy).

Voiding studies in women

Women have a higher Q_{max} (maximal flow), for a given voided volume than that of men. Women with BOO have lower Q_{max} than those without BOO. There are no universally accepted urodynamic criteria for diagnosing BOO in women.

Treatment of BOO in women

Treat the cause (e.g., dilatation of a urethral stricture; repair of a pelvic prolapse). Where this is not possible (because of a neurological cause such as MS or spinal cord injury), the options are as follows:

- Intermittent self-catheterization (ISC) or intermittent catheterization by a caregiver
- Indwelling catheter (preferably suprapubic rather than urethral)
- Mitrofanoff catheterizable stoma

Where urethral intermittent self-catheterization is technically difficult, a catheterizable stoma can be constructed between the anterior abdominal wall and the bladder, using the appendix, Fallopian tube, or a narrowed section of small intestine, known collectively as the Mitrofanoff procedure. It is simply a new urethra that has an abdominal location, rather than a perineal one, and is therefore easier to access for ISC.

For women with a suprasacral spinal cord injury with preserved detrusor contraction and urinary retention due to detrusor-sphincter dyssynergia (DSD), sacral deafferentation combined with a Brindley stimulator can be used to manage the resulting urinary retention.

Fowler syndrome

Fowler syndrome is a primary disorder of sphincter relaxation (as opposed to secondary to, for example, SCI). Increased electromyographic (EMG) activity (repetitive discharges on external sphincter EMG) can be recorded in the external urethral sphincters of these women (which on ultrasound are of increased volume) and is hypothesized to cause impaired relaxation of external sphincter.

It occurs in premenopausal women, typically aged 15–30, often in association with polycystic ovaries (50% of patients), acne, hirsutism, and menstrual irregularities. It may also be precipitated by childbirth, gynecological or other surgical procedures.

Patients report no urgency with bladder volumes >1000 mL, but when attempts are made to manage their retention by ISC, they experience pain, especially on withdrawing the catheter.

Pathophysiology

Fowler may be due to a channelopathy of the striated urethral sphincter muscle leading to involuntary external sphincter contraction.

Treatment

Treatment is with ISC, sacral neuromodulation with Medtronic InterStim (90% void post-implantation and 75% are still voiding at 3-year follow-up). The mechanism of action of sacral neuromodulation in urinary retention is unknown.

Further reading

Swinn MJ, Fowler C, et al. (2002). The cause and treatment of urinary retention in young women. *J Urol* 167:151–156.

1 Madersbascher S, Pycha A, Klingler CH, et al. (1998). The aging lower urinary tract: a comparative urodynamic study of men and women. *Urology* 51:206–212.

Urethral stricture disease

A *urethral stricture* is an area of narrowing in the caliber of the urethra due to formation of scar tissue in the tissues surrounding the urethra. The disease process of anterior urethral stricture disease is different from that in the posterior urethra.

Anterior urethra

The process of scar formation occurs in the spongy erectile tissue (corpus spongiosum) of the penis that surrounds the urethra (spongiofibrosis). Causes include the following:

- Inflammation (e.g., balanitis xerotica obliterans [BXO]), gonococcal infection leading to gonococcal urethritis (less common today because of prompt treatment of gonorrhea)
- Trauma
  - Straddle injuries—blow to bulbar urethra (e.g., cross-bar injury)
  - Iatrogenic—instrumentation (e.g., traumatic catheterization, traumatic cystoscopy, TURP, bladder neck incision)

The role of nonspecific urethritis (e.g., *Chlamydia*) in the development of anterior urethral strictures has not been established.

Posterior urethra

Fibrosis of the tissues around the urethra results from trauma—pelvic fracture or surgical (radical prostatectomy, TURP, urethral instrumentation). These are essentially *distraction* injuries, where the posterior urethra has been pulled apart, and the subsequent healing process results in the formation of a scar, which contracts and thereby narrows the urethral lumen.

Symptoms and signs of urethral stricture

- Voiding symptoms—hesitancy, poor flow, post-micturition dribbling
- Urinary retention—acute, or high-pressure acute-on-chronic
- Urinary tract infection—prostatitis, epididymitis

Management of urethral strictures

When the patient presents with urinary retention, the diagnosis is usually made following a failed attempt at urethral catheterization. In such cases, avoid the temptation to blindly dilate the urethra. Dilatation may be the wrong treatment option for this type of stricture—it may convert a short stricture that could have been cured by urethrotomy or urethroplasty into a longer and denser stricture, thus committing the patient to more complex surgery and a higher risk of recurrent stricturing. Place a suprapubic catheter instead, and image the urethra with retrograde and antegrade urethrography to establish the precise position and the length of the stricture.

Similarly, avoid the temptation to inappropriately dilate a urethral stricture diagnosed at flexible cystoscopy (urethroscopy). Arrange retrograde urethrography so appropriate treatment can be planned.

Treatment options

Urethral dilatation

This is designed to stretch the stricture without causing more scarring; bleeding post-dilatation indicates tearing of the stricture (i.e., further injury has been caused) and restricturing is likely.

Internal (optical) urethrotomy

This procedure involves stricture incision, with an endoscopic knife or laser. The stricture is divided, followed by epithelialization of the incision. If deep spongiofibrosis is present, the stricture will recur.

It is best suited for short (<1.5 cm) bulbar urethral strictures with minimal spongiofibrosis.[1] Leave a catheter for 3–5 days (longer catheterization does not reduce long-term restricturing).

Consider ISC for 3–6 months, starting several times daily, reducing to once or twice a week toward the end of this period.

Excision and reanastomosis or tissue transfer

Treatment involves excision of the area of spongiofibrosis with primary reanastomosis or closure of defect with buccal mucosa or pedicled skin flap; this has best chance of cure.

A stepwise progression up this reconstructive ladder (the process of starting with a simple procedure and moving onto the next level of complexity when this fails) is not appropriate for every patient. For the patient who wants the best chance of long-term cure, offer excision and reanastomosis or tissue transfer up front.

For the patient who is happy with lifelong management of his stricture (with repeat dilatation or optical urethrotomy), offer dilatation or optical urethrotomy.

Balanitis xerotica obliterans (BXO)

BXO is genital lichen sclerosis and atrophicus in the male. Hyperkeratosis is seen histologically. BXO appears as a white plaque on the foreskin, glans of the penis, or within the urethral meatus. It is the most common cause of stenosis of the meatus.

The foreskin becomes thickened and adheres to the glans, leading to phimosis (a thickened, nonretractile foreskin). Patients with long-standing BXO and meatal stenosis often have more proximal urethral strictures.

---

1 Pansadoro V, Emiliozzi P (1996). Internal urethrotomy in the management of anterior urethral strictures: long term follow-up. *J Urol* 156:73–75.

Incontinence

Classification *110*
Causes and pathophysiology *112*
Evaluation *114*
Treatment of sphincter weakness incontinence: injection
    therapy *116*
Treatment of sphincter weakness incontinence: retropubic
    suspension *117*
Treatment of sphincter weakness incontinence: pubovaginal
    slings *118*
Treatment of sphincter weakness incontinence: the artificial
    urinary sphincter *120*
Overactive bladder: conventional treatment *122*
Overactive bladder: options for failed conventional
    therapy *124*
"Mixed" incontinence *126*
Post-prostatectomy incontinence *128*
Vesicovaginal fistula (VVF) *130*
Incontinence in the elderly patient *132*

Classification

Definition

The International Continence Society (ICS) defines incontinence as "involuntary loss of urine that is a social or hygienic problem and is objectively demonstrable." Urinary incontinence (UI) is a failure to store urine usually due to either abnormal bladder smooth muscle or a deficient urethral sphincter. Urine loss may also be extraurethral, secondary to anatomical abnormalities such as ectopic ureter or vesicovaginal fistula.

Prevalence

UI has been reported to affect 12–43% of adult women and 3–11% of adult men. Severe incontinence has a low prevalence in young women, but rapidly increases at ages 70 through 80. Incontinence in men also increases with age, but severe incontinence in 70- to 80-year-old men is about half that in women.

Classification

Stress urinary incontinence (SUI) is involuntary urinary leakage during effort, exertion, sneezing, or coughing, due to hypermobility of the bladder base, pelvic floor, and/or intrinsic urethral sphincter deficiencies. In females SUI is usually associated with multiparity. In males, SUI is most commonly the result of prostatectomy.
- **Type 0**—report of urinary incontinence, but without clinical signs
- **Type I**—leakage that occurs during stress with <2 cm descent of the bladder base below the upper border of the symphysis pubis
- **Type II**—leakage on stress accompanied by marked bladder base descent (>2 cm) that occurs only during stress (II_a) or is permanently present (II_b)
- **Type III**—bladder neck and proximal urethra are open at rest (with or without descent). Also known as intrinsic sphincter deficiency (ISD)

Urge urinary incontinence (UUI) is involuntary urine leakage accompanied or immediately preceded by a sudden, strong desire to void (urgency).

Mixed urinary incontinence is urine leakage that has characteristics of both SUI and UUI.

Overflow incontinence is leakage of urine when the bladder is abnormally distended with large post-void residual volumes. Typically, men present with chronic urinary retention and dribbling incontinence. This can lead to hydronephrosis and renal failure in 30% of patients.

Nocturnal enuresis describes any involuntary loss of urine during sleep. The prevalence in adults is 0.5%. Approximately 750,000 children over age 7 years will regularly wet the bed. Childhood enuresis can be further classified into primary (never been dry for longer than a 6-month period) or secondary (re-emergence of bed wetting after a period of being dry for at least 6–12 months).

Post-micturition dribble is the complaint of a dribbling loss of urine that occurs after voiding. It predominantly affects males and is due to pooling of urine in the bulbous urethra after voiding. It affects approximately 20% of healthy adults[1] and 60–70% of those with existent LUTS.[2]

1 Furuya S, Ogura H, Tanaka M, et al. (1997). Incidence of postmicturition dribble in adult males in their twenties through fifties. *Hinyokika Kiyo* 43(6):407–410.
2 Paterson J, Pinnock CB, Marshall VR (1997). Pelvic floor exercises as a treatment for post-micturition dribble. *Br J Urol* 79(6):892–897.

Causes and pathophysiology

Risk factors
Predisposing factors
- Gender (female > males)
- Race (Caucasian > African American/Asian)
- Genetic predisposition
- Neurological disorders (spinal cord injury, stroke, MS, Parkinson disease)
- Anatomical disorders (vesicovaginal fistula, ectopic ureter, urethral diverticulum)
- Childbirth
- Anomalies in collagen subtype
- Prostate or pelvic surgery (radical prostatectomy; radical hysterectomy; TURP) leading to pelvic muscle and nerve injury
- Pelvic radiotherapy

Promoting factors
- Smoking (associated with chronic cough and raised intra-abdominal pressure)
- Obesity
- UTI
- Increased fluid intake
- Medications
- Poor nutrition
- Aging
- Cognitive deficits
- Poor mobility

Pathophysiology
Bladder abnormalities
Detrusor overactivity is a urodynamic observation characterized by involuntary bladder muscle (detrusor) contractions during the filling phase of the bladder, which may be spontaneous or provoked, and can consequently cause urinary incontinence. The underlying cause may be neurogenic, where there is a relevant neurological condition, or idiopathic, where there is no defined cause.

Low bladder compliance is characterized by a decreased volume-to-pressure relationship during a cystometrogram and is often associated with upper tract damage. High bladder pressures occur during filling because of alterations in the viscoelastic properties of the bladder wall, or changes in bladder muscle tone (secondary to myelodysplasia, spinal cord injury, radical hysterectomy, interstitial or radiation cystitis).

Sphincter abnormalities
Urethral hypermobility is due to a weakness of pelvic floor support causing a rotational descent of the bladder neck and proximal urethra during increases in intra-abdominal pressure. If the urethra opens concomitantly, there will be urinary leaking.

Intrinsic sphincter deficiency (ISD) describes an intrinsic malfunction of the sphincter, regardless of its anatomical position, which is responsible for type III SUI. Causes include inadequate urethral compression (previous urethral surgery; aging; menopause; radical pelvic surgery) or deficient urethral support (pelvic floor weakness; childbirth; pelvic surgery; menopause).

Evaluation

History

Inquire about LUTS (storage or voiding symptoms), triggers for incontinence (cough, sneezing, exercise, position, urgency), and frequency and severity of symptoms. Establish risk factors (abdominal/pelvic surgery; neurological diseases; obstetric and gynecological history; medications).

A validated patient-completed questionnaire may be helpful (e.g., IPSS; see Fig. 1.1, p. 11).

Physical examination

Women

Perform a pelvic examination in the supine and standing position with a speculum while the patient has a full bladder. Ask the patient to cough or strain, and inspect for vaginal wall prolapse (cystocele, rectocele, enterocele), uterine or perineal descent, and urinary leakage (stress test). Eighty percent of SUI patients will leak with a brief squirt during cough in the supine position, while another 20% will leak only in an inclined or standing position.

Urethral hypermobility is assessed with the Q-tip test. A lubricated cotton-tipped applicator is introduced through the urethra to bladder neck level. *Hypermobility* is defined as a resting or straining angle of >30° from horizontal.

The Bonney test is used to assess continence with manual repositioning of the urethra and vesicle neck. Using one or two fingers to elevate the anterior vaginal wall laterally without compressing the urethra, relief of incontinence during cough suggests that surgical correction will be successful.

Both sexes

Examine the abdomen for a palpable bladder (indicating urinary retention). A neurological examination should include assessment of anal tone and reflex, perineal sensation, and lower limb function.

Inspect the underwear for the status of urinary collection pads; for men, a standing or squatting "cough test" gives a good indicator of the presence and severity of stress incontinence.

Investigation

Bladder diaries

Record the frequency and volume of urine voided, incontinent episodes, pad usage, fluid intake, and degree of urgency. Alternatively, pads can be weighed to estimate urine loss (pad testing).

Urinalysis can exclude UTIs.

Blood tests, X-ray imaging, cystoscopy

These are indicated for persistent or severe symptoms, bladder pain, and voiding difficulties. Cystoscopy is useful for evaluating men who have had prostatectomy—it will show the presence of clips, stones, and strictures that may develop after surgery that might need to be addressed concomitantly with anti-incontinence surgery.

Screening tests

Uroflow testing measures the ability of the bladder to empty; a minimum bladder volume of 150 cc is desired. A low flow rate indicates bladder outflow obstruction or reduced bladder contractility. The volume of urine remaining in the bladder after voiding (post-void residual) is also important (<50 mL is normal; >200 mL is abnormal; 50–200 mL requires clinical correlation).

Urodynamic investigations

Valsalva leak point pressure (VLPP) measures the abdominal pressure at which a half-full bladder leaks during straining—normal individuals should not leak. VLPP readings <60 cm H_2O suggest ISD; VLPP readings >100 cm H_2O suggest hypermobility, while readings of 60–100 cm are indeterminant.

Detrusor leak point pressure (DLPP) measures the bladder pressure at which leakage occurs without valsalva—DLPP >40 cm H_2O puts the upper tract at risk.

Videourodynamics can visualize movement of the proximal urethra and bladder neck, and establish the precise anatomical etiology of UI.

Sphincter electromyography (EMG)

EMG measures electrical activity from striated muscles of the urethra or perineal floor and provides information on synchronization between bladder muscle (detrusor) and external sphincter.

Treatment of sphincter weakness incontinence: injection therapy

The injection of bulking materials into the bladder neck and periurethral muscles is used to increase outlet resistance. Bulking substances include silicone polymers (Macroplastique); cross-linked bovine collagen (Contigen); Teflon; PTFE; and carbon-coated zirconium beads (Durasphere).

Indications

These include stress incontinence secondary to demonstrable intrinsic sphincter deficiency (ISD), with normal bladder muscle function. Injection therapy is used in adults and children.

Contraindications

These include UTI, untreated bladder dysfunction, and bladder neck stenosis. There is improved outcome in patients without urethral hypermobility (which is better treated with a sling or, less commonly, an artificial urinary sphincter).

Preinjection evaluation

Conduct a stress test and Q-tip test. Use videourodynamics to diagnose ISD and exclude detrusor overactivity.

Injection techniques

Either a local block or a general anesthetic is required, with full antibiotic coverage. Usually a series of injections are given via a transurethral (retrograde) route using a cystoscopically guided injection needle. The bulking agent is injected suburethrally with the aim of achieving urethral muscosal apposition and closure of the lumen.

In men, injection treatment following radical prostatectomy is associated with success rates <10%. In women, a periurethral (percutaneous) technique can also be used, with endoscopic or ultrasound guidance: overall success rate in women is ~50–70%.[1,2]

Complications

Complications include urinary urgency, urinary retention (which may need ISC or SPC insertion), hematuria, cystitis, migration of the injected particles (PTFE, Macroplastique), and risk of granuloma formation (PTFE). Repeat treatments are the norm.

1 Koelbl H (1998). Transurethral injection of silicone microimplants for intrinsic urethral sphincter deficiency. *Obstet Gynaecol* 92:332–336.
2 Appell RA (1994). Collagen injection therapy for urinary incontinence. *Urol Clin North Am* 21:177–182.

Treatment of sphincter weakness incontinence: retropubic suspension

Retropubic suspension procedures are used to treat female stress incontinence caused by urethral hypermobility. The aim of surgery is to elevate and fix the bladder neck and proximal urethra in a retropubic position, to support the bladder neck, and to regain continence.

It is contraindicated in the presence of significant intrinsic sphincter deficiency (ISD).

Types of surgery

Surgery is considered after conservative methods have failed. The main types of operation are via a Pfannenstiel or lower midline abdominal incision to approach the bladder neck and develop the retropubic space. Better results are seen in patients with pure stress incontinence and primary repair (as opposed to "redo" surgery).

Marshall–Marchetti–Krantz (MMK) procedure

Sutures are placed either side of the urethra around the level of the bladder neck and then tied to the hyaline cartilage of the pubic symphysis. Short-term success is about 90%,[1] but declines over time.

Complications include osteitis pubis (3%), typically presenting up to 8 weeks postoperatively, with pubic pain radiating to the thigh. Treatment is with simple analgesia, bed rest, and steroids.

Burch colposuspension

This requires good vaginal mobility, to allow the vaginal wall to be elevated and attached to the lateral pelvic wall where the formation of adhesions over time secures its position. The paravaginal fascia is exposed and approximated to the iliopectineal (Cooper) ligament of the superior pubic rami.

Initial success rates are 90%.[1] Better long-term results compare with those for other retropubic repairs. A laparoscopic approach can also be performed, but long-term results have proven to be poor.

Vagino-obturator shelf/paravaginal repair

Sutures are placed by the vaginal wall and paravaginal fascia and then passed through the obturator fascia to attach to part of the parietal pelvic fascia below the tendinous arch (arcus tendoneus fascia). Cure rates are up to 85%.

Complications of retropubic suspension procedures

- Urinary retention (5%)
- Bladder overactivity
- Vaginal prolapse

1 Jarvis GJ (1994). Stress incontinence. In Mundy AR, Stephenson TP, Wein AJ (Eds.), *Urodynamics: Principles, Practice and Application*, 2nd ed. New York: Churchill-Livingstone, pp. 299–326.

Treatment of sphincter weakness incontinence: pubovaginal slings

Indications

Sling procedures were developed mainly for female stress incontinence associated with poor urethral function (type III or ISD) or when previous surgical procedures have failed. The success of sling procedures, however, has resulted in expanded applications in women with hypermobility. It is essential that urethral and bladder function is evaluated prior to surgical repair.

Types of sling

- **Autologous**—rectus fascia, fascia lata (from the thigh), vaginal wall slings
- **Nonautologous**—allograft fascia lata from donated cadaveric tissue
- **Synthetic**—monofilament "macropore" polypropylene mesh (via transobturator, transabdominal, or transvaginal needles)

Autologous and allograft slings

The tissue strip is inserted via an abdominal incision and tunneled through the endopelvic fascia on one side, behind the proximal urethra and into the anterior vagina, and then guided out the other side. The two ends are sutured to rectus fascia, using the minimal amount of tension needed to prevent urethral movement. Alternative methods of fixation include bone anchoring; however, this is associated with increased risk of osteitis pubis.

Synthetic slings

Synthetic slings have become extremely popular worldwide—these procedures are less invasive, can be inserted under local anesthetic as a day case, and have few complications. The slings are inserted using either suprapubic (TVT™, SPARC™) or transobturator (Monarch™, TVT-O™) needles and tunneled into a mid-urethral location. "Macropore" polypropylene slings have been widely recognized as being more resistant to infectious complications

Cystoscopy is often used to detect bladder perforation during sling placement. Postoperatively, patients may temporarily require ISC until post-void residuals are <100 mL.

Outcomes

Overall, long-term cure rates for slings are 80%, with improvement seen in 90%.[1] Complication rates are low but include voiding disorders (urinary retention, de novo bladder overactivity); vaginal, urethral, and bladder erosions; bowel and bladder perforation; and pelvic bleeding.

1 Abrams P, Cardozo L, Khoury S, et al. (Eds.) (2002) *Incontinence*, 2nd International Consultation on Incontinence, 2nd ed, Health Publications Ltd, pp. 825–863.

Treatment of sphincter weakness incontinence: the artificial urinary sphincter

The artificial urinary sphincter (AUS; AMS800™) consists of an inflatable cuff placed around the bulbar urethra in men, via either a perineal or high scrotal incision. Good coaptation of the cuff around the proximal corpus spongiosum provides the best outcomes.

Other components include a pressure-regulating balloon placed extra-peritoneally, and an activating pump placed in the scrotum. The cuff, when activated, provides a constant pressure to compress the urethra. To void, the pump is squeezed, which transfers all fluid to the reservoir balloon, thereby deflating the cuff. The cuff then automatically refills within 3 minutes. Voiding takes place in the interval taken for the cuff to refill.

In women, a lower abdominal incision (midline or Pfannenstiel) may be used to place a cuff around the bladder.

Indications and patient selection

Indications include incontinence secondary to urethral sphincter deficiency in patients with normal bladder capacity and compliance. In men, it is used almost always for sphincter damage due to prostatectomy (radical prostatectomy for prostate cancer or TURP). In women it can be used for neuropathic sphincter weakness (e.g., spinal cord injury, spina bifida) if the incontinence is not due to bladder overactivity.

If there is combined bladder overactivity and sphincter weakness, treat the bladder first (i.e., trial of anticholinergics)—in some cases this will be enough to achieve continence. If incontinence persists, proceed with AUS at a later date.

Good manual dexterity is required to manipulate the pump. Patients must also have sufficient cognitive function to operate the sphincter by themselves, several times daily.

Patient evaluation

Patients should undergo a careful history and physical exam to evaluate voiding function and severity of incontinence. Although urodynamics and/or cystoscopy are often used to further identify anatomical abnormalities within the lower urinary tract in complex cases, "garden variety" SUI can often be diagnosed reliably on the basis of careful history and physical alone.

Results

An AUS can function well for many years. Overall long-term success (continued continence, no device malfunction) is 80%. Revision rates are about 20%, usually due to subcuff atrophy.

Complications and long-term outcomes

Recurrent incontinence

This is secondary to urethral atrophy under the cuff (10% over the first 5 years post implantation); mechanical failure; urethral erosion (due to chronic pressure/ischemia from the cuff, often due to urethral catheterization during nonurological procedures without prior cuff deactivation); bladder overactivity or reduced compliance causing reflux; hydronephrosis; and renal failure.

Investigate recurrent incontinence by cystoscopy (to exclude erosion) and urodynamics (to detect high bladder pressures).

Erosion

Erosion is most common at 3–4 months, with 75% occurring in the first year. Patients present with pain and swelling of the scrotum, sudden worsening of incontinence, UI, and bloody discharge. Cuff erosion usually occurs if the AUS is not deactivated during catheterization or instrumentation—this dreaded complication results in prompt surgical removal of the entire device.

Use of an indwelling urethral catheter for more than 24 hours should be avoided in men with an AUS to prevent erosion—if long-term urinary diversion is required, consider SP tube placement.

Infection

Primary implant infection rates are 1–3%. With infection or erosion, remove the entire device and wait 3–6 months before reinsertion.

Salvage of an infected AUS may be accomplished via removal of the infected device, followed by copious washout with antiseptic solutions and immediate replacement with a new device

Overactive bladder: conventional treatment

Definition

Overactive bladder (OAB) is a symptom syndrome that includes urgency, with or without urge incontinence, frequency, and nocturia. The symptoms are usually caused by bladder (detrusor) overactivity, but can be due to other forms of voiding dysfunction. Roughly 17% of the population >40 years old in Europe has symptoms of OAB.[1]

Conventional treatment

Conservative

Patient management involves a multidisciplinary team approach (urologists, gynecologists, continence nurse specialists, physiotherapists, and community-based health care workers). Treat underlying causes (urethral obstruction, bladder stones, spinal disease, tumor).

TURP for bladder outlet obstruction due to BPH can provide symptomatic relief in >66% of men. Treatment of the SUI component includes pelvic floor exercises, biofeedback, and high-frequency electrical stimulation (which strengthens the pelvic floor and sphincter by increasing tone through sacral neural feedback systems).

Behavioral modification

This involves modifying fluid intake, avoiding stimulants (caffeine, alcohol), and bladder training for urgency (delay micturition for increasing periods of time by inhibiting the desire to void).

Medication

Most patients will benefit from medication.

- **Anticholinergic drugs** act to inhibit bladder contractions and increase capacity (oxybutynin, tolterodine, trospium chloride, solifenacin, darifenicin, fesoteridine). Oxybutynin also exerts a direct muscle effect and can be administered directly into the bladder (intravesically) in patients performing intermittent catheterization (5 mg in 30 mL normal saline q8h after emptying the bladder).
  - *Contraindications* include closed angle glaucoma.
  - *Side effects* are dry mouth, constipation, and blurred vision.
- **Tricyclic antidepressants** (imipramine) exert a direct relaxant effect on bladder muscle as well as produce sympathomimetic and central effects.
- **Desmopressin (DDAVP)** is a synthetic vasopressin analog that acts as an antidiuretic. It is used intranasally to alleviate nocturia in adults. Oral DDAVP is effective for nocturnal polyuria.
- **Baclofen** is a GABA receptor agonist, used orally or via intrathecal pump in patients with bladder dysfunction and limb spasticity.

---

1 Milsom I, Abrams P, Cardozo L, et al. (2001). How widespread are the symptoms of an overactive bladder and how are they managed? A population-based prevalence study. *Br J Urol Int* 87(9):760–766.

Overactive bladder: options for failed conventional therapy

Neuromodulation (see also p. 528)

This involves electrical stimulation of the bladder's nerve supply to suppress reflexes responsible for involuntary bladder muscle (detrusor) contraction.

The Interstim device stimulates the S3 afferent nerve, which then inhibits detrusor activity at the level of the sacral spinal cord. An initial percutaneous nerve evaluation is performed, followed by surgical implantation of permanent electrode leads into the S3 foramen, with a pulse generator that is programmed externally.

Surgery

The aim is to increase functional bladder capacity, decrease maximal detrusor pressure, and protect the upper urinary tract (also see p. 512).

Augmentation enterocystoplasty ("clamshell" ileocystoplasty)

This procedure is the gold-standard method of providing a high-volume low-pressure storage system for the pathological bladder. It relieves intractable frequency, urge, and UUI in 90% of patients.

The bladder dome is bivalved and a U-shaped detubularized segment of ileum is patched into the defect, creating a larger bladder volume that can store urine at lower pressures.

Many patients will void spontaneously but most will need to perform intermittent catheterization periodically to empty completely.

Conduit diversion

This is a noncontinent urinary outlet in which the ureters are anastomosed to a short ileal segment, which is brought out cutaneously as a stoma in the right lower quadrant.

Ileocystoplasty: acts like an ileal conduit attached to the bladder, performed in conjunction with bladder neck closure to provide conduit drainage without the need for ureteral reconstruction.

Auto-augmentation (detrusor myectomy)

Detrusor muscle is excised from the dome of the bladder, leaving the underlying bladder endothelium intact. A large epithelial bulge is created which augments bladder capacity.

Intravesical pharmacotherapy

Botulinum toxin A (BTX-A) injection therapy acts by inhibiting calcium-mediated release of ACh at the neuromuscular junction, reducing muscle contractility. It is used predominantly for neuropathic bladder dysfunction, but increasingly is being used for failed medical therapy of the OAB in non-neuropaths. It is injected directly into detrusor muscle under cystoscopic guidance (flexible cystoscopy or rigid under regional or general anesthetic) at 20–30 random sites, excluding the trigone (dose dependent on supplier's recommended dose schedule).

Repeat treatments are required (6–12 months between injections), and ISC may be needed to empty residuals (5% of non-neuropaths).

Mild flu-like reactions lasting a week or so can occur. Generalized weakness, swallowing or breathing difficulty are rarely reported. Allergic reactions are uncommon.

"Mixed" incontinence

Definition

Mixed incontinence is involuntary urinary leakage associated with both urgency and exertion, effort, sneezing, or coughing (UUI + SUI). Roughly 30–50% of women with SUI also have symptoms of frequency, urgency, or UUI.

Underlying etiologies and evaluation remain the same as for SUI and UUI (see p. 20).

SUI component

Risk factors for women include childbirth (increased with forceps delivery); aging; estrogen withdrawal; previous pelvic surgery; and obesity. There also appears to be an intrinsic loss of urethral strength, often associated with urethral hypermobility. Neurological disorders (SCI, MS, spina bifida) also cause sphincter weakness.

Investigation and management

This mixed UI patient group needs further investigation to rule out pathologies such as bladder cancer, stones, and interstitial cystitis. Voiding records and urodynamic studies are most useful.

- **Behavioral** and pelvic floor exercises with vaginal weights (Kegel exercises) are important and can improve symptoms in 30% of women with mild SUI.
- **Biofeedback** is the technique by which information on ability and strength of pelvic floor muscle contraction is presented back to the patient as a visual, auditory, or tactile signal. Patients may also be helped by the perineometer, which measures pelvic floor contraction.
- Correct pelvic organ prolapse with a pessary.

When stress symptoms predominate, surgical repair via a sling can alleviate symptoms. However, if UUI is also a significant symptom, surgery may be less helpful, and a trial of pharmacotherapy should be used first.

Post-prostatectomy incontinence

Incidence

After TURP or open prostatectomy (OP) performed for benign prostate disease, <1% of patients will have significant SUI.[1]

Results after radical prostatectomy (RP) for malignant disease are more variable—up to 40% suffer mild urinary leakage requiring pads, but this usually improves over 12–18 months post-surgery, with severe UI persisting in 2–10%.[2,3]

Risk factors

Risk factors include increasing age; pre-existing bladder dysfunction; previous radiotherapy (TURP following brachytherapy has a 40% risk of severe UI); prior TURP; advanced stage of disease; and surgical technique.

Earlier recovery of continence after RP is achieved using nerve-sparing techniques and sphincter- and bladder neck–preserving procedures.

Pathophysiology

The proximal sphincter mechanism is removed at prostatectomy. Post-prostatectomy continence therefore requires a functioning distal urethral sphincter mechanism and low bladder pressure during bladder filling. Direct damage to the external sphincter can occur during prostatectomy (at TURP it occurs particularly during resection between the 11 and 2 o'clock position, when the reference point for the position of the distal sphincter—the verumontanum—cannot be seen).

Damage to the innervation of the sphincter can occur during both open prostatectomy and TURP. Urodynamic studies before and after RP show that maximal urethral closure pressure (MUCP) and functional urethral length (the length of urethra over which the sphincter functions to maintain high pressures) both fall predictably.

Nerve-sparing RP (where the neurovascular bundles are specifically identified and preserved) produces better continence rates and longer functional urethral lengths and MUCPs.

A substantial proportion of men also have overactive bladders (detrusor instability) before prostatectomy, and this may remain so after prostatectomy, often taking months to resolve after successful surgery for BPH. The main cause of post-RP incontinence is sphincter dysfunction.

Evaluation

Wait for up to 12 months' spontaneous improvement unless incontinence is severe.

- **History:** stress-induced leakage (cough, standing from a sitting position) suggests sphincter dysfunction.
- **Examination:** observe for leakage while patient is coughing in standing position and note the severity.
- **Tests:** post-void residual volume measurement on ultrasound (to exclude retention with overflow); urodynamic studies allow determination of bladder overactivity and sphincter function

- Cystoscopy allows identification of strictures (this is particularly important if artificial sphincter implantation is contemplated, since it is preferable to stabilize the stenotic vesicourethral anastomosis prior to undertaking AUS placement).

Treatment

Sphincter dysfunction

The AdVance transobturator male urethral sling is an effective new transobturator polypropylene sling that has recently been developed for men with mild to moderate incontinence (1–3 pads per day). Alternatively, pelvic floor exercises, urethral bulking agents, and bone-anchored slings may be used.

Artificial urinary sphincter insertion is usually deferred until 1 year post-prostatectomy and is the most effective long-term treatment (80% success rate). It is used primarily in men with considerable leakage (>3 pads per day).

Bladder dysfunction

Conservative treatment for bladder overactivity includes behavioral therapy, pelvic floor exercises, and anticholinergic medication.

Surgery for intractable cases includes augmentation cystoplasty or urinary diversion. Catheterization may be considered in the older patient.

1 Agency for Health Care Policy and Research (AHCPR) (1994). Benign Prostatic Hyperplasia: Diagnosis and Treatment. Clinical Practice Guidelines No. 8 Feb. www.ncbi.nlm.nih.gov.
2 Catalona WJ, Carvalhal GF, Mager DE, et al. (1999). Potency, continence and complication rates in 1,870 consecutive radical retropubic prostatectomies. *J Urol* 162(2):433–438.
3 Walsh PC, Marschke P, Ricker D, et al. (2000). Patient-reported urinary incontinence and sexual function after anatomic radical prostatectomy. *Urology* 55(1):58–61.

Vesicovaginal fistula (VVF)

A *fistula* is an abnormal communication between two epithelial surfaces, in the case of a VVF, between the bladder and vagina. In 10% of patients there is a coexisting ureterovaginal fistula.

Etiology

In developing countries, most cases are associated with obstructed or prolonged childbirth, causing tissue pressure necrosis between the vagina and bladder. In developed countries, 75% of cases follow hysterectomy (0.1–0.2% risk)[1,2] (Fig. 4.1).

Other causes include pelvic surgery (e.g., bowel resection); radiotherapy; pessaries; advanced pelvic malignancy (cervical carcinoma); pelvic endometriosis; inflammatory bowel disease; trauma (pelvic fracture); childbirth (5%); low estrogen states; infection (urinary TB); and congenital abnormalities.

Symptoms

These include immediate or delayed onset of urinary leakage from the vagina postoperatively, prolonged bowel ileus (due to leak of urine into the peritoneal cavity as well as through the vagina), and suprapubic pain or flank pain.

Examination

- Vaginal examination may demonstrate the VVF, if large (the examining finger can reach inside the bladder).
- 3-swab test—oral phenazopyridine turns urine orange. After 1 hour, place 3 swabs into the vagina and instill methylene blue into the bladder. If the proximal swab turns blue, it indicates VVF; if it is orange, it suggests ureterovaginal fistula.
- Cystogram (or voiding cystourethrography [VCUG]). This is the best test for identifying fistulae.
- Fistula track may be seen at cystoscopy and can help in determining its proximity to the ureteric orifices. Biopsy the tract if there is a history of malignancy.
- IVP and/or bilateral retrograde pyelograms are essential to assess ureteral involvement.

Management

Most cases require surgery. Conservative methods include urethral catheterization combined with anticholinergics and antibiotics for small, uncomplicated VVF. Alternatively, de-epithelization of the tract can be attempted with silver nitrate or electrocoagulation.

If there is a coexisting ureterovaginal fistula, a ureteric stent alone is often successful.

Surgery

Early repair (within 2–3 weeks) is advocated in simple cases, but traditionally, surgery is delayed 3–6 months. The transvaginal approach has success rates of 82–100%. The fistula tract is closed with two layers of sutures and covered by an anterior vaginal wall flap.

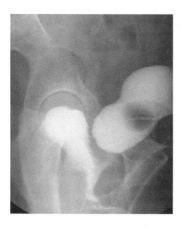

Figure 4.1 Cystogram showing leak of contrast from the bladder and into the vagina due to a VVF. This followed a hysterectomy.

Additionally, interpositional tissue grafts should be mobilized between the bladder and vagina (Martius fat pad graft from labia majora; peritoneal flap; gracilis flap).

The abdominal approach is reserved for complex cases. The bladder is bisected to the level of the fistula tract, which is then completely excised (85–90% success). The bladder is closed and an interpositional omentum graft created. In complex cases, urinary diversion procedures may be needed.

Postoperatively, maximal urinary drainage is prudent using a large-bore Foley catheter and possibly a suprapubic catheter and/or ureteral catheter. Antibiotic coverage and anticholinergics are maintained for 2 weeks until catheters are removed. A VCUG should be performed to document the absence of extravasation. Give estrogen replacement to postmenopausal women. Patients should avoid use of tampons or sexual intercourse for 2–3 months.

Postoperative complications include vaginal bleeding; infection; bladder pain; dyspareunia due to vaginal stenosis; graft ischemia; ureteric injury; and recurrence.

1 Tancer ML (1992). Observations on prevention and management of vesicovaginal fistula after total hysterectomy. *Surg Gynaecol Obstet* 175(6):501–506.
2 Harris WJ (1995). Early complications of abdominal and vaginal hysterectomy. *Obstet Gynaecol Survey* 50(11):795–805.

Incontinence in the elderly patient

Prevalence

UI increases markedly with advancing age, affecting 10–20% of women and 7–10% of men >65 years who are living at home. These figures escalate if older people are institutionalized, as follows: residential home, 25%; nursing home, 40%; long-stay hospital ward, 50–70%.

Functional incontinence is often associated with factors outside of the urinary tract, such as permanent immobility, cognitive impairment, and environmental changes.

Transient causes of UI ("DIAPPERS")

- **D**ementia/delirium
- **I**nfection
- **A**trophic vaginitis or urethritis
- **P**harmaceuticals (opiates and calcium antagonists cause urinary retention and constipation; anticholinergics cause increased PVR and retention;
- **P**sychological problems—depression; neurosis; anxiety
- **E**xcess fluid input or output (diuretics; CHF; nocturnal polyuria)
- **R**estricted mobility
- **S**tool impaction (constipation)

Management

Simple measures such as timed voids or laxative use may be helpful and should be attempted initially. Biofeedback and behavioral methods are appropriate only if cognition is intact.

Treat any vaginitis (0.01% estriol cream topically) in postmenopausal females.

Absorbent appliances include bed pads and body-worn pad products (pull-up adult diapers); body-worn external urine collection devices (condom catheter) or compression devices (Cunningham clamp) may be helpful for severe leakage in males.

Indwelling catheters are initially preferable when UI is due to obstruction or no alternative intervention is suitable. Suprapubic tube placement is preferable to long-term indwelling urethral catheterization, which is often associated with pressure necrosis and/or erosion of the urethra.

Chapter 5

Infections and inflammatory conditions

Urinary tract infection: definitions, incidence, and
    investigations *134*
Urinary tract infection: microbiology *138*
Lower urinary tract infection *140*
Recurrent urinary tract infection *142*
Urinary tract infection: treatment *146*
Acute pyelonephritis *148*
Pyonephrosis and perinephric abscess *150*
Other forms of pyelonephritis *152*
Chronic pyelonephritis *154*
Septicemia and urosepsis *156*
Fournier gangrene *160*
Epididymitis and orchitis *162*
Periurethral abscess *164*
Prostatitis: epidemiology and classification *166*
Prostatitis: presentation, evaluation, and treatment *168*
Other prostate infections *170*
Interstitial cystitis *172*
Tuberculosis *176*
Parasitic infections *178*
HIV in urological surgery *180*
Inflammatory and other disorders of the penis *182*

Urinary tract infection: definitions, incidence, and investigations

Definitions

Urinary tract infection (UTI) is currently defined as the inflammatory response of the urothelium to bacterial invasion. UTI due to other organisms is less common and addressed elsewhere.

This inflammatory response causes a constellation of clinical symptom. In bladder infection this is described as *cystitis*—frequent small-volume voids, urgency, suprapubic pain or discomfort, and urethral burning on voiding (dysuria).

In acute kidney infection (acute pyelonephritis) the symptoms are fever, chills, malaise, and flank pain, often with associated LUTS of frequency, urgency, and urethral pain on voiding.

Bacteriuria is the presence of bacteria in the urine and may be asymptomatic or symptomatic and varies by age and sex (Table 5.1). Bacteriuria without pyuria indicates the presence of bacterial *colonization* of the urine, rather than the presence of active infection, where "active" implies an inflammatory response to bacterial invasion of the urothelium.

Risk factors for bacteriuria include female sex; increasing age; low estrogen states (menopause); pregnancy; diabetes mellitus; previous UTI; institutionalized elderly; indwelling catheters; urolithiasis; genitourinary malformation; and voiding dysfunction (including obstruction).

Pyuria is the presence of white blood cells (WBCs) in the urine in dipstick or 10 WBC/HPF (400×) in resuspended sediment of centrifuged urine. Pyuria implies an inflammatory response of the urothelium to bacterial infection or, in the absence of bacteriuria, some other pathology such as carcinoma in situ, TB infection, bladder stones, or other inflammatory conditions.

An uncomplicated UTI is one occurring in a patient with a structurally and functionally normal urinary tract. The majority of such patients are women who respond quickly to a short course of antibiotics.

A complicated UTI is one occurring in the presence of an underlying anatomical or functional abnormality (e.g., functional problems causing incomplete bladder emptying, such as bladder outlet obstruction due to BPH, DSD in spinal cord injury), urolithiasis, fistula between bladder and bowel, etc. Most UTIs in men occur in association with a structural or functional abnormality and are therefore defined as complicated UTIs.

Complicated UTIs take longer to respond to antibiotic treatment than uncomplicated UTIs, and if there is an underlying anatomical or structural abnormality they are at increased risk of recurrence within days, weeks, or months.

UTI may also be classified as isolated, recurrent, or unresolved.

Isolated UTI has an interval of at least 6 months between infections.

Recurrent UTI is >2 infections in 6 months, or 3 within 12 months. Recurrent UTI may be due to reinfection (i.e., infection by a different

Table 5.1 Prevalence of bacteriuria

Age	Female	Male
Infants (<1 year)	1%	3%
School (<15 years old)	1–3%	<1%
Reproductive	4%	<1%
Elderly	20–30%	10%

bacteria) or bacterial persistence (infection by the same organism originating from a focus within the urinary tract).

Bacterial persistence is caused by the presence of bacteria within calculi (e.g., struvite calculi), a chronically infected prostate (chronic bacterial prostatitis), or an obstructed or atrophic infected kidney, or it occurs as a result of a bladder fistula (with bowel or vagina) or urethral diverticulum.

Unresolved infection is failure of the initial treatment course to eradicate bacteria from the urine. It is usually due to pre-existing or acquired antimicrobial resistance, patient noncompliance with therapy, insufficient antibiotic dosing, or disorders that decrease drug bioavailability (i.e., azotemia, urinary calculus)

UTI incidence

- *Newborns <1 year:* Male children have a slightly higher risk of UTI than females, which is thought to be caused by foreskin contamination and congenital structural abnormalities.
- *Children 1–5 years:* Females have approximately a 5% incidence of UTI compared to 0.5% in males, and anatomic anomalies account for the majority of UTIs in both sexes.
- *Children 6–15 years:* Functional voiding abnormalities account for the increased incidence of UTIs (about 5% in females) with a low rate (<0.5–1%) in males.
- *Adolescents and adults 16–35 years:* Females have a much higher risk of UTI related to sexual activity and the use of intravaginal contraceptives.
- *Adults >35 years:* The incidence of UTI gradually increases in both sexes until the incidence is similar above age 65 (40% incidence in females vs. 35% in males)

UTI investigations

Urine dipstick
Urine dipstick, obtained from a mid-stream sample, is used as a first-line screening. Urine dipstick has the following performance characteristics: leukocyte esterase, 50% positive predictive value and 92% negative predictive value; nitrate, sensitivity 35%–85%. Best performance for dipstick is when urine culture colony counts are >100,000 CFU/HPF.

However, if the dipstick is negative for blood, protein, leukocyte esterase, and nitrite, <2% of urine samples will be positive for cultured bacteria.

Leukocyte esterase

Leukocyte esterase activity detects the presence of white blood cells in the urine. Leukocyte esterase is produced by neutrophils and causes a color change in a chromogen salt on the dipstick.

- **False positive** (pyuria present but negative dipstick test): concentrated urine, glycosuria, presence of urobilinogen, consumption of large amounts of ascorbic acid
- **False positive** (pyuria absent, but positive dipstick test): contamination (vaginal, etc.)

There are many causes for pyuria and a positive leukocyte esterase test occurring in the absence of bacteria on urine microscopy. This is so-called *sterile pyuria* and it occurs with TB infection, renal calculi, bladder calculi, glomerulonephritis, interstitial cystitis, and carcinoma in situ. Thus, the leukocyte esterase dipstick test may be truly positive and suggest a significant disease process, in the absence of infection.

Nitrites

Nitrates are not normally found in urine and are produced by the dietary breakdown of nitrates in the urine by various gram-negative bacteria. *Nitrite testing* is therefore indirect testing for bacteriuria but may miss gram-positive infections.

Many species of gram-negative bacteria can convert nitrates to nitrites, and these are detected in urine by a reaction with the reagents on the dipstick that form a red azo dye.

The specificity of the nitrite dipstick for detecting bacteriuria is >90% with sensitivity of 35–85% (i.e., false negatives are common—a negative dipstick in the presence of active infection) and is less accurate in urine containing fewer than 10^5 organisms/mL. So, if the nitrite dipstick test is positive, the patient probably has a UTI, but a negative test can occur in the presence of infection.

- **False positive:** with contamination (i.e., vaginal)
- **False negative:** common in setting of low dietary nitrate, diuretics, and with certain species of bacteria (e.g., *Enterococcus, Staphylococcus, Pseudomonas*)

Urine microscopy

Microscopic examination of the urine sediment is also helpful. After centrifugation of the sample, the observation of bacteria and >3 WBC/HPF is diagnostic of a urinary tract infection. Occasionally, a Gram stain of an uncentrifuged urine may demonstrate gram-positive or gram-negative bacteria.

If the urine specimen contains large numbers of squamous epithelial cells (cells derived from the foreskin, vaginal, or distal urethral epithelium), this suggests contamination of the specimen, and the presence of bacteria in this situation may indicate a false-positive result.

Urine culture and collection

Urine culture is the gold standard for the diagnosis of a bacterial UTI. Urine samples must be properly collected, the method of collection documented, and samples cultured immediately or, if this is not possible, stored in a refrigerator (not frozen) for up to 24 hours.

The diagnosis of UTI is based on symptomatology, urinalysis, and urine culture findings. The traditional strict definition of >105 bacteria/mL of urine is no longer required to make a diagnosis of UTI. Treatment is usually indicated if ≥102 CFU/mL in a patient with symptoms of UTI, particularly with associated pyuria.

The method of collection and sex of the patient can influence the results of the urine culture; see Table 5.2.

Further investigation
Based on the initial clinical evaluation, further diagnostic testing may be necessary to evaluate the *cause* of the urinary tract infection. While most cases of simple UTI do not require further investigation, complicated or recurrent UTI may require imaging (plain abdominal film, CT, ultrasound) or functional studies (uroflow, post void residual urine determination, urodynamics studies) Further workup is needed if the following occur:
• Symptoms and signs of upper tract infection (flank pain, malaise, fever) that suggest acute pyelonephritis, a pyonephrosis, or perinephric abscess
• Recurrent UTIs develop (see p. 142).
• The patient is pregnant.
• Unusual infecting organism (e.g., *Proteus*), suggesting the possibility of an infection stone

Table 5.2 Probability of UTI based on urine culture and collection method

Collection	CFU	Probability of infection (%)
Suprapubic	Gram negative any	>99
	Gram positive >1000	
Catheterization	>10^5	95
	10^{4-5}	Likely
	10^{3-4}	Repeat
	<10^3	Unlikely
Clean catch		
Male	>10^4	Likely
Female	3 specimens: >10^5	95
	2 specimens: >10^5	90
	1 specimen: >10^5	80
	5×10^4–10^5	Repeat
	1–5×10^4 symptomatic	Repeat
	1–5×10^4 nonsymptomatic	Unlikely
	<10^4	Unlikely

CFU, colony-forming unit.
Reproduced with permission from Chapter 13. Bacterial infections of the genitourinary tract. In *Smith's General Urology*, 17th Edition, 2008. Emil A. Tanagho and Jack W. McAninch, Eds. New York: McGraw Hill.

Urinary tract infection: microbiology

Most UTIs are caused by fecal-derived bacteria that are facultative anaerobes (i.e., they can grow under both anaerobic and nonanaerobic conditions)—see Table 5.3.

Uncomplicated UTI

Most UTIs are bacterial in origin. The most common cause is *Escherichia coli (E. coli)*, a gram-negative bacillus, which accounts for 85% of community-acquired and 50% of hospital-acquired infection.

Other common causative organisms include *Staphylococcus saprophyticus* and *Enterococcus faecalis* (also known as *Streptococcus faecalis*—gram positive), *Proteus mirabilis, Klebsiella,* and other gram-negative *Enterobacteriaceae.*

Complicated UTI

E. coli is responsible for up to 50% of cases. Other causes include Enterococci (e.g., *Streptococcus faecalis*), *Staph. aureus, Staph. epidermidis* (gram positive) and *Pseudomonas aeruginosa* (gram negative).

Route of infection

Ascending

The vast majority of UTIs result from ascending or retrograde infections up the urethra. The bacteria, derived from the large bowel, colonize the perineum, vagina, and distal urethra. They ascend along the urethra to the bladder (risk is increased in females as the urethra is shorter), causing cystitis, and from the bladder they may ascend, via the ureters, to involve the kidneys (pyelonephritis).

Reflux is not necessary for infection to ascend to the kidneys, but the presence of reflux facilitates ascending infection, as will any process that impairs ureteric peristalsis (e.g., ureteric obstruction, gram-negative organisms and endotoxins, pregnancy).

Infection that ascends to involve the kidneys is also more likely where the infecting organism has P pili (filamentous protein appendages—also known as fimbriae—which allow binding of bacteria to the surface of epithelial cells).

Hematogenous is uncommon, but is seen with *Staph. aureus*, Candida fungemia, and TB.

Infection via lymphatics is seen rarely in inflammatory bowel disease and retroperitoneal abscess.

Factors increasing bacterial virulence

Adhesion factors

Many gram-negative bacteria contain pili on their surface, which aid attachment to urothelial cells of the host. A typical piliated cell may contain 100–400 pili. Pili are 5–10 nm in diameter and up to 2 μm long.

E. coli produces a number of antigenically and functionally different types of pili on the same cell; other strains may produce only a single type, and, in some isolates, no pili are seen.

Pili are defined functionally by their ability to mediate hemagglutination (HA) of specific types of erythrocytes. Mannose-sensitive (type 1) pili are

Table 5.3 Bacterial classification: uropathogens

Cocci	**Gram-positive**
	Staphylococcus, Enterococcus faecalis (also known as *Streptococcus faecalis*) e.g., *S. saprophyticus* causes approximately 10% of symptomatic lower UTIs in young, sexually active women
	Gram-negative
	Aerobes: *Neisseria*
Bacilli (rods)	**Gram-positive**
	Anaerobes*: *Clostridium, Lactobacillus* (usually a vaginal commensal)
	Gram-negative
	Aerobes: Enterobacteria (*Escherichia, Klebsiella, Proteus*), *Pseudomonas*
	Anaerobes*: Bacteroides
Others	Filamentous bacteria: *Mycobacterium* (*M. tuberculosis*—acid-fast, aerobic, gram-positive)
	Chlamydiae: *Chlamydia trachomatis* Fungi: *Candida albicans*
	Mycoplasma: *Mycoplasma* species, *Ureaplasma urealyticum* (cause UTI in patients with indwelling catheters)

*Anaerobic infections of the bladder and kidney are uncommon—anaerobes are normal commensals of the perineum, vagina, and distal urethra. However, infections of the urinary system that produce pus (pyogenic) (e.g., scrotal, prostatic, or perinephric abscesses) are often caused by anaerobic organisms (e.g., *Bacteroides* species such as *Bacteroides fragilis*, *Fusobacterium* species, anaerobic cocci, and *Clostridium perfringens*).

produced by all strains of *E. coli*. Certain pathogenic types of *E. coli* also produce mannose-resistant (P) pili (associated with pyelonephritis).

Avoidance of host defense mechanisms:
An extracellular capsule reduces immunogenicity and resists phagocytosis (*E. coli*). *M. tuberculosis* resists phagocytosis by preventing phagolysosome fusion.

Toxins
E. coli releases cytokines with direct effect on host tissues.

Enzyme production
Proteus species produce ureases, which causes breakdown of urea in the urine to ammonia. This contributes to disease processes (struvite stone formation).

Host defenses

Factors protecting against UTI are the following:
- Mechanical flushing effect of urine through the urinary tract (i.e., antegrade flow of urine)
- A mucopolysaccharide coating of the bladder (Tamm–Horsfall protein, glucose amino glycan [GAG layer]) helps prevent bacterial adherence.
- Low urine pH and high osmolarity reduce bacterial growth.
- Urinary immunoglobulin (IgA) inhibits bacterial adherence.

Lower urinary tract infection

Cystitis

Cystitis is infection and/or inflammation of the bladder.

Presentation

There is frequent voiding of small volumes, dysuria, urgency, offensive urine, suprapubic pain, hematuria, fever (uncommon), and incontinence. Up to 33% of women experience an episode of bacterial cystitis by age 24, and 50% of women will have an episode in their lifetime. Bacterial cystitis in healthy men is rare.

Investigation

Dipstick of midstream specimen of urine (MSU)

Not all patients with bacteriuria have significant pyuria (sensitivity of 75–95% for detection of infection, that is, 5–25% of patients with infection will have a negative leukocyte esterase test suggesting, erroneously, that they have no infection). Cloudy urine that is positive for WBCs on dipstick and is nitrite positive is very likely infected.

Microscopy of midstream specimen of urine (MSU)

- **False negatives:** Low bacterial counts may make it very difficult to identify bacteria, and the specimen of urine may therefore be deemed negative for bacteriuria, when in fact there is active infection.
- **False positives:** Bacteria may be seen in the MSU in the absence of infection. This is most often due to contamination of the MSU with commensals from the distal urethra and perineum (urine from a woman may contain thousands of lactobacilli and corynebacteria, and these organisms are derived from the vagina). These bacteria are readily seen under the microscope, and although they are gram-positive, they often appear gram-negative (gram-variable) if stained.

The finding of pyuria and red blood cells suggests the presence of active infection.

Noninfective hemorrhagic cystitis

While bacterial cystitis can result in hemorrhagic cystitis, pelvic radiotherapy (radiation cystitis—bladder capacity is reduced and multiple areas of mucosal telangiectasia are seen cystoscopically) and drug-induced cystitis (e.g., cyclophosphamide treatment) are types of noninfectious hemorrhagic cystitis.

Urethritis

Urethritis is inflammation of the urethra. Urethritis in men is a sexually transmitted disease, which presents with dysuria and urethral discharge.

Gonococcal urethritis (GU)

GU is caused by the gram-negative diplococcus *Neisseria gonorrhoea* (incubation 3–10 days) and commonly associated with concomitant infection with *Chlamydia trachomatis*. Diagnosis is based on cultures from urethral swab.

Treatment involves ceftriaxone 125 mg IM in a single dose or cefixime 400 mg orally in a single dose or 400 mg by suspension (200 mg/5 mL) plus treatment for chlamydia if chlamydial infection is not ruled out. Quinolones are no longer recommended in the United States because of resistant strains).[1]

Sexual contacts must be informed and treated.

Nongonococcal urethritis (NGU)

NGU is mainly caused by *Chlamydia trachomatis* (incubation 1–5 weeks). Treat with azithromycin, 1 g as a single oral dose; or doxycycline, 100 mg orally twice a day for 7 days.

Transmission to females results in increased risk of pelvic inflammatory disease, abdominal pain, ectopic pregnancy, infertility, and perinatal infection.

Urethral syndrome

Urethral syndrome is a condition of uncertain etiology that only affects women. It manifests as dysuria, frequency, and urgency without evidence of infection, although some cases improve with antibiotics.[2]

Further reading

Foster RT Sr (2008). Uncomplicated urinary tract infections in women [review]. *Obstet Gynecol Clin North Am* 35(2):235–248, viii.

1 *MMWR Morbid Mortal Wkly Rep* April 13, 2007; 56(14);332–336.
2 Kaur H, Arunkalaivanan AS (2007). Urethral pain syndrome and its management. *Obstet Gynecol Surv* 62(5):348–351.

Recurrent urinary tract infection

Recurrent UTI is defined as >2 infections in 6 months, or 3 within 12 months. It may be due to *reinfection* (i.e., infection by different bacteria) or *bacterial persistence* (infection by the same organism originating from a focus within the urinary tract).

Bacterial persistence

This implies the presence of bacteria within a site in the urinary tract, the presence of which leads to repeat episodes of infection. Such sites include urolithiasis anywhere in the urinary tract, chronically infected pro-state (chronic bacterial prostatitis), bacteria within an obstructed or atrophic kidney, bacteria gaining access to the urinary tract via a fistula (bowel or vagina), and bacteria within a urethral diverticulum.

Thus, recurrent urinary infection due to bacterial persistence implies a *functional or anatomical problem*. The recurrent UTIs will not resolve until this underlying problem has been addressed.

Reinfections

Reinfections usually occur after a *prolonged interval* (months) from the previous infection and are often caused by a *different* organism than the previous infecting bacterium. Bacterial persistence often leads to *frequent recurrence* of infection (within days or weeks) and the infecting organism is usually the *same* organism as that causing the previous infection(s).

Women with reinfection do not usually have an underlying functional or anatomical abnormality. Reinfections in women are associated with increased vaginal mucosal receptivity for uropathogens and ascending colonization from the fecal flora. These women cannot be cured of their predisposition to recurrent UTIs, but they can be managed by a variety of techniques (see below).

Men with reinfection may have underlying BLADDER OUTLET OBSTRUCTION (due to prostate enlargement or urethral stricture), which makes them more likely to develop a repeat infection, but between infections their urine is sterile (i.e., they do not have bacterial persistence between symptomatic UTIs). A urethrogram, flexible cystoscopy, post-void bladder ultrasound for residual urine volume, and, in some cases, urodynamics may be helpful in establishing the potential causes.

Both men and women with bacterial persistence usually have an underlying functional or anatomical abnormality and they can potentially be cured of their recurrent UTIs if this abnormality is identified and corrected.

Management of women with recurrent UTIs from reinfection

Most urologists will arrange a series of screening tests (KUB radiograph, renal ultrasound, CT scan, flexible cystoscopy) to evaluate for a potential source of bacterial persistence. In the absence of finding an underlying functional or anatomic abnormality, many of these patients cannot be cured of their tendency to recurrent UTI, but they can be managed in one of the following ways.

Avoidance of spermicides used with the diaphragm or on condoms

Spermicides containing nonoxynol-9 reduce vaginal colonization with lacto-bacilli and may enhance *E. coli* adherence to urothelial cells. Recommend an alternative form of contraception.

Estrogen replacement therapy

Lack of estrogen in postmenopausal women causes loss of vaginal lacto-bacilli and increased colonization by *E. coli*. In postmenopausal women, estrogen replacement, locally or systemically, has been shown to decrease the rate of recurrent UTI by recolonization of the vagina with lactobacilli and to eliminate colonization with bacterial uropathogens.[1]

Low-dose antibiotic prophylaxis

Oral antimicrobial therapy with full-dose oral tetracyclines, ampicillin, sulfonamides, amoxicillin, and cephalexin causes resistant strains in the fecal flora and subsequent resistant UTIs. However, trimethoprim, nitro-furantoin, low-dose cephalexin, and the fluoroquinolones appear to have minimal adverse effects on the fecal and vaginal flora.

Efficacy of prophylaxis

Recurrences of UTI may be reduced by as much as 90% when compared with placebo.[2] Prophylactic therapy requires only a small dose of an anti-microbial agent, generally given at bedtime for 6 to 12 months.

Symptomatic reinfection during prophylactic therapy is managed with a full therapeutic dose with the same prophylactic antibiotic or another antibiotic. Prophylaxis can then be restarted.

Symptomatic reinfection immediately after cessation of prophylactic therapy is managed by restarting nightly prophylaxis.

Trimethoprim

The gut is a reservoir for organisms that colonize the periurethral area and that may subsequently cause episodes of acute cystitis in young women. Trimethoprim eradicates gram-negative aerobic flora from the gut and vaginal fluid (i.e., it eliminates the pathogens from the infective source). Trimethoprim is also concentrated in bactericidal concentrations in the urine following an oral dose.

Dosage for trimethoprim is 100 mg/day.

Adverse reactions include blood dyscrasias due to bone marrow depres-sion; rarely, Stevens–Johnson syndrome; allergic reactions; and rarely, erythema multiforme, toxic epidermal necrolysis (photosensitivity).

Nitrofurantoin

Nitrofurantoin is completely absorbed and/or degraded or inactivated in the upper intestinal tract and therefore has no effect on gut flora. It is present for brief periods at high concentrations in the urine and leads to repeated elimination of bacteria from the urine. Nitrofurantoin prophy-laxis therefore does not lead to a change in vaginal or introital colonization with *Enterobacteria*.

1 Perrotta C, Aznar M, Mejia R, Albert X, Ng CW (2008). Oestrogens for preventing recurrent urinary tract infection in postmenopausal women. *Cochrane Database Syst Rev* 16;(2):CD005131.
2 Kaur H, Arunkalaivanan AS (2007). Urethral pain syndrome and its management. *Obstet Gynecol Surv*. 62(5):348–351

The bacteria colonizing the vagina remain susceptible to nitrofurantoin because of the lack of bacterial resistance in the fecal flora.

Dosage of nitrofurantoin is 50 mg/day or nitrofurantoin macrocrystals 100 mg/day.

Adverse reactions include acute pulmonary reactions (pulmonary fibrosis has been reported), allergic reactions (angioedema, anaphylaxis, urticaria, rash and pruritus), peripheral neuropathy, blood dyscrasias (agranulocytosis, thrombocytopenia, aplastic anemia), liver damage, lupus erythematosus–like syndrome, and chronic pulmonary reactions.

The risk of an adverse reaction increases with age, with the greatest number occurring in patients older than 50 years.

Cephalexin

Cephalexin at low dose is an excellent prophylactic agent because fecal resistance does not develop at this low dosage.

Dosage of cephalexin is 125–250 mg/day.

Adverse reactions include allergic reactions.

Fluoroquinolones (e.g., Ciprofloxacin)

Short courses can eradicate *Enterobacteria* from fecal and vaginal flora.

Dosage of ciprofloxacin is 125 mg/day.

Adverse reactions to quinolones include tendon damage (including rupture), which may occur within 48 hours of starting treatment (quinolones are contraindicated in patients with a history of tendon disorders related to quinolone use; elderly patients are more prone, and risk is increased by concomitant use of corticosteroids).

Other adverse reactions are arthropathy in children, Stevens–Johnson syndrome, allergic reactions, and pseudomembranous colitis.

Alternative therapies

Natural yogurt

Yogurt applied to the vulva and vagina can help restore normal vaginal flora, and some believe that this improves the natural resistance to recurrent infections. Immunoactive prophylaxis using various products such as vaginal vaccines are under study, and the use of probiotic such as lactobacillus remains unproven.[3]

There is some evidence from four randomized controlled trails (RCTs) that cranberry juice may decrease the number of symptomatic UTIs over a 12-month period in women with recurrent UTI.

Post-intercourse antibiotic prophylaxis

Sexual intercourse has been established as an important risk factor for acute cystitis in women, and women who use the diaphragm have a significantly greater risk of UTI than women who use other contraceptive methods. Post-intercourse therapy with antimicrobials such as nitrofurantoin, cephalexin, or trimethoprim, taken as a single dose, effectively reduces the incidence of reinfection.

3 Naber KG, Cho YH, Matsumoto T, Schaeffer AJ (2009). Immunoactive prophylaxis of recurrent urinary tract infections: a meta-analysis. *Int J Antimicrob Agents* 33(2):111–119.

"Self-start therapy"

Women keep a home supply of an antibiotic (e.g., trimethoprim, nitro-furantoin, a fluoroquinolone) and start treatment when they develop symptoms suggestive of UTI. This program should be limited to those who have been completely evaluated and are knowledgeable in the appropriate use of self-directed therapy.

Management of men and women with recurrent UTIs due to bacterial persistence

Investigations

These are directed at identifying the potential causes of bacterial persist-ence, outlined above.

- KUB radiograph to detect radio-opaque renal calculi.
- Renal ultrasound to detect hydronephrosis and renal calculi. If hydro-nephrosis is present, but the ureter is not dilated, consider the possibility of a radio-opaque stone obstructing the PUJ (this will usually be seen as an acoustic shadow on the ultrasound; arrange a CT urogram if no stone is seen) or a PUJO (arrange a MAG3 renogram to determine the presence or absence of PUJO).
- Determination of post-void residual urine volume by bladder ultrasound
- IVP or CT urogram where a stone is suspected but not identified on plain X-ray or ultrasound
- Flexible cystoscopy to identify possible causes of recurrent UTIs such as bladder stones, an underlying bladder cancer (rare), urethral or bladder neck stricture, or fistula

Treatment

Treatment depends on the functional or anatomical abnormality identi-fied as the cause of the bacterial persistence. If a stone or multiple stones are identified, they should be removed. If there is obstruction (e.g., BPO, PUJO, DSD in spinal injured patients), this should be corrected.

Further reading

Schooff M, Hill K (2005). Antibiotics for recurrent urinary tract infections [review]. *Am Fam Physician* 1;71(7):1301–1302.

Urinary tract infection: treatment

Antimicrobial drug therapy

The aim is to eliminate bacterial growth from the urine. Empirical treatment involves the administration of antibiotics according to the clinical presentation and most likely causative organism, before culture sensitivities are available (see Table 5.4).

Men are often affected by complicated UTI and may require longer treatments, as may patients with uncorrectable structural or functional abnormalities (e.g., indwelling catheters, neuropathic bladders).

Bacterial resistance to drug therapy

Organisms susceptible to concentrations of an antibiotic in the urine (or serum) after the recommended clinical dosing are termed *sensitive*, and those that do not respond are *resistant*. Bacterial resistance may be intrinsic (e.g., Proteus is intrinsically resistant to nitrofurantoin), via selection of a resistant mutant during initial treatment, or genetically transferred between bacteria by R plasmids.

Definitive treatment

Once urine or blood culture results are available, antimicrobial therapy should be adjusted according to bacterial sensitivities. Underlying abnormality should be corrected if feasible (i.e., extraction of infected calculus; removal of catheter; nephrostomy drainage of an infected, obstructed kidney).

Table 5.4 Recommendations for antimicrobial therapy

Infection	Bacteria	Initial empirical drug	Duration
Acute, uncomplicated cystitis	E. coli, Klebsiella, Proteus, Staphylococcus	Trimethoprim/ co-trimoxazole quinolone (ciprofloxacin) or **Nitrofurantoin (not for Proteus)	3 days 3 days 7 days
Acute, uncomplicated pyelonephritis	E. coli, Proteus, Klebsiella, other Enterobacter, Staphylococcus	Ciprofloxacin Cephalosporin or Aminopenicillin (ampicillin) with Aminoglycoside (gentamicin)	7–10 days
Complicated UTI	E. coli, Enterococcus	Ciprofloxacin Aminopenicillin	Continue for 3–5 days after elimination of underlying factor
Nosocomial (hospital acquired) UTI	Staphylococcus, Klebsiella, Proteus	Cephalosporin Aminoglycoside	
Acute complicated pyelonephritis	Enterobacter, Pseudomonas, Candida	For Candida: Fluconazole Amphotericin B	

These are general recommendations only; therapy should be guided by local microbiology bacterial sensitivities and resistance and specific culture and sensitivities. **Avoid nitrofurantoin in the elderly because of the potential for renal impairment.

Further reading

Rubenstein J, et al. (2003). Managing complicated urinary tract infections. The urologic review. *Infect Dis Clin N Am* 17:333–351.

Acute pyelonephritis

A clinical diagnosis is based on the presence of fever, flank pain, and tenderness, often with an elevated white count. It may affect one or both kidneys. There are usually accompanying symptoms suggestive of a lower UTI (frequency, urgency, suprapubic pain, urethral burning or pain on voiding) responsible for the ascending infection that resulted in the subsequent acute pyelonephritis. Nausea and vomiting are common.

Differential diagnosis

This includes cholecystitis, pancreatitis, diverticulitis, and appendicitis.

Risk factors

These include vesicoureteric reflux (VUR), urinary tract obstruction, calculi, spinal cord injury (neuropathic bladder), diabetes mellitus, congenital malformation, pregnancy, and indwelling catheters.

Pathogenesis and microbiology

Initially, there is patchy infiltration of neutrophils and bacteria in the parenchyma. Later changes include the formation of inflammatory bands extending from renal papilla to cortex, and small cortical abscesses. 80% of infections are secondary to *E. coli* (possessing P pili virulence factors). Other infecting organisms include enterococci (*Streptococcus faecalis*), *Klebsiella, Proteus,* and *Pseudomonas*.

Urine culture will be positive for bacterial growth, but the bacterial count may not necessarily be >10^5 CFU/mL of urine Thus, if you suspect a case of acute pyelonephritis based on symptoms, but there are <10^5 CFU/mL of urine, manage the case as acute pyelonephritis.

Investigation and treatment

For those patients who have a fever but are not systemically ill, outpatient management is reasonable. Culture the urine and start oral antibiotics according to your local antibiotic policy (which will be based on the likely infecting organisms and their likely antibiotic sensitivity). Common primary oral agents include the following:

- Fluoroquinolones (ciprofloxacin 500 mg PO bid, or levofloxacin 750 mg PO qd) empiric treatment
- Trimethoprim-sulfamethoxazole (TMP-SMZ) alternative

Therapy should be continued for 10–14 days and milder cases may be treated for 7 days. Recent studies suggest an increase in quinolone resistance as well as susceptibility to TMP-SMZ.

If the patient is systemically ill, obtain culture urine and blood and start IV fluids and IV antibiotics, selecting the antibiotic according to your local antibiotic policy. Treat patient until afebrile for 24 hours, then switch to oral agents based on sensitivities as above for a total of 14 days of antibiotic therapy. Empiric choices include the following:

- Ampicillin (2 g IV q6h) and gentamicin (1.5 mg/kg IV q8h or 3 mg/kg daily dosing)
- Ceftriaxone (1 g IV qd)
- Intravenous fluoroquinolones (e.g., ciprofloxin 200–400 mg IV q12h)
- Aztreonam (2 g IV q8h)

Arrange a KUB radiograph and renal ultrasound to see if there is an under-lying upper tract abnormality, unexplained hydronephrosis, or (rarely) gas surrounding the kidney (suggesting emphysematous pyelonephritis). Some centers will use a CT urogram as the first screening tool. However, if the patient does not respond within 3 days to this regimen of IV antibiotics (confirmed on sensitivities), a CT urogram is essential.

The lack of response to treatment suggests the possibility of a pyoneph-rosis (i.e., pus in the kidney, which, like any abscess, will only respond to drainage), a perinephric abscess (which again will only respond to drain-age), or emphysematous pyelonephritis.

The CT may demonstrate an obstructing calculus that may have been missed on the KUB X-ray, and ultrasound may show a perinephric abscess.

A pyonephrosis should be drained by insertion of a percutaneous neph-rostomy tube. A perinephric abscess should also be drained by insertion of a drain percutaneously.

Further reading

Drekonja DM, Johnson JR (2008). Urinary tract infections. *Prim Care* 35(2):345–367.

Wagenlehner FM, Pilatz A, Naber KG, Perletti G, Wagenlehner CM, Weidner W (2008). Anti-infective treatment of bacterial urinary tract infections. *Curr Med Chem* 15(14):1412–1427.

Pyonephrosis and perinephric abscess

Pyonephrosis

Pyonephrosis is an infected hydronephrosis. Pus accumulates within the renal pelvis and calyces. The causes are essentially those of hydronephrosis, where infection has supervened (e.g., ureteric obstruction by stone, URETEROPELVIC JUNCTION OBSTRUCTION).

Patients with pyonephrosis are usually very ill, with a high fever, flank pain, and tenderness. Patients with this combination of symptoms and signs will usually be investigated urgently by a renal ultrasound or CT urogram, where the diagnosis of a pyonephrosis is usually obvious.

Treatment consists of IV antibiotics as for acute pyelonephritis, IV fluids, and percutaneous nephrostomy insertion for drainage.

Perinephric abscess

Perinephric abscess develops as a consequence of extension of infection outside the parenchyma of the kidney in acute pyelonephritis or, more rarely today, from hematogenous spread of infection from a distant site. The abscess develops within Gerota (perinephric) fascia. These patients are often diabetic, and associated conditions such as an obstructing ureteric calculus may be the precipitating event leading to development of the abscess.

Failure of a seemingly straightforward case of acute pyelonephritis to respond to IV antibiotics within a few days arouses suspicion that there is an accumulation of pus in or around the kidney or obstruction with infection.

Imaging studies will establish the diagnosis and allow radiographically controlled percutaneous drainage of the abscess. If the pus collection is large, formal open surgical drainage under general anesthetic will provide more effective drainage.

Other forms of pyelonephritis

Emphysematous pyelonephritis

This is a rare, severe form of acute pyelonephritis caused by gas-forming organisms. It is characterized by high fever and abdominal pain, with radiographic evidence of gas within and around the kidney (on plain radiography or CT).

It usually occurs in diabetics and, in many cases, is precipitated by urinary obstruction by, for example, ureteral stones. The high glucose levels of the poorly controlled diabetic provide an ideal environment for fermentation by *Enterobacteria*, with carbon dioxide being produced during this process.

The presentation is usually as severe acute pyelonephritis (high fever and systemically very ill) that fails to respond within 2–3 days with conventional IV therapy. It is commonly caused by *E. coli,* less frequently by *Klebsiella* and *Proteus*.

On KUB radiograph, crescent- or kidney-shaped distribution of gas may been seen around the kidney. Renal ultrasonography often demonstrates strong focal echoes, indicating gas within the kidney. Intrarenal gas is seen on CT scan.

Patients with emphysematous pyelonephritis are usually very unwell and mortality is high. In selected cases, it can be managed conservatively, by IV antibiotics and fluids, percutaneous drainage, and careful control of diabetes. In those where sepsis is poorly controlled, emergency nephrectomy is sometimes required.

Xanthogranulomatous pyelonephritis

This is a severe renal infection usually, although not always, occurring in association with underlying renal calculi and renal obstruction. The severe infection results in destruction of renal tissue, leading to a non-functioning kidney. *E. coli* and *Proteus* are common causative organisms.

Macrophages full of fat become deposited around abscesses within the parenchyma of the kidney, hence the description xanthogranulomatous. The infection may be confined to the kidney or extend to the perinephric fat. The kidney becomes grossly enlarged and macroscopically contains yellowish nodules, pus, and areas of hemorrhagic necrosis.

It can be very difficult to distinguish the radiological findings from a renal cancer on imaging studies such as CT. Indeed, in many cases the diagnosis is made after nephrectomy for what was presumed to be a renal cell carcinoma.

Presentation is with acute flank pain, fever, and a tender flank mass. Bacteria *(E. coli, Proteus)* may be found on culture urine.

Renal ultrasonography shows an enlarged kidney containing echogenic material, and on CT, renal calcification is usually seen within the renal mass. Non-enhancing cavities are seen, containing pus and debris. On radioisotope scanning, there may be some or no function in the affected kidney.

On presentation these patients are usually started on IV fluids and antibiotics, as the constellation of symptoms and signs suggests infection. When imaging studies are done, the appearances often suggest the possibility of a renal cell carcinoma, and when signs of the acute infection have resolved, most patients undergo radical nephrectomy.

Only following pathological examination of the removed kidney will it become apparent that the diagnosis was one of infection (xanthogranulomatous pyelonephritis) rather than tumor.

Acute pyelonephritis, pyonephrosis, perinephric abscess, and emphysematous pyelonephritis—making the diagnosis

Maintaining a high degree of suspicion in all cases of presumed acute pyelonephritis is the single most important factor in allowing an early diagnosis of these complicated renal infections. If the patient is very ill, is diabetic, or has a history suggestive of stones, they may have something more than simple acute pyelonephritis.

Specifically ask about a history of sudden onset of severe flank pain a few days earlier, suggesting the possibility that a stone passed into the ureter, with later infection supervening. Renal imaging (KUB, ultrasound or CT urogram) should be done in all patients with suspected renal infection to rule out hydronephrosis, pyonephrosis, abscess or pus, or stones.

Clinical indicators suggesting a more complex form of renal infection are length of symptoms prior to treatment and time taken to respond to treatment. Most patients with uncomplicated acute pyelonephritis have been symptomatic for <5 days; often with a perinephric abscess patients are sick for >5 days prior to hospitalization.

Patients with acute pyelonephritis became afebrile within 2–3 days of treatment with an appropriate antibiotic, whereas those with perinephric abscesses remain febrile and systemically ill.

Chronic pyelonephritis

Chronic pyelonephritis is a confusing term. It can be a radiological or pathological diagnosis or a description. It is not a specifically clinically based
diagnosis. The appearance, either pathologically or radiologically, is one
of renal *scarring*. The scarring can be due to previous infection or it can
occur from the long-term effects of reflux (with or without superimposed
infection).

A child with reflux, particularly where there is reflux of infected urine,
will develop reflux nephropathy (if bilateral, it may cause renal impairment
or renal failure). If the child's kidneys are examined radiologically (or pathologically if they are removed by nephrectomy), the radiologist or pathologist will describe the appearances as those of "chronic pyelonephritis."

An adult may also develop radiological and pathological features of
chronic pyelonephritis, due to the presence of reflux, or bladder outlet
obstruction combined with high bladder pressures, again particularly when
the urine is infected. This was a common occurrence in male patients with
spinal cord injuries and detrusor-sphincter dyssynergia before the advent
of effective treatments for this condition.

Essentially, chronic pyelonephritis is the end result of longstanding reflux
(nonobstructive chronic pyelonephritis) or of obstruction (obstructive
chronic pyelonephritis). These processes damage the kidneys, leading to
scarring. The degree of damage and subsequent scarring is more marked
if infection has supervened.

The scars are closely related to a deformed renal calyx. Distortion and
dilatation of the calyces are due to scarring of the renal pyramids. These
scars typically affect the upper and lower poles of the kidneys, because
these sites are more prone to intrarenal reflux. The cortex and medulla in
the region of a scar are thin. The kidney may be so scarred that it becomes
small and atrophic. Scars can be seen radiologically on a renal ultrasound,
an IVP, renal isotope scan, or a CT.

Septicemia and urosepsis

Urosepsis is a form of sepsis that results from bacterial, fungal, or other infections originating from the genitourinary system Urosepsis accounts for approximately 25% of all sepsis cases and may develop from a community or nosocomial acquired urinary tract infection.

Bacteremia is the presence of pathogenic organisms in the blood stream. True rigors with fever and chills almost always indicate bacteremia and can lead to sepsis.

Septicemia or *sepsis*, the clinical syndrome caused by bacterial infection of the blood, is confirmed by positive blood cultures for a specific organism and accompanied by a systemic response to the infection known as the systemic inflammatory response syndrome (SIRS)[1]

SIRS is defined by at least two of the following:
- Fever (>38°C) or hypothermia (<36°C)
- Tachycardia (>90 beats/min in patients not on β-blockers)
- Tachypnea (respiratory >20/min or $PaCO_2$ <4.3 kPa or a requirement for mechanical ventilation)
- White cell count >12,000cells/mm³, <4000cells/mm³ or 10% immature (band) forms

Severe sepsis is sepsis associated with organ dysfunction.

Septic shock is sepsis, plus hypotension despite adequate fluid resuscitation, plus hypoperfusion changes, such as lactic acidosis, oliguria, or alteration in mental status.

Septicemia is often accompanied by *endotoxemia*, the presence of circulating bacterial endotoxins. Hypotension in septic shock is defined as a sustained systolic BP <90 mmHg, or a drop in systolic pressure of >40 mmHg for >1 hour, when the patient is normovolemic and other causes have been excluded or treated.

It results from gram-positive bacterial toxins or gram-negative endotoxins that trigger release of cytokines (TNF, IL-1), vascular mediators, and platelets, resulting in vasodilatation (manifest as hypotension) and disseminated intravascular coagulation (DIC).

Causes of urosepsis

In the hospital setting, the most common causes are the presence or manipulation of indwelling urinary catheters, urinary tract surgery (particularly endoscopic procedures such as TURP, TURBT, ureteroscopy, PCNL), and urinary tract obstruction (particularly that due to stones obstructing the ureter).

Septicemia has been reported to occur in up to 1.5% of men undergoing TURP. Diabetic patients, patients in ICUs, and patients on chemotherapy and steroids are more prone to urosepsis.

Common causative organisms in urosepsis
- *E. coli*, enterococci (*Streptococcus faecalis*), staphylococci, *Pseudomonas aeruginosa*, *Klebsiella*, and *Proteus mirabilis*.

---

1 Bone R, Back RA, Cerra FB, et al. (1992). Definition for sepsis and organ failure and guidelines for the use of innovative therapies in sepsis. *Chest* 101(6):1644–1655.

Management

The principles of management include early recognition, resuscitation, localization of the source of sepsis, early and appropriate antibiotic administration, and removal of the primary source of sepsis. From a urological perspective, the clinical scenario is a de novo presentation of patient with a clinical picture of sepsis or, as is sometimes seen, a postoperative patient who has undergone TURP or surgery for stones.

On return to the floor bed, they become febrile, develop rigors, and are tachycardic and tachypnea, resulting in initial respiratory alkalosis. They may be confused and oliguric and initially be peripherally vasodilatated (flushed appearance with warm peripheries).

It is also important to consider the possibility of a nonurological source of sepsis (such as pneumonia). If there are no indications of infection elsewhere, assume the urinary tract is the source of sepsis.

Investigations

- Urine culture. An immediate gram-stain of an unspun urine may aid in deciding which antibiotic to use.
- Full blood count. The white blood count is usually elevated. The platelet count may be low—a possible indication of impending DIC.
- Coagulation screen. This is important if surgical or radiological drainage of the source of infection is necessary.
- Creatine, blood urea nitrogen (BUN), and electrolytes as a baseline determination of renal function
- Arterial blood gases to identify hypoxia and the presence of metabolic acidosis, although respiratory alkalosis may be present initially due to tachypnea.
- Blood cultures
- Chest X-ray (CXR) to evaluate for pneumonia, atelectasis, and effusions
- Depending on the clinical situation, a renal ultrasound may be helpful to demonstrate hydronephrosis or pyonephrosis, and CT urography may be used to establish the presence or absence of other urological pathology.

Treatment

Immediate support care is necessary with attention to the basic **A** (**A**irway), **B** (**B**reathing), and **C** (**C**irculation) and to prevent cardiovascular collapse through coordinated-goal directed therapy.

- Give 100% oxygen via a facemask and monitor with use of oximetry.
- Establish IV access with a wide-bore intravenous cannula.
- Intravenous crystalloid (e.g., normal saline). Maintain adequate hemoglobin levels and transfuse if needed (>10 g/dL) to normalize blood pressure.
- Catheterize to monitor urine output.
- Obtain cultures before administering antibiotic therapy. Give empiric antibiotic therapy (see below) and adjust when cultures are available.

If there is septic shock, then the patient needs to be transferred to the intensive care unit (ICU), as ionotropic support may be needed. Steroids may have an adjunctive role in gram-negative infections and refractory septic shock. All of these steps should be coordinated with an intensivist.

Treat the underlying cause. Drain any urinary obstruction and remove any foreign body if possible. If there is a stone obstructing the ureter, insert a nephrostomy tube to relieve the obstruction or take the patient to the operating room and insert a double J-stent.

Send any urine specimens obtained for microscopy and culture.

Empirical antibiotic recommendations for treatment of urosepsis

This use of antibiotics is based on an educated guess of the most likely pathogen that has caused the urosepsis. Gram-negative aerobic rods are common causes of urosepsis (e.g., *E. coli*, *Klebsiella*, *Citrobacter*, *Proteus*, and *Serratia*). The enterococci (gram-positive aerobic nonhemolytic streptococci) may sometimes cause urosepsis.

In urinary tract operations involving the bowel, anaerobic bacteria may be the cause of urosepsis, and in wound infections, staphylococci (e.g., *Staph. aureus* and *Staph. epidermidis*) are the usual cause.[2]

There are no uniform published guidelines to the initial and empiric treatment of urosepsis. The following are some recommendations:

- Gentamicin is used in conjunction with other antibiotics such as ampicillin. Gentamicin has a relatively narrow therapeutic spectrum against gram-negative organisms. Close monitoring of therapeutic levels and renal function is important. It has good activity against enterobacteria and *Pseudomonas*, with poor activity against streptococci and anaerobes and, therefore, should ideally be combined with beta-lactam antibiotics (ampicillin) or ciprofloxacin.
- A third-generation cephalosporin (e.g., IV cefotaxime or ceftriaxone). These are active against gram-negative bacteria but have less activity against staphylococci and gram-positive bacteria. Ceftazidime also has activity against *Pseudomonas aeruginosa*.
- Fluoroquinolones (e.g., ciprofloxacin) are an alternative to cephalosporins. They exhibit good activity against *Enterobacteriaceae* and *P. aeruginosa* but less activity against staphylococci and enterococci.
- Monotherapy with suspected enterococci (*E. faecalis*) is with ampicillin 2 g IV q4h or vancomycin (if penicillin-allergic).
- Add metronidazole if there is a potential anaerobic source of sepsis.
- If *Candida* sepsis suspected, fluconazole 6 mg/kg/d or 400 mg IV q24h should be initiated.

If there is no clinical response to the above antibiotics, consider a combination of piperacillin and tazobactam. This combination is active against enterobacteria, enterococci, and *Pseudomonas*.

---

2 Wagenlehner FM, Weidner W, Naber KG (2007). Optimal management of urosepsis from the urological perspective. Int J Antimicrob Agents 30(5):390–397.

If there is clinical improvement, IV treatment should continue for at least 48 hours and then be changed to oral medication. Make appropriate adjustments when sensitivity results are available from urine cultures (which may take about 48 hours).

Further reading

Bugano DD, Camargo LF, Bastos JF, Silva E (2008). Antibiotic management of sepsis: current concepts. *Expert Opin Pharmacother* 9(16):2817–2828.

Mackenzie I, Lever A (2007). Management of sepsis. *BMJ* 335(7626):929–932.

Naber KG, Bergman B, Bishop MC, et al. (2001). Guidelines on urinary and male genital tract infections. European Association of Urology, *Eur Urol* 40:576–588.

Fournier gangrene

Fournier gangrene is a necrotizing fasciitis of the genitalia and perineum primarily affecting males and causing necrosis and subsequent gangrene of infected tissues. Culture of infected tissue reveals a mixed polymicrobial infection with aerobic (*E. coli*, enterococcus, *Klebsiella*) and anaerobic organisms (*Bacteroides, Clostridium*, microaerophilic streptococci), which are believed to grow in a synergistic fashion.

Conditions predisposing to the development of Fournier gangrene include diabetes, local trauma to the genitalia and perineum (e.g., zipper injuries to the foreskin, periurethral extravasation of urine following traumatic catheterization or instrumentation of the urethra), and surgical procedures such as circumcision.

Presentation

This is one of the most dramatic and rapidly progressing infections in medicine. A previously well patient may become critically ill over a very short time course (hours). It may follow a seemingly trivial injury to the external genitalia.

A fever is usually present, the patient looks very ill, with marked pain in the affected tissues, and the developing sepsis may alter the patient's mental state. The genitalia and perineum are edematous, and on palpation of the affected area, tenderness and crepitus may be present, indicating presence of subcutaneous gas produced by gas-forming organisms.

As the infection advances, blisters (bullae) appear in the skin and, within a matter of hours, areas of necrosis may develop on the genitalia and perineum that spread to involve adjacent tissues (e.g., the lower abdominal wall).

The condition advances rapidly—hence its alternative name of *spontaneous fulminant gangrene of the genitalia.*

Diagnosis

The diagnosis is a clinical one and is based on awareness of the condition and a high index of suspicion. CT will demonstrate areas of subcutaneous areas of necrosis and gas.

Treatment

Do not delay. While IV access is obtained, blood taken for culture, IV fluids started, and oxygen administered, broad-spectrum antibiotics are given to cover both gram-positive and gram-negative aerobes and anaerobes (e.g., ampicillin, gentamicin, and metronidazole or clindamycin). Monitor for signs of septic shock and manage as noted on p. 156.

Make arrangements to transfer the patient to the operating room emergently so that debridement of necrotic tissue (skin, subcutaneous fat) can be carried out. Extensive areas of tissue may have to be removed, but it is unusual for the testes or deeper penile tissues to be involved, and these can usually be spared.

A suprapubic catheter is inserted to divert urine and allow monitoring of urine output.

Where facilities allow, consider treatment with hyperbaric oxygen therapy.[1] There is some evidence that this may be beneficial. Repeated débridements to remove residual necrotic tissue are usually required with subsequent skin grafting required.

A VAC (vacuum-assisted closure) dressing can be used or wet-to-dry dressing changes are performed 2–3 times a day. Repeat operative debridement every 24–72 hours may be necessary to remove newly necrotic tissue.

Mortality is on the order of 20–30%. There is debate about whether diabetes increases the mortality rate.

Further reading

Chawla SN, Gallop C, Mydlo JH (2003). Fournier's gangrene: an analysis of repeated surgical debridement. *Eur Urol* 43:572–575.

Sorensen MD, Broghammer JA, Rivara FP, et al. (2008). Fournier's gangrene—contemporary population-based incidence and outcomes analysis: a HCUP database study. *J Urol* 179(4):13.

1 Mindrup SR, Kealey GP, Fallon B (2005). Hyperbaric oxygen for the treatment of Fournier's gangrene. *J Urol* 173:1975–1977.

Epididymitis and orchitis

This is an inflammatory condition of the epididymis, often involving the testis, and caused usually caused by bacterial infection. It has an acute onset and a clinical course lasting <6 weeks. It presents with pain, swelling, and tenderness of the epididymis.

It should be distinguished from chronic epididymitis, where there is long-standing pain in the epididymis but usually no swelling. Untreated, bacterial epididymitis can extend to the testicle, resulting in epididmo-orchitis.

Infection ascends from the urethra or bladder. In men aged <35 years, the infective organism is usually N. gonorrhoeae, C. trachomatis, or coliform bacteria (causing a urethritis that then ascends to infect the epididymis).

In children and older men, the infective organisms are usually coliforms (such as E coli, Pseudomonas, Proteus, and Klebsiella species). Occasionally, Ureaplasma urealyticum, Corynebacterium, or Mycoplasma is the cause. Mycobacterium tuberculosis (TB) is a rarer cause—the epididymis feels like a beaded cord.

A rare, noninfective cause of epididymitis is the antiarrhythmic drug amiodarone, which causes inflammation and resolves on discontinuation of the drug. Vasculitis, sarcoidosis, and more rare infections (coccidioidomycosis, blastomycosis) can be seen in immunocompromised men.

Differential diagnosis

Torsion of the testicle is the leading differential diagnosis. A preceding history of symptoms suggestive of urethritis, STD or urinary infection (dysuria, frequency, urgency, and suprapubic pain) suggest that epididymitis is the cause of the scrotal pain, but these symptoms may not always be present in epididymitis.

In epididymitis pain, tenderness and swelling may be confined to the epididymis, whereas in torsion, the pain and swelling are localized to the testis. However, there may be overlap in these physical signs.

Where the diagnosis is not clear between torsion or epididymitis, exploration is the safest option. Though radionuclide scanning can differentiate between a torsion and epididymitis, this is not available in many hospitals.

Color Doppler ultrasonography, which provides a visual image of blood flow, can differentiate between a torsion and epididymitis, but its sensitivity for diagnosing torsion is only 80% (i.e., it 'misses' the diagnosis in as many as 20% of cases—these 20% have torsion but normal findings on Doppler ultrasonography of the testis). Its sensitivity for diagnosing epididymitis is about 70%.

Again, if in doubt, explore. Complications of acute epididymitis abscess formation, infarction of the testis, chronic pain, and infertility.

Treatment of epididymitis

Culture urine, any urethral discharge, and blood (if the patient appears systemically ill). Urine cultures are often sterile. Management consists of bed rest, analgesia, anti-inflammatories, ice packs and antibiotics. Any form of urethral instrumentation should be avoided.

- With suspected gonorrhea infection: Ceftriaxone 125 mg IM in a single dose or Cefixime 400 mg orally in a single dose or 400 mg by suspension (200 mg/5 mL) with treatment for chlamydia if chlamydial infection is not ruled out.
- Where *C. trachomatis* is a possible infecting organism, prescribe a 10–14 day course of tetracycline 500 mg 4 times a day or doxycycline 100mg twice daily.
- For non-STD related epididymitis, prescribe antibiotics empirically (until culture results are available). Typically levofloxin or ofloxacin × 14 days.
- When the patient is systemically ill, IV gentamicin and ampicillin are often used. When afebrile complete a 14 day total antibiotic course based on sensitivities.

Chronic epididymitis

Chronic epididymitis is diagnosed in patients with long-term pain in the epididymis and testicle. It can result from recurrent episodes of acute epididymitis. Clinically, the epididymis is thickened and may be tender. Treatment is with the appropriate antibiotics (guided by cultures), or epididymectomy in severe cases.

Supportive therapy with gabapentin and tricyclic antidepressants has shown to sometimes control symptoms.

Orchitis

Orchitis is inflammation of the testis, although it often occurs with epididymitis (epididymo-orchitis). Causes include mumps; *M. tuberculosis*; syphilis; autoimmune processes (granulomatous orchitis). The testis is swollen and tense, with edema of connective tissues and inflammatory cell infiltration. Treat the underlying cause.

Mumps orchitis occurs in 30% of infected post-pubertal males. It manifests 3–4 days after the onset of parotitis, and can result in tubular atrophy. 10–30% of cases are bilateral and are associated with infertility.

Periurethral abscess

This can occur in patients with urethral stricture disease, in association with gonococcal urethritis and following urethral catheterization. These conditions predispose to bacteria (gram-negative rods, enterococci, anaerobes, gonococcus) gaining access through Buck fascia to the periurethral tissues. If not rapidly diagnosed and treated, infection can spread to the perineum, buttocks, and abdominal wall.

The majority (90%) of patients present with scrotal swelling and a fever. Up to 20% will have presented with urinary retention, 10% with a urethral discharge, and 10% having spontaneously discharged the abscess through the urethra.

The abscess should be incised and drained, a suprapubic catheter placed to divert the urine away from the urethra, and broad-spectrum antibiotics commenced (gentamicin and cefuroxime) until antibiotic sensitivities are known.

Prostatitis: epidemiology and classification

Prostatitis is infection and/or inflammation of the prostate.

Classification of prostatitis

Given the variation in the descriptions of prostatitis clinically, in 1999 the National Institutes of Health (NIH) developed a classification system for prostatitis:[1]

I	Acute bacterial prostatitis (ABP)
II	Chronic bacterial prostatitis (CBP)
III	Chronic pelvic pain syndrome (CPPS)
III$_A$	Inflammatory CPPS (chronic nonbacterial prostatitis): WBC in expressed prostatic secretions (EPS), VB3, or semen
III$_B$	Noninflammatory CPPS (prostatodynia): no WBC in EPS, VB3 or semen
IV	Asymptomatic inflammatory prostatitis (histological prostatitis)

Acute and chronic bacterial (NIH I and II) forms of prostatitis are defined by documented bacterial infections of the prostate.

Chronic pelvic pain syndrome (NIH III) is characterized primarily by urological pain complaints in the absence of urinary tract infection.

Asymptomatic inflammatory prostatitis (NIH IV) is the incidental finding of prostatic inflammation on a biopsy specimen without any specific symptoms.

Epidemiology

The most common type of prostatitis is NIH III chronic pelvic pain syndrome, accounting for 90–95% of cases of prostatitis. Acute and chronic bacterial prostatitis (NIH I and II) each makes up another 2–5% of cases.

Pathogenesis

The tissues surrounding the prostatic acini become infiltrated with inflammatory cells (lymphocytes). The most common infective agents are gram-negative *Enterobacteriaceae* (*Escherichia coli, Pseudomonas aeruginosa, Klebsiella, Serratia, Enterobacter aerogenes*). From 5% to 10% of infections are caused by gram-positive bacteria (*Staphylococcus aureus* and *saprophyticus, Streptococcus faecalis*).

The etiology of inflammatory and noninflammatory forms of prostatitis is not well understood. Theories include the presence of functional or structural bladder pathology failure of the external sphincter to relax during voiding or some form of primary bladder neck obstruction.

Appropriate prostatic antimicrobial choice is critical because the prostate has an epithelial lining and a pH gradient that inhibits antimicrobials from entering the acini. The best agents have a high dissociation constant that allows diffusion of their unionized components into the prostate. If the antibiotic is basic, it can concentrate much higher in prostatic fluid because of the pH gradient.

Risk factors

These include UTI; acute epididymitis; urethral catheters; transurethral surgery; intraprostatic ductal reflux; phimosis; prostatic stones (corpora amylacea that can provide a nidus of infection for chronic prostatitis).

Segmented urine cultures

Also known as the Meares-Stamey or 4-glass test, segmented urine cultures are useful in the clinical evaluation of prostatitis syndromes and allow the localization bacteria to a specific part of the urinary tract by sampling different parts of the urinary stream, with or without prostatic massage (which produces EPS).

- **VB_1**—first 10 mL of urine voided. Positive culture indicates urethritis or prostatitis.
- **VB_2**—midstream urine. Positive culture indicates cystitis.
- **VB_3**—first 10 mL of urine voided following prostatic massage. Positive culture indicates bacterial prostatitis.
- **EPS**—Positive culture indicates bacterial prostatitis.

An alternative approach has been described that relies on a voided specimen before and after prostatic massage.[2]

1 Krieger JN, Nyberg LJ, Nickel JC (1999). NIH consensus definition and classification of prostatitis. *JAMA* 282:236–237.
2 Nickel JC (1997). The Pre and Post Massage Test (PPMT): a simple screen for prostatitis [review]. *Tech Urol.* 3(1):38–43.

Prostatitis: presentation, evaluation, and treatment

Evaluation

- History of previous urological disease and conditions
- NIH-CPSI questionnaire (National Institute of Health Chronic Prostatitis Symptom Index). This scores three main symptom areas: pain (location, frequency, severity), voiding (obstructive and irritative symptoms), and impact on quality of life. It can be useful in guiding response to therapy.
- Segmented urine cultures and EPS. When cultures are negative, increased leukocytes per high-powered field (>10) favor a diagnosis of inflammatory chronic pelvic pain syndrome.

Acute bacterial prostatitis

Acute bacterial prostatitis (NIH I) is infection of the prostate associated with lower urinary tract infection and generalized sepsis. *E. coli* is the most common cause; *Pseudomonas, Serratia, Klebsiella*, and enterococci are less common causes.

Acute onset of fevers, chills, nausea and vomiting; perineal and suprapubic pain; irritative urinary symptoms (urinary frequency, urgency, and dysuria); and obstructive urinary symptoms (hesitancy, strangury, intermittent stream or urinary retention) are the hallmarks. Signs of systemic toxicity (fever, tachycardia, hypotension) may be present.

Suprapubic tenderness and a palpable bladder will be present if there is urinary retention. On digital rectal examination, the prostate is extremely tender and aggressive manipulation of the prostate is to be discouraged.

Treatment

If the patient is not systemically ill, use an oral quinolone such as ciprofloxacin 500 mg bid for at least 3 weeks.

For a patient who is ill, use IV gentamicin with a third-generation cephalosporin or ampicillin, pain relief, anti-inflammatory medications, and relief of retention if present. Traditional teaching was that a suprapubic (rather than urethral) catheter should be inserted to avoid the potential obstruction of prostatic urethral ducts by a urethral catheter. However, in-and-out catheterization or a short period with an indwelling catheter probably does no harm and is certainly an easier way of relieving retention than suprapubic catheterization.

A total course of 3 weeks of antibiotics is essential to minimize the chance for the development of chronic bacterial prostatitis. A negative culture should be confirmed after treatment.

Chronic bacterial prostatitis

NIH II classification of chronic bacterial prostatitis typically presents with history of documented recurrent UTI. *E coli* is responsible for 75–80% of cases, with enterococci and other gram-negative aerobes responsible.

Chronic episodes of genitourinary pain and voiding dysfunction may be a feature. DRE may show a tender, enlarged, and boggy prostate, or it may be entirely normal.

This condition is characterized by bacterial growth in culture of the expressed prostatic fluid, semen, or post-massage urine specimen. The EPS usually contains >10 WBCs/HPF and macrophages. The recurrent organism is usually the same each time.

Treatment

An empiric trial of antibiotics is used if the evaluation suggests chronic bacterial prostatitis and is administered long term (4–6 weeks).

- Trimethoprim-sulfamethoxazole (TMP-SMZ) 80/400 mg PO bid given twice a day
- Fluoroquinolone (e.g., ciprofloxacin 500 mg or ofloxacin 400 mg) PO bid. Ofloxin may be the best choice in men <35 years because of increased activity against *Chlamydia*.

Chronic pelvic pain syndrome (CPPS)

Both inflammatory (III_A) and noninflammatory (III_B) types present with >3-month history of localized pain (perineal, suprapubic, penile, groin, or external genitalia); pain with ejaculation; LUTS (frequency, urgency, poor flow); and erectile dysfunction. *Prostadynia* is an older term that should no longer be used.

Etiology is not clear. Symptoms can recur over time and severely affect the patient's quality of life.

There is no evidence of pyuria and bacteriuria, but excess WBCs in EPS may be found in III_A but are absent in III_B.

Treatment

- While there is not a defined role for antibiotics, an empiric trial of a quinolone or TMP-SMX is often tried with variable results.
- α-Blockers (doxazosin, terazosin, tamsulosin) have become the mainstay of therapy. These act on prostate and bladder neck α-receptors, causing smooth muscle relaxation, improved urinary flow, and reduced intraprostatic ductal reflux.[1]
- Anti-inflammatory drugs
- Sitz baths, more frequent ejaculation, dietary modifications (avoid caffeine, tobacco, spicy foods), biofeedback, and significant psychological support all may have potential benefits in this group of patients.
- Microwave thermotherapy is considered when severe symptoms are refractory to all treatments.

Asymptomatic inflammatory prostatitis

There is incidental histological diagnosis of prostatic inflammation from prostate tissue taken for other indications (i.e., biopsy for raised PSA). No specific therapy is usually indicated for this incidental finding.

Further reading

Habermacher GM, Chason JT, Schaeffer AJ (2006). Prostatitis/chronic pelvic pain syndrome. *Annu Rev Med* 57:195–206.

1 Nickel JC (2005). Alpha-blockers for treatment of the prostatitis syndromes. *Rev Urol.* 7(Suppl 8):S18–25.

Other prostate infections

Prostatic abscess

Failure of acute bacterial prostatitis to respond to an appropriate anti-biotic treatment regimen (i.e., persistent symptoms and fever while on antibiotic therapy) suggests the development of a prostatic abscess.

A transrectal ultrasound or CT scan (if the former proves too painful) is the best way of diagnosing a prostatic abscess. This may be drained by a transurethral incision.

Granulomatous prostatitis

This is a very uncommon form of prostatitis and can result from bacterial, viral, or fungal infection, systemic granulomatous diseases, and the use of BCG to treat bladder cancer. Most often it is idiopathic.

Patients can present as with bacterial prostatitis. Rectal examination is similar to prostate cancer (hard, indurated, nodular). The diagnosis is usu-ally made after prostate biopsy to rule out cancer.

Some patients respond to antibiotic therapy and temporary bladder drainage. With histological evidence of eosinophilic granulomatous pros-tatitis, steroids may be useful.

TURP may be necessary if there is no response to treatment and the patient has bladder outlet obstruction.

Interstitial cystitis

Interstitial cystitis (IC) is a refractory bladder disorder of unknown etiology. Also known as *painful bladder syndrome*, IC is characterized by daytime and nighttime urinary frequency, urgency, suprapubic and pelvic pain of unknown etiology, and no identifiable pathological cause.

The presence of glomerulations on cystoscopic examination (petechiae seen after bladder wall distention) or Hunner's ulcers may help confirm clinical suspicion. Only 5% of cases are associated with Hunner's ulcers (focal regions of panmural inflammation).

The symptom complex is similar to that of prostatitis type III_B noninflammatory CPPS (prostatodynia).

IC is a diagnosis of exclusion (see Table 5.5). It is diagnosed once other causes for these symptoms have been excluded (e.g., TB, radiation cystitis, bladder tumor, overactive bladder). The presence of uninhibited bladder contractions on urodynamics excludes a diagnosis of IC.

In 1988, the National Institute of Diabetes, Digestive, and Kidney Diseases (NIDDK) described criteria for IC. However, originally developed for research purposes, it identifies patients with more severe disease and some experts do not recommended it for use in clinical practice.

Epidemiology

IC predominantly affects females (~90%). Estimated female prevalence is 18.1 cases per 100,000 from European studies. American data suggest higher rates of 52–67 per 100,000.

Associated disorders

A higher prevalence of allergies, irritable bowel syndrome, fibromyalgia, focal vulvitis, lupus, and Sjögren syndrome has been reported in IC. Anxiety, depression, and adjustment reactions are also found.

Pathogenesis

IC appears to be a multifactorial syndrome. Possible contributing factors include the following:
- Increased mast cells. Studies have demonstrated increased mast cells in bladder smooth muscle (detrusor). Activated mast cells release histamine, which can cause pain, hyperemia, and fibrosis in tissues.
- Defective bladder epithelium. An abnormal glycosaminoglycan (GAG) layer may allow urine to leak past the luminal surface, causing inflammation in muscle layers.
- Neurogenic mechanisms. Abnormal activation of sensory nerves causes release of neuropeptides, resulting in neurogenic inflammation.
- Reflex sympathetic dystrophy of the bladder. Excessive sympathetic activity
- Urinary toxins or allergens
- Bladder autoimmune response

Evaluation

Exclude other causes for symptoms (see Table 5.5). History, examination (including pelvic in women and DRE in men), urinalysis, and culture are

Table 5.5 NIDDK* diagnostic criteria for interstitial cystitis

Diagnosis criteria	1. Cystoscopic evidence of Hunner's ulcer or petechiae (glomerulations)
	2. Bladder/pelvic pain or urinary urgency
Exclusion criteria	1. Bladder capacity >350 mL, measured by awake cystometry
	2. Lack of urgency with a 150mL injection in cystometry
	3. Uninhibited contractions during cystometry
	4. <9 months from onset
	5. Absence of nocturia
	6. Symptoms improved by antibiotics, anticholinergics, or antispasmodics
	7. Daytime voids <8
	8. Bacterial cystitis or prostatitis within 3 months
	9. Bladder or ureteral calculi
	10. Genital herpes
	11. Uterine, cervical, vaginal, or urethral cancer
	12. Urethral diverticulum
	13. Cyclophosphamide- or drug-induced cystitis
	14. Tuberculous cystitis
	15. Radiation cystitis
	16. Bladder tumor
	17. Vaginitis
	18. <18 years old

* National Institute of Diabetes and Digestive and Kidney Diseases.

mandatory. The IC symptom index questionnaire and voiding diaries are useful. Urodynamics has limited role. Diagnostic studies are as follows.

Cystoscopy

Ten percent of patients will have pink ulceration of bladder mucosa (Hunner's ulcer). Under anesthesia, the bladder should be distended twice (to 80–100 cmH$_2$O for 1–2 min) and then inspected for diffuse glomerulations (>10 per quadrant in ¾ bladder quadrants).

Bladder biopsy is only indicated to rule out other pathologies such as carcinoma in situ. In conscious patients, bladder filling causes pain and reproduces symptoms.

Intravesical KCl challenge

In 75% of IC patients, installation of 0.4 M KCl into the bladder will provoke pain and symptoms.

Treatment

Patients should understand that there is no known cure, and treatment is
for symptom control. The Interstitial Cystitis Association, at www.ichelp.
org, is a useful patient resource. Stress reduction, exercise, and diet modification may be helpful.

There are only two FDA-approved medications:
- Pentosan polysulfate sodium: 100 mg PO tid; augments protective
  GAG layer of bladder to minimize irritative effects
- 50% Dimethylsulfoxide (DMSO), weekly intravesical instillation × 6
  weeks; often used as cocktail with triamcinolone, heparin sodium,
  $NaHCO_3$

All other medications are off-label.

Oral medications

Tricyclics (amitriptyline) have anticholinergic, antihistamine, and sedative
effects. Narcotics are to be avoided.

Nerve stimulation

Transcutaneous electrical nerve stimulation (TENS) or sacral neuromodulation can be used.

Surgery

Transurethral resection, laser coagulation or diathermy of Hunner's
ulcers, and bladder hydrodistention under anesthesia may be beneficial,
otherwise surgery should only be considered after failed conservative
treatments. Rarely, urinary diversion cystectomy or enterocystoplasty may
be required.

Further reading

Moldwin RM, Evans RJ, Stanford EJ, et al. (2007). Rational approaches to the treatment of patients
  with interstitial cystitis. *Urology* 69(Suppl 4A):73.

Payne CK, Joyce GF, Wise M, et al. (2007). Interstitial cystitis and painful bladder syndrome. *J Urol*
  177:2042.

Tuberculosis

Tuberculosis (TB) of the genitourinary (GU) tract is caused by *Mycobacterium tuberculosis*. TB predominantly affects Asian populations, with a higher incidence in males than females.

Pathogenesis

Primary TB

The primary granulomatous lesion forms in the mid to upper zone of the lung. It consists of a central area of caseation surrounded by epithelioid and Langhans giant cells, accompanied by caseous lesions in the regional lymph nodes.

There is early spread of bacilli via the bloodstream to the GU tract; however, immunity rapidly develops, and the infection remains quiescent. Acute diffuse systemic dissemination of tubercle bacilli can result in symptomatic military TB.

Post-primary TB

Reactivation of infection is triggered by immune compromise (including HIV). It is at this point that patients develop clinical manifestations.

Kidney

Hematogenous spread causes granuloma formation in the renal cortex, associated with caseous necrosis of the renal papillae and deformity of the calyces, leading to release of bacilli into the urine. This is followed by healing fibrosis and calcification, which causes destruction of renal architecture and autonephrectomy.

Ureters

Spread is directly from the kidney and can result in stricture formation (vesicoureteric junction, pelviureteric junction, and mid-ureteric) and ureteritis cystica.

Bladder

Infection is usually secondary to renal infection, although iatrogenic TB can be caused by intravesical BCG treatment for carcinoma in situ. The bladder wall becomes edematous, red, and inflamed, with ulceration and tubercles (yellow lesions with a red halo).

Disease progression causes fibrosis and contraction (resulting in a small capacity 'thimble' bladder), obstruction, and calcification.

Prostate and seminal vesicles

Hematogenous spread causes cavitation and calcification, with palpable, hard-feeling structures. Fistulae may form to the rectum or perineum.

Epididymis

Hematogenous spread results in a "beaded" cord. Infection may spread to the testis.

Presentation

Early symptoms include fever, lethargy, weight loss, night sweats, and UTI not responding to treatment. Later manifestations include LUTS, hematuria, and flank pain.

Investigations

- **Urine:** At least 3 early morning urines (EMUs) are required, but often many more EMU specimens will be needed before a positive culture for TB is obtained. A typical finding is sterile pyuria (leukocytes, but no growth). Ziehl–Neelsen staining will identify these acid- and alcohol-fast bacilli (cultured on Lowenstein–Jensen medium).
- **CXR and sputum**
- **Tuberculin skin test**
- **IVP or CT urogram:** Findings include renal calcification (nephrocalcinosis), irregular calyces ("moth-eaten kidney"), infundibular stenosis, cavitation, pelviureteric and vesicoureteric obstruction, and a contracted, calcified bladder.
- **Cystoscopy and biopsy**

Treatment

Treatment is with 6 months of isoniazid, rifampicin, and pyrazinamide. Regular follow-up imaging with IVP is recommended to monitor for ureteric strictures, which may need stenting, nephrostomies, or ureteric reimplantation.

Severe bladder disease may require surgical augmentation, reconstruction, or urinary diversion.

Parasitic infections

Schistosomiasis (bilharziasis)

Urinary schistosomiasis is caused by the trematode (or fluke) *Schistoma haematobium*. It is endemic in Africa, Egypt, and the Middle East. Fresh water snails release the infective form of the parasite (cercariae), which can penetrate skin, and migrate to the liver (as schistosomules), where they mature. Adult flukes couple, migrate to vesical veins, and lay eggs (containing miracidia larvae), which leave the body by penetrating the bladder and entering the urine.

The disease has two stages: active (when adult worms are actively laying eggs) and inactive (when the adult has died, and there is a reaction to the remaining eggs). The development of squamous cell carcinoma of the bladder is result of the chronic inflammation.

Presentation

The first clinical sign is "swimmer's itch"—a local inflammatory response. Other early manifestations include Katayama fever, a generalized allergic reaction, which includes fever, urticaria, lymphadenopathy, hepatosplenomegaly, and eosinophilia. Active inflammation results in hematuria, frequency, and terminal dysuria.

Investigation

- Midday urine specimen; bladder and rectal biopsies may contain eggs (distinguished by having a terminal spine).
- Serology tests (ELISA).
- Cystoscopy identifies eggs in the trigone ("sandy patches").
- IVP or CT urogram may show a calcified, contracted bladder, and obstructive uropathy.

Treatment

Give praziquantel 40 mg/kg in 2 divided doses 4–6 hours apart. Alternative medications include metrifonate or niridazole.

Complications

Chronic infection can lead to obstructive uropathy, ureteric stenosis, renal failure, and bladder contraction, or ulceration. The most significant and concerning complication is the development of squamous cell carcinoma of the bladder that often presents at an advanced stage.

Hydatid disease

Infection occurs after ingestion of the dog parasite *Echinococcus granulosus* (tapeworm). Sheep are the intermediate hosts. Cases occur in the Middle East, Australia, and Argentina, with 3% affecting the kidneys. Large cysts form, which can be asymptomatic or present with flank pain. A peripheral eosinophilia is seen with a positive hydatid complement-fixation test. X-rays and CT scans show a thick-walled, fluid-filled spherical cyst with a calcified wall.

Medical treatment is with albendazole. Where surgical excision is indicated, cysts can be first sterilized with formalin or alcohol. Praziquantel is also recommended preoperatively or if cyst contents are spilt (which can provoke systemic anaphylaxis).

Genital filariasis

Lymphatic filariasis is caused by *Wuchereria bancrofti* nematode infection and is common in the tropics. Manifestations include funiculoepididymitis, orchitis, hydrocele, scrotal and penile elephantiasis, and lymph scrotum (edema).

Diagnosis is made on capillary finger-prick, or venous blood is used for thick blood microscopic thick film and serology.

Medical treatments include diethylcarbamazine, ivermectin, and albendazole.

HIV in urological surgery

Human immunodeficiency virus (HIV)

HIV disease results from the acquired deficiency of cellular immunity caused by the human immunodeficiency virus (HIV). The signature hallmark of the disease is the reduction of the helper T-lymphocytes in the blood and the lymph nodes, the development of opportunistic infections (*Pneumocystis carinii* pneumonia, cytomegalovirus (CMV) infections, tuberculosis, candida infections, cryptococcosis, others), and the development of malignancy such as lymphoma and Kaposi sarcoma.

The spectrum HIV infections range from asymptomatic seropositivity, thru AIDS-related complex (ARC), to acquired immunodeficiency syndrome (AIDS). HIV-1 is pandemic and accounts for significant mortality in developing countries.

HIV-2 has less pathogenicity and is predominant in West Africa. Transmission is via sexual intercourse, contaminated needles, mother-to-fetus transmission, and infected blood and blood products (blood transfusion risks are now minimal).

Urological manifestations of HIV/AIDS include bacterial and nonbacterial infections, urolithiasis, increased risk of malignancy, renal impairment, and voiding dysfunction.

Pathogenesis

HIV is a retrovirus. It possesses the enzyme reverse transcriptase that enables viral RNA to be transcribed into DNA, which is then incorporated into the host cell genome. HIV binds to CD4 receptors on helper T-lymphocytes (CD4 cells), monocytes, and neural cells. After an extended latent period (8–10 years), CD4 counts decline.

AIDS is defined as HIV positivity and CD4 lymphocyte counts <200 × 10^6/L. The associated immunosuppression increases the risk of opportunistic infections and tumors.

Diagnosis

Screening HIV-1 antibody titer, if positive, is confirmed by Western blot or immunofluorescence. Separate consent for HIV testing is required. Informed consent is required for the test.

Urological sequelae

- **Urinary tract infections:** Common bacterial pathogens are most common in HIV: *E. coli*, *Enterobacter* (enterococci), *Pseudomonas aeruginosa*, *Proteus* spp, *Klebsiella*, *Acinetobacter*, *Staphylococcus aureus*, group D streptococcus, *Serratia*, and *Salmonella* spp. If UTI is suspected and C&S are negative, consider atypical organisms such as fungi, parasites, or viruses
- **Kidneys:** cytomegalovirus, *Aspergillus*, *Toxoplasma gondii* infections, which can cause acute tubular necrosis and abscess formation; renal failure; HIV-associated nephropathy (HIVAN): nephrotic disease with proteinuria >3.5 g/day and edema, hypertension. Progresses to dialysis in <10 months; renal stones (secondary to indinavir treatment). Up to 8-fold risk of renal cell carcinoma.
- **Ureters:** calculi associated with indinavir therapy

- **Bladder:** voiding dysfunction and retention (hypo- and hyperreflexia, acontractile hypoactive bladder, and detrusor-sphincter dyssynergia); UTI (opportunistic organisms); squamous cell carcinoma
- **Urethra:** Reiter syndrome (urethritis, conjunctivitis, arthritis); bacterial urethritis
- **Prostate:** bacterial prostatitis and abscesses (opportunistic organisms)
- **External genitalia:** chronic or recurrent genital herpes; atypical syphilis; opportunistic infections of testicle and epididymis (*Salmonella* epididymitis); scrotal and penile Kaposi sarcoma; Fournier gangrene. Testicular tumors are up to 50 times more common, usually seminoma.

Needle stick injury

The risk of seroconversion following needle stick injury from a seropositive patient is ~0.3%. Risks are increased if the patient has terminal ARC illness and if the needle is hollow bore with visible blood contamination, inserted deeply or directly into a vein.

The seroconversion rate after cutaneous exposure to HIV-infected blood is 0.09%. Immediately wash the area well, report to occupational health, and where appropriate, commence antiviral prophylaxis as soon as possible.

Health care workers exposed to infected blood from non-AIDS or acute HIV should be given zidovudine plus lamivudine.

For increased-risk exposure use a three-drug regimen including a protease inhibitor (lopinavir and ritonavir).

Further reading

Cohen MS, Hellmann N, Levy JA, DeCock K, Lange J (2008). The spread, treatment and prevention of HIV-1: evolution of a global pandemic. *J Clin Invest* 118:1244–1254.

Lebovitch S, Mydlo JH (2008). HIV-AIDS: urologic considerations. *Urol Clin North Am* 35(1):59–68.

Inflammatory and other disorders of the penis

See Table 5.6 for dermatologic descriptors. Most penile ulcers and vesicobullous lesions are associated with a sexually transmitted disease.

Premalignant lesions associated with penile cancer are discussed in Chapter 6.

Balanitis

This is a condition seen most commonly in uncircumcised men with poor hygiene. *Balanitis* is the inflammation of the glans penis. When the foreskin and prepuce are involved it is termed *balanoposthitis*. The most common complication of balanitis is phimosis.

Daily hygiene is most critical in treatment, with careful cleaning after retraction of the foreskin. Clotrimazole can be used in adults with probable candidal balanitis. Betamethasone 0.05% applied bid is useful, with some reports of success with topical 1% pimecrolimus cream.

Circumcision may sometimes be necessary.

Paraphimosis

This is a true urological emergency where in an uncircumcised male the foreskin is pulled behind the glans and cannot be brought back to the normal position. If not immediately reduced, swelling ensues and the tight band of tissue can compromise lymphatic and vascular flow to the distal, resulting in pain, edema, and possible tissue loss.

Manual reduction is preferred using ice packs, elastic compression, and topical anesthetic such as 2% lidocaine gel. Operative dorsal slit may be required in refractory cases.

Phimosis

Phimosis is when the foreskin cannot be retracted behind the glans. A physiological phimosis is present at birth due to adhesions between the foreskin and glans. As the penis develops, epithelial debris (smegma) accumulates under the foreskin, causing gradual separation.

Ninety percent of foreskins are retractile at age 3; few persist into adulthood (<1% phimosis at age 17). Recurrent balanitis in uncircumcised males can cause new phimosis.

Treatment

Older children with phimosis, suffering recurrent infection (balanitis), can be treated with a 6-week course of topical 0.1% dexamethasone cream, which acts to soften the phimosis and allow foreskin retraction (avoid circumcision where possible).

Adults may require a dorsal slit or circumcision for recurrent balanitis, voiding obstruction, or difficulties with sexual intercourse.

Complications

These include recurrent balanitis; balanoposthitis (severe balanitis where inflammatory secretions and pus are trapped in the foreskin by the phimotic band); paraphimosis; chronic inflammation; and squamous cell carcinoma of the penis.

Table 5.6 Dermatologic descriptions of skin lesions useful in examination of the penis

Blister, bulla	Vesicle >1 cm
Crust	Lesion covered with drying exudate (serum, blood, pus)
Erosions	Loss of epidermis
Erythema	Redness of skin (usually blanches on pressure)
Macule	Flat, discrete lesion; different color to surrounding skin; <1 cm diameter
Maculopapular	Raised spots different in color to surrounding skin
Nodule	Solid dermal or hypodermal lesion >0.5 cm
Papule	Raised palpable lesion <0.5 cm
Patch	Macule >1 cm diameter
Plaque	Coalesced papules (larger, raised, flat areas)
Pustule	Circumscribed pus-filled lesion
Scale	Flake of hard skin
Ulcer	Break in epithelium (+superficial dermis)
Vesicle	Small, fluid-filled lesion <1 cm

Urological neoplasia

Pathology and molecular
biology *188*

Prostate cancer: epidemiology and
etiology *190*

Prostate cancer: incidence,
prevalence, and mortality *192*

Prostate cancer pathology:
premalignant lesions *193*

Prostatic-specific antigen
(PSA) and prostate cancer
screening *194*

Counseling before prostate cancer
screening *195*

Prostate cancer: clinical
presentation *196*

PSA and prostate cancer *198*

PSA derivatives: free-to-total ratio,
density, and velocity *200*

Prostate cancer: transrectal
ultrasonography and
biopsies *202*

Prostate cancer staging *206*

Prostate cancer grading *212*

Risk stratification in management
of prostate cancer *214*

General principles of management
of localized prostate cancer *215*

Management of localized prostate
cancer: watchful waiting and
active surveillance *216*

Management of localized
prostate cancer: radical
prostatectomy *218*

Postoperative course after radical
prostatectomy *222*

Prostate cancer control with
radical prostatectomy *224*

Management of localized prostate
cancer: radical external beam
radiotherapy (EBRT) *226*

Management of localized prostate
cancer: brachytherapy (BT) *228*

Management of localized and
radiorecurrent prostate cancer:
cryotherapy and HIFU *230*

Management of locally advanced
nonmetastatic prostate cancer
(T3–4 N0M0) *232*

Management of advanced prostate
cancer: hormone therapy I *233*

Management of advanced prostate
cancer: hormone therapy II *234*

Management of advanced prostate
cancer: hormone therapy III *238*

Management of advanced prostate
cancer: androgen-independent/
castration-resistant disease *240*

Palliative management of prostate
cancer *242*

Prostate cancer: prevention;
complementary and alternative
therapies *244*

Bladder cancer: epidemiology and
etiology *246*

Bladder cancer: pathology and
staging *248*

Bladder cancer: presentation *252*

Bladder cancer: diagnosis and
staging *254*

Management of superficial UC:
transurethral resection of
bladder tumor (TURBT) *256*

Management of superficial
UC: adjuvant intravesical
chemotherapy and BCG *258*

Muscle-invasive bladder cancer:
surgical management of
localized (pT2/3a) disease *260*

Muscle-invasive bladder
cancer: radical and palliative
radiotherapy *263*

Muscle-invasive bladder cancer:
management of locally advanced
and metastatic disease *264*

Bladder cancer: urinary diversion after cystectomy 266

Transitional cell carcinoma (UC) of the renal pelvis and ureter 270

Radiological assessment of renal masses 274

Benign renal masses 276

Renal cell carcinoma: epidemiology and etiology 278

Renal cell carcinoma: pathology, staging, and prognosis 280

Renal cell carcinoma: presentation and investigations 284

Renal cell carcinoma: active surveillance 286

Renal cell carcinoma: surgical treatment I 288

Renal cell carcinoma: surgical treatment II 290

Renal cell carcinoma: management of metastatic disease 292

Testicular cancer: epidemiology and etiology 294

Testicular cancer: clinical presentation 296

Testicular cancer: serum markers 299

Testicular cancer: pathology and staging 300

Testicular cancer: prognostic staging system for metastatic germ cell cancer 303

Testicular cancer: management of non-seminomatous germ cell tumors (NSGCT) 304

Testicular cancer: management of seminoma, IGCN, and lymphoma 308

Penile neoplasia: benign, viral-related, and premalignant lesions 310

Penile cancer: epidemiology, risk factors, and pathology 314

Squamous cell carcinoma of the penis: clinical management 318

Carcinoma of the scrotum 320

Tumors of the testicular adnexa 321

Urethral cancer 322

Retroperitoneal fibrosis 326

Wilms tumor and neuroblastoma 328

Pathology and molecular biology

Neoplasia may be benign or malignant. Malignant neoplasms, characterized by local invasion of normal tissue or distant spread (metastasis) via lymphatic or vascular channels, may be primary or secondary.

Primary urological neoplasms most commonly arise from the lining epithelium of the genitourinary tract—benign (less commonly) or malignant. Neoplasms are considered to arise from a single abnormal cell, through successive aberrant divisions. This is called clonal expansion.

Malignant epithelial neoplasms are termed **carcinomas**; carcinomas may be further characterized histologically by prefixing either **adeno-** if the neoplasm is glandular, or **squamous cell** or **urothelial cell** (formerly transitional cell) according to the epithelium from which it has arisen.

Benign epithelial neoplasms from glandular or transitional epithelium are respectively termed **adenoma** or papillary neoplasm of low malignant potential (PNLMP) (formerly papilloma).

Connective tissue neoplasms are described according to their components, adding benign (*-oma*) or malignant (*-sarcoma*) suffixes. For example, a benign neoplasm composed of blood vessels, fat, and smooth muscle is an **angiomyolipoma**; a malignant neoplasm composed of smooth muscle is a **leiomyosarcoma**. Sarcomas are rare in urological organs, constituting 1% of all neoplasms.

In the early stages of tumorigenesis, an identifiable precursor lesion may exist. Several invasive carcinomas are considered to arise from non-invasive epithelial lesions. As an example in the bladder it is known as *carcinoma in situ* (CIS) may progress and become muscle invasive and metastatic bladder cancer.

There are exceptions and rarities. The most common primary testicular neoplasms arise from testicular tubules and are collectively described as **germ cell tumors**. Rarely, primary malignant lymphoma can arise in the testis.

In the kidney, the childhood **Wilms tumor** arises from the embryonic mesenchyme of the metanephric blastema, while the relatively common benign **oncocytoma** is thought to arise from cells of the collecting ducts.

Secondary neoplasms within urological tissues are uncommon; they may arise by direct invasion from adjacent tissues (e.g., adenocarcinoma of the sigmoid colon may invade the bladder) or hematogenous spread from another site in the genitourinary (GU) system or more remote site such as breast cancer involving the kidney.

Like all neoplasia, urological neoplasia is a result of molecular genetic alterations. It may be **hereditary** or **sporadic**, depending on whether the genetic abnormalities are partly constitutional (germ-line) or wholly somatic (acquired).

Hereditary tumors tend to appear at a younger age than their sporadic counterparts and are often multifocal, due to an underlying constitutional genetic abnormality such as von Hipple–Lindau syndrome and renal cell carcinoma. Tumor formation results from loss of the balance between cell division and withdrawal from the cell cycle by differentiation or programmed cell death (apoptosis). Signals regulating cell proliferation and interactions come from proteins, encoded by messenger RNA that is in turn transcribed from genomic DNA.

Genetic abnormalities may promote tumor development or growth in a number of ways:

- Activation (overexpression) of **oncogenes** encoding transcription factors (e.g., c-myc)
- Inactivation (reduced expression) of **tumor suppressor genes** (e.g., pp. 190, 246, 279)
- Overexpression of **peptide growth factors** (e.g., insulin-like growth factor 1 [IGF-1])
- Overexpression of **angiogenic factors** (e.g., vascular endothelial growth factor [VEGF])

The diverse proteins encoded by **tumor suppressor genes** stabilize the cell, ensuring differentiation and a finite lifespan in which the cell performs its function. Inactivation of such genes by deletion or mutation may result in loss of this negative growth control.

For example, the gene for phosphatase and tensin homologue *(PTEN)* is a prostate tumor suppressor gene encoding a phosphatase that is active against protein and lipid substrates. It is present in normal epithelium but is commonly reduced in prostate cancer. It inhibits one of the intracellular signaling pathways, PI3 kinase-Akt, that is essential for cell cycle progression and cell survival. Inactivation of *PTEN* would therefore promote cell immortalization and proliferation.

Interest in the molecular genetics of urological neoplasia will lead to improved screening tests for hereditary diseases, enhanced diagnostic testing, and expanded choice for "targeted" treatment strategies. As an example, the newer multikinase receptor inhibitors such as sunitinib, sorafenib and temsirolimus are based on the latest understanding of the molecular biology of renal cell carcinoma.

Prostate cancer: epidemiology and etiology

Hormonal influence

Growth of prostate cancer (PC), like benign prostatic epithelium, is under the influence of *testosterone* and its potent metabolite, *dihydrotestosterone*. Removal of these androgens by castration largely results in programmed cell death (apoptosis) and involution of the prostate. PC is not seen in eunuchs or people with congenital deficiency of 5-α-reductase (5AR), which converts testosterone to dihydrotestosterone (DHT).

Estrogens, including phytoestrogens found in foodstuffs used in Asian and Oriental cuisine, have a similar negative growth effect on PC. This is one explanation why individuals in this part of the world are less likely to develop clinical disease and have lower death rates from prostate cancer.

Other proposed dietary inhibitors of PC growth include vitamins E and D, and the antioxidants lycopene (present in cooked tomatoes) and the trace element selenium (see also p. 244). A very large U.S. trial (SELECT Trial) failed to demonstrate that formulations of vitamin E and selenium, used alone or in combination, could reduce the risk of PC.

Genetics

The multifocal and heterogeneous nature of PC makes clinical genetic studies difficult, as this cancer exhibits numerous genetic abnormalities, increasing with more advanced stage and grade.

Identified genetic changes include inactivation of tumor suppressor genes *PTEN* (chromosome 10q) and *p53* (chromosome 17p), activation of c-myc and bcl-2 proto-oncogenes, and PC susceptibility genes such as *ELAC2/HPC2*, *SR-A/MSR1*, *CHEK2*, *BRCA2*, and others. Shortened CAG repeat length in the androgen receptor gene is associated with an increased risk of the disease.

Risk factors

Age

This is an important risk factor for development of histological PC. Less than 10% of cases are diagnosed in men <54 years of age, with 64% of cases diagnosed between 55 and 74 years of age. Autopsy prevalence of PC rises from 31% for men in their 30's to 83% in their 80's.

This rise is paralleled several years earlier by a premalignant lesion—high-grade prostatic intraepithelial neoplasia (HGPIN). However, most prostate cancer does not achieve a clinically recognizable and aggressive state.

Geographic variation

The disease appears to be more common in Western nations, particularly Scandinavian countries and the United States. The clinical diagnosis of the disease is less common in Asia and the Far East, but immigrants to the United States from Asia and Japan have a 20-fold increased risk. This suggests an environmental etiology, such as the Western diet (higher levels of meat, dairy, and saturated fat), may be important.

Race

Black men are at greater risk than Caucasians; Asians and Oriental races have a low risk of prostate cancer unless they migrate to the West. The world's highest incidence is among U.S. and Jamaican Blacks, although there are few reliable data available regarding African and European Blacks.

Family history

From 5% to 10% of prostate cancer cases are thought to be inherited. Hereditary PC tends to occur in younger (<55 years) men who have a family history of multiple relatives afflicted; genetic abnormalities on chromosomes 1q, 8p, Xp and mutations of the *BRCA2* gene are reported.

The risk of a man developing PC is doubled if there is one affected first-degree relative and can be further increased if there are two. A familial association between breast cancer and prostate cancer has also been suggested.

HPC-1 gene on chromosome 1 is strongly associated with familial PC; *HPC-1* mutation results in defective RNase L and accumulation of genetic defects, and eventually prostate cancer.

Familial PC tends to follow a similar clinical course to sporadic PC.

Other factors

Some controversy surrounds the possible increased risk of developing PC conferred by sexual overactivity, viral infections, and vasectomy. The balance of data and opinion currently go against these putative risk factors. Exposure to cadmium has been suggested to raise the risk of PC, but convincing contemporary data are lacking.

Prostate cancer: incidence, prevalence, and mortality

Incidence

The widespread use of prostatic-specific antigen (PSA)-based screening led to a sharp increase in the incidence of prostate cancer that peaked the early 1990s in the United States.

In 2010 men were diagnosed with prostate cancer in the United States. This exceeds the number of men diagnosed with lung cancer (116,759), placing prostate cancer as the most commonly diagnosed male cancer (excluding basal and squamous cell skin cancers). It accounts for about 33% of all male cancers diagnosed.

Prevalence

Currently, it is estimated that a man in the United States has a 1 in 6 (16.6%) lifetime risk of being diagnosed with prostate cancer as a result of clinical symptoms, signs, or PSA testing. However, the true prevalence of the disease is hinted at by postmortem studies carried out on men who have died of other causes.

There is a significant number of men with so-called autopsy cancers. This concept of latent prostate cancer—a biologically nonaggressive and slow-growing form of the disease, may be unnecessarily detected by aggressive PSA screening (p. 216).

Mortality

It is estimated that prostate cancer accounts for 9% of male cancer deaths. Mortality increased slowly in the UK and United States during the 1970s and 1980s, peaking in the 1990s and slowly decreasing thereafter. Mortality has declined 4% per year between 1999 and 2003.

In 2009, 27,360 deaths were attributed to prostate cancer in the United States, the second-most common form of male cancer death. This compares with 25,240 deaths due to colorectal cancer and 88,900 due to lung cancer.

The explanation for the reduced prostate cancer mortality is highly controversial. The potential reasons for this decline include improved diagnosis and treatment of localized disease, the early use of hormonal therapy, and PSA-based screening.

The concept of screening for prostate cancer detecting earlier stages and possibly more curable disease remains highly controversial, with various studies supporting and refuting the effectiveness of screening based on PSA testing and rectal examination (see p. 194).

Prostate cancer pathology: premalignant lesions

Two histological lesions are currently regarded as either premalignant or "perimalignant" (related to the presence of cancer)—prostatic intraepithelial neoplasia (PIN) and atypical small acinar proliferation (ASAP).

Prostatic intraepithelial neoplasia

PIN consists of architecturally benign prostatic acini and ducts lined by cytologically atypical cells and confined within the epithelium. The basal cell layer is present, although the basement membrane may be fragmented.

PIN was formerly known as *ductal dysplasia* or reported by pathologists as "suspicious for cancer." PIN was classified into low-grade (mild) and high-grade (moderate to severe) forms, based on the presence of prominent nucleoli. Subsequently, pathologists have agreed to report only high-grade PIN, since low-grade PIN has no prognostic value.

High-grade PIN is believed by many to be to be a precursor to intermediate- or high-grade prostate cancer and its finding in sextant peripheral zone prostate biopsies carries a 30–40% prediction of prostate cancer at subsequent biopsy. However, with the widespread use of more extensive biopsy protocols, the significance of isolated high-grade PIN has become less clear.

High-grade PIN is reported in 5–10% of prostate needle biopsies. It does not appear to affect the serum PSA value. The site of the PIN is not indicative of the site of subsequently diagnosed cancer, nor is PIN always present in a prostate containing cancer.

Most authors recommended that repeat systematic biopsies be performed in 3–6 months if multifocal high-grade PIN is reported on initial needle biopsy or transurethral resection of the prostate (TURP). Studies also suggest that a repeat biopsy may be unnecessary in the setting of isolated high-grade PIN without other clinical indicators of cancer.

Atypical small acinar proliferation

ASAP is a histological finding suggesting that a focus of atypical glands is suspicious for cancer. ASAP and HGPIN are distinct entities and the two should not be used interchangeably. The ASAP acini are small, lined with cytologically abnormal epithelial cells. The columnar cells have prominent nuclei containing nucleoli, while the basal layer may be focally absent. The basement membrane is intact.

Prostate cancer has been identified in specimens from subsequent biopsies in up to 60% of cases of ASAP, indicating that this finding is a significant predictor of cancer. Identification of ASAP (with or without high-grade PIN) warrants repeat biopsy for concurrent or subsequent invasive prostate carcinoma.

Prostatic-specific antigen (PSA) and prostate cancer screening

Screening men aged 50–70 years with PSA and digital rectal examination (DRE), and subsequent early detection and treatment, may reduce the significant mortality and morbidity caused by prostate cancer. Supporters of screening say these acceptable and relatively inexpensive tests will detect clinically significant disease before it leaves the prostate.

The lead time, estimated at 6–12 years, between the screened diagnosis and the clinical diagnosis should enable more organ-confined cancers to be diagnosed and cured. However, because of the low specificity of PSA (40%) and the high prevalence of latent or autopsy prostate cancer, opponents argue that many men would suffer unnecessary anxiety, biopsies, overdiagnosis (25–50%), and overtreatment.

Two long-awaited screening studies were reported in 2009 with conflicting data. The U.S. PLCO (Prostate Lung Colorectal and Ovarian) screening study did not demonstrate a reduction in prostate cancer mortality.[1] However, the study was considered "contaminated" by many, as a large number of men were prescreened and the control group was contaminated by this screening outside of the study. The ERSPC (European Randomized Study of Screening for Prostate Cancer) trial demonstrated a 20% reduction in mortality and a 25% reduction in metastatic disease due to screening.[2]

Decisions regarding early detection of prostate cancer should be individualized, and benefits and consequences should be discussed with the patient before PSA testing occurs. Not all men are appropriate candidates for screening efforts for this disease. Ideally, physicians should consider a number of factors, including patient age and comorbidity, as well as preferences for the relevant potential outcomes.

The practice of screening in men with less than a 10-year life expectancy (due to age or comorbidity) should generally be discouraged.[4] Informed consent prior to PSA testing has been recommended by some groups. The American Urological Association (AUA) 2009 guideline recommends that early detection and risk assessment of prostate cancer be offered to asymptomatic men 40 years of age or older who wish to be screened and have an estimated life expectancy of more than 10 years.

If the patient and clinician are interested in the best objective data on determining the risk of biopsy-detectable prostate cancer, the National Cancer Institute (NCI) has published a risk calculator[3] based on the Prostate Cancer Prevention Trial.

---

1 Andriole G, et al. (2009). Mortality results from a randomized prostate-cancer screening trial. *N Engl J Med* 360:1310–1319.

2 Schröder F, et al. (2009). Screening and prostate-cancer mortality in a randomized European study. *N Engl J Med* 360:1320–1328.

3 Available at: http://deb.uthscsa.edu/URORiskCalc/Pages/uroriskcalc.jsp. (Accessed July 2009). Race, age, PSA level, family history, prior prostate biopsy, and the use of finasteride are factors that are entered into the system.

4 Smith, RA, et al (2010). Cancer Screening in the United States, 2010: A Review of Current American Cancer Society Guidelines and Issues in Cancer Screening *CA Cancer J Clin* 60:70–98.

Counseling before prostate cancer screening

Discussing the risks and benefits of prostate cancer screening is considered mandatory before offering a PSA and DRE to *asymptomatic* men. Such counseling is less controversial when evaluating a *symptomatic* patient, because a diagnosis of prostate cancer could alter the management. However, all patients should be informed when PSA testing is being considered.

The following points should be considered when counseling *asymptomatic* men:

- Cancer will be identified in up to 5% men screened.
- Screening enables earlier cancer detection and has the potential to decrease mortality rates.
- Early detection and treatment may avoid future cancer–related illness.
- DRE and PSA measurements can have both false-positive and false-negative results.
- Prostatic biopsy can be uncomfortable and carries a small risk of sepsis or significant bleeding.
- Repeat biopsy may be recommended (PIN, ASAP, or rising PSA).
- Treatment may not be necessary, or may not be curative.
- Aggressive therapy is necessary to realize any benefit from screening if cancer is found based on the screening biopsy.
- Treatment-related morbidity could lead to a reduction in quality of life.
- Active surveillance may be recommended if a low-risk cancer is found.

Prostate cancer: clinical presentation

Since the widespread use of serum PSA testing, the majority of patients now have organ-confined disease at presentation. Shown below are the possible presentations, grouped by disease stage.

Localized prostate cancer (T1–2)
- Asymptomatic, detected through screening serum PSA (most common) or incidental digital rectal examination (DRE)
- Lower urinary tract symptoms (LUTS) (probably due to coexisting benign hyperplasia causing bladder outflow obstruction)
- Hematospermia
- Hematuria (probably due to coexisting benign hyperplasia)
- Perineal discomfort (probably due to coexisting prostatitis)

Locally advanced cancer (T3–4)
- Asymptomatic, with screening serum PSA or incidental DRE
- Lower urinary tract symptoms
- Hematospermia
- Hematuria
- Perineal discomfort
- Symptoms of renal failure/anuria due to ureteral obstruction
- Malignant priapism (rare)
- Rectal obstruction (rare)

Metastatic disease (N+, M+)
- Asymptomatic ("occult disease"), with screening serum PSA or incidental DRE
- Swelling of lower limb due to malignant lymphatic obstruction
- Anorexia, weight loss
- Bone pain, pathological fracture
- Neurological symptoms/signs in lower limbs (spinal cord compression)
- Anemia

Box 6.1 A note about DRE

Since most prostate cancers arise in the peripheral, posterior part of the prostate, they may be palpable on DRE. An *abnormal DRE* is defined by asymmetry, a nodule, or a fixed, "rock hard" mass. Less than 50% of abnormal DREs are associated with prostate cancer, the remainder being benign hyperplasia, prostatic calculi, chronic prostatitis, or post-therapy changes (TURP, biopsy, radiation therapy).

Only 40% of cancers diagnosed by DRE will be organ confined. The fact that an abnormal DRE in the presence of a low PSA carries a 20–30% chance of predicting prostate cancer rules out any suggestion that the DRE could be abandoned as part of our screening approach.

The utility of the DRE in men on 5α-reductase inhibitors is maintained and in some cases may actually be enhanced through the volume effects of reduction in the overall size of the gland.

PSA and prostate cancer

See p. 39 for an introduction to the serum PSA test. Until the development of commercial serum PSA assays in the late 1980s, the only serum marker for prostate cancer was acid phosphatase. This was highly specific for prostate cancer metastatic to bone, but lacked sensitivity in detecting less advanced disease and was even normal in >20% patients with bone metastases.

PSA is a glycoprotein produced primarily by the prostatic acini and disruption of the prostatic architecture by disease states appears to allow more PSA to leak into the bloodstream.

Prior to the PSA era, most men with newly diagnosed prostate cancer had advanced and mostly incurable disease. PSA has revolutionized the diagnosis and management of prostate cancer, although its use in screening and early detection remains controversial.

The predictive values of PSA and DRE for diagnosing prostate cancer in biopsies are shown in Table 6.1. The Prostate Cancer Prevention Trial (PCPT) has forever changed our definition of what a "normal" PSA is. A surprising finding in this study was the high prevalence of prostate cancer among men without clinical suspicion for prostate cancer, including men with PSA levels fewer than 4 ng/mL.

AUA PSA Best Practice Policy 2009 no longer recommends a single, threshold value of PSA that should prompt prostate biopsy. The decision should be based primarily on PSA and DRE results, but should take into account multiple factors, including free and total PSA, patient age, PSA velocity, PSA density, family history, ethnicity, prior biopsy history, and comorbidities. In addition to its use as a serum marker for the diagnosis of prostate cancer, PSA elevations may help in staging, counseling, and monitoring prostate cancer patients.

PSA derivatives (see p. 200) are also useful. Here are some examples:

PSA generally increases with advancing stage and tumor volume, although a small proportion of poorly differentiated tumors fail to express PSA. In men taking 5α-reductase inhibitors such as finasteride or dutasteride for benighn prostatic hyperplasia (BPH) or taking finasteride to treat alopecia, the production of PSA will be suppressed by about 50% at 6 months. Therefore, a corrected PSA should be twice the measured value when these drugs are used. This maintains the utility of PSA as a screening tool for prostate cancer detection.

PSA is used, along with clinical (DRE) T stage and Gleason score, to predict pathological tumor staging and outcome after radical treatments, using statistically derived nomograms and tables as noted on p. 208.

- >50% of patients have extraprostatic disease if PSA >10 ng/mL.
- <5% of patients have lymph node metastases and only 1% have bone metastases if PSA <20 ng/mL.
- 66% of patients have lymphatic involvement and 90% have seminal vesicle involvement if PSA >50 ng/mL.

- PSA should be virtually undetectable following radical prostatectomy for gland-confined disease (usually < 0.2 ng/mL). A progressive rise in PSA (continuing to rise above 0.5 ng/mL) after radical prostatectomy precedes the development of clinical metastatic disease by a mean time of 8 years.

PSA falls to within the normal range in 80% of patients with metastatic disease on hormone therapy within 4 months; the PSA rises in a mean time of 18 months after starting hormone therapy, signaling progressive hormone refractory (castrate resistant) disease.

PSA is prostate specific, but unfortunately not prostate cancer specific. Other causes of elevated serum PSA include recent instrumentation (cystoscopy, catheterization for retention), prostate surgical intervention (biopsy, TRUP, laser or microwave ablation), urinary tract infection, including acute (NIH I) or chronic (NIH II) bacterial prostatitis.

In the presence of infection or instrumentation, PSA should not be measured until at least 28 days after the event, to avoid a false-positive result. Ideally, PSA should not be requested within 2 days of ejaculation, as a small number of men may have a transient rise. Routine DRE does not appear to cause any significant changes in PSA levels.

Table 6.1 Predictive value of PSA and DRE for biopsy diagnosis of prostate cancer

PSA (ng/mL)	≤0.5	0.6–1.0	1.1–2.0	2.1–3.0	3.1–4.0	4.1–10	>10.0
DRE normal	6.6%	10%	17%	24%	27%	27%	>50%
DRE abnormal	—	15%	15%	30%	30%	45%	>75%

PSA derivatives: free-to-total ratio, density, and velocity

Measurement of the **free-to-total (F:T) PSA ratio** can increase the specificity of total PSA because the ratio is lower in men with prostate cancer than in men with benign hyperplasia. Most urologists use this in deciding whether to rebiopsy a patient with previous benign biopsies, instead of using this to decide about the need for a first-time biopsy.

As an example, a man with a normal DRE and a PSA of 4–10 ng/mL has a 27% risk of prostate cancer. This risk rises to 60% if the F:T ratio is 10% and falls to 10% if his ratio is >25%. The F:T ratio is most useful in the total PSA range 2.5–10 ng/mL.

Consideration may be given to the prostate volume, since large benign prostates are the most common cause of mildly elevated PSA. Serum PSA/prostate volume = **PSA density**, and serum PSA/prostate transition-zone volume = **PSA-TZ density**. Various cutoff densities have been proposed to raise the specificity of total PSA, possibly to reduce the need for prostatic biopsy, but the issue remains controversial.

Short-term variations in serum PSA occur in the presence or absence of cancer, the cause of which may be technical or physiological. Longer term, the PSA tends to rise slowly due to BPH and faster due to prostate cancer—**PSA velocity**.

A PSA velocity >0.75 ng/mL per year with at least three determinations over at least 18 months is suggestive of the presence of PC. Recent studies have lowered this threshold significantly and some authorities believe it should no longer be considered as an indication for biopsy. A high pretreatment PSA velocity (>2.0 ng/mL/year) has been shown to correlate with a worse prognosis after radiotherapy or radical surgery.

PSA doubling time (PSADT) is the time it takes for a PSA value to double, based on an exponential growth pattern. Pretreatment PSADT has little diagnostic value. PSADT is an important predictor of tumor progression, therapeutic outcome, and tumor-specific mortality. Following surgery or radiotherapy for prostate cancer, PSADT <6 months indicates distant disease progression, whereas a more delayed PSADT suggests local recurrence.

Other markers are being studied for the diagnosis of prostate cancer. Urine-based analysis of PCA3 is promising. The biomarker known as early prostate cancer antigen-2 (EPCA-2) is also showing promise in identifying which patients with an elevated PSA may have cancer.

Prostate cancer: transrectal ultrasonography and biopsies

The most common diagnostic modality for prostate cancer is currently transrectal ultrasonography (TRUS) with guided biopsies (Fig. 6.1). TRUS provides imaging of the prostate and seminal vesicles using a 7.5 mHz biplane intrarectal probe measuring approximately 1.5 cm in diameter.

While TRUS imaging may be performed for other reasons (e.g., evaluation of infertility, sizing for treatment planning), a TRUS without biopsy is considered an inadequate way to evaluate for prostate cancer. Many advocate use of an enema before the biopsy to enhance visualization.

The ultrasound-guided periprostatic injection of local anesthetic (1% lidocaine) has become the standard in the United States when biopsy is planned. Rarely, general or regional anesthesia may be necessary, especially in the presence of anal stenosis or if saturation (>20) biopsies are planned.

A careful DRE precedes insertion of the probe. Broad-spectrum antimicrobials (e.g., quinolone antibiotic) are given before and after the procedure.

TRUS can image the outline of the prostate, cysts, abscesses, and calcifications within the prostate. Hypoechoic and hyperechoic lesions in the peripheral zone may be due to prostate cancer or inflammatory conditions, although most prostate cancers are in fact isoechoic and are not visualized on ultrasound.

Advanced biopsy techniques that use microbubble contrast agents with and without color Doppler are being actively investigated to improve yield. There are no convincing data that color Doppler alone can improve the yield of prostate biopsy over the standard grayscale biopsy.

Indications for TRUS without biopsy

- Accurate measurement of prostate volume for treatment planning (e.g., microwave, needle ablation, brachytherapy)
- Male infertility with azoospermia, to look for seminal vesicle and ejaculatory duct obstruction due to calculus or Müllerian cyst
- Suspected prostatic abscess (can be drained by needle aspiration)
- Investigation of chronic pelvic pain, looking for prostatic cyst or calculi

Indications for TRUS with biopsies

- An abnormal DRE and/or an elevated PSA (exceptions include very elderly men with massively elevated PSA and abnormal DRE, or those in whom a TURP is indicated for severe LUTS/retention where histology will be obtained). See Table 6.1 (p. 199).
- Previous biopsies showing multifocal high-grade PIN or ASAP
- Previous biopsies normal, but PSA rising or DRE abnormal
- To confirm viable prostate cancer following treatment if further treatment is being considered

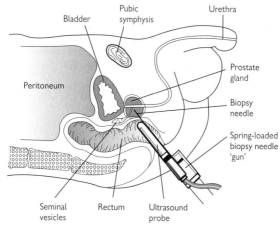

Figure 6.1 Transrectal ultrasound scanning (TRUS). An ultrasound probe is inserted into the rectum to guide the biopsy needle into the correct position so that multiple core biopsies can be taken from different areas of the prostate.

Biopsy protocol

Ten to 12 18 French Tru-Cut needle biopsies are taken in a systematic fashion to include any palpable or sonographic target lesion. The traditional sextant protocol (a parasagittal base, mid-gland, and apex from each side) is no longer considered an adequate technique. To the 10–12 biopsy regimen, add samples from the far lateral peripheral zones (Fig. 6.2). Studies have demonstrated that these extra biopsies detect up to 15% more cancers.

Additional biopsies of each transition zone may be taken if a transition zone cancer is suspected or if a patient is undergoing repeat biopsies due to a rising PSA. Seminal vesicles biopsies occasionally add staging information if they appear abnormal on DRE, TRUS, or MRI.

Complications of prostatic biopsy

- Occasional vasovagal reaction (fainting) immediately after procedure
- Small risk of urinary tract infection and rarely urosepsis, which may be life threatening
- Small risk of significant rectal bleeding
- Mild hemospermia or hematuria, for several weeks after the procedure

Prostate cancer may also be diagnosed by transurethral resection of the prostate (TURP) histology or clinically (without histology) in certain circumstances. For example, it could be viewed as unnecessarily invasive to biopsy an elderly and frail symptomatic patient with a rock-hard prostate and a PSA of >100 ng/mL prior to commencing hormone therapy.

Box 6.2

It is not safe to biopsy a patient who is anticoagulated on warfarin; biopsying patients on low-dose aspirin remains controversial but is not considered unsafe by many. Other antiplatelet drugs (e.g., clopidogrel) are usually stopped for 7–10 days prior to biopsy.

It is important that the patient appreciates that negative biopsies do not exclude the possibility of prostate cancer, and that a positive result will not necessarily result in the recommendation of immediate treatment.

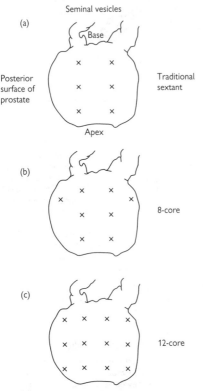

Figure 6.2 Biopsy protocols. A 10- to 12-core biopsy regimen is considered the standard of care today. Obtaining 4 apical cores can often be difficult.

Prostate cancer staging

Tumor staging uses the most current 2002 TNM (tumor, nodes, malignancy) classification (see Table 6.2 and Fig. 6.3). As with all cancer, prostate cancer staging may be considered clinical (prefixed with c) or pathological (prefixed with p), dependent on available data. (Note: In 2010 the American Joint Committee on Cancer (AJCC) will begin to incorporate PSA and Gleason Score into the staging system for prostate cancer.)

T stage

T stage is assessed primarily by digital rectal examination (see Fig. 6.3). Current imaging resolution limits reliability in detection of focal and microscopic extraprostatic extension of disease by means of MRI or TRUS. Recent prostatic biopsy may also confuse the interpretation of MRI images, particularly regarding the seminal vesicles.

Table 6.2 TNM (2002) staging of adenocarcinoma of the prostate

T0	No tumor (pT0 if no cancer found by histological examination)
Tx	T stage uncertain
T1a	Cancer nonpalpable on digital rectal examination (DRE), present in <5% of TURP specimens (in up to 18% of TURPs)
T1b	Cancer nonpalpable on DRE, present in >5% of TURP specimens
T1c	Cancer nonpalpable on DRE, present in needle biopsy taken because of elevated PSA
T2a	Palpable tumor, feels confined, in <half of one lobe on DRE
T2b	Palpable tumor, feels confined, in >half of one lobe on DRE
T2c	Palpable tumor, feels confined, in both lobes on DRE
T3a	Palpable tumor, locally advanced into periprostatic fat, uni- or bilateral and mobile on DRE
T3b	Palpable tumor, locally advanced into seminal vesicle(s) on DRE
T4a	Palpable tumor, locally advanced into adjacent structures, feels fixed on DRE
T4b	Palpable tumor, locally advanced into pelvic side-wall, feels fixed on DRE
Nx	Regional lymph not assessed
N0	No regional lymph node metastasis
N1	Tumor involves regional (pelvic) lymph nodes
Mx	Distant metastases not assessed
M0	No distant metastasis
M1a	Nonregional lymph node metastasis
M1b	Tumor metastasis in bone
M1c	Tumor metastasis in other sites

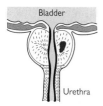

T1

Early (non-palpable) prostate cancer only detectable under the microscope; found at TURP or by needle biopsy

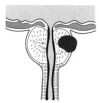

T2

Early (palpable) prostate cancer

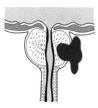

T3

Locally advanced prostate cancer—into peri-prostate fat or seminal vesicles

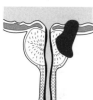

T4

Locally advanced prostate cancer—invades the bladder, rectum, penile urethra, or pelvic side wall

Figure 6.3 The T stages of prostate cancer. (2002 TNM System)

N stage

N stage is assessed by imaging (CT/MRI) or biopsy as necessary. Pelvic lymph node dissection is the gold-standard assessment of N stage. MRI or CT scanning may image enlarged nodes and most radiologists report nodes of >5 mm in maximal diameter.

However, nodes larger than this often contain no cancer, while micrometastases may be present in normal-sized nodes.

M stage

M stage is assessed by use of physical examination, imaging (MRI or iso-tope bone scan, chest radiology), and biochemical investigations (e.g., alka-line phosphatase).

Nomograms

Based on several thousand radical prostatectomies, these are used widely to predict pathological T and N stage by combining clinical T stage, PSA, and biopsy Gleason score. Nomograms, developed by Kattan and asso-ciates (www.nomograms.org), may be able to predict final pathological stage on the basis of preoperative parameters.

Higher pathological stage (i.e., pT3 disease) found at radical prostatec-tomy may also be predicted by the following:[1]

- Higher percentages (>66%) of positive biopsies
- Cancer invading adipose in the biopsies (there is no fat in the prostate)
- Possibly the presence of perineural cancer invasion within the prostate

Partin tables

These tables are useful to predict the stage of prostate cancer treated by radical prostatectomy (Table 6.3). Table 6.3 reflects an updated ver-sion of the 2001 Partin tables with a contemporary patient cohort (5730 men treated with prostatectomy and no additional therapy from 2000 to 2005 at the Johns Hopkins Hospital). This cohort demonstrated trends in presentation and pathological stage for men diagnosed with clinically localized prostate cancer and was used to correct for the effects of stage migration.

Table 6.3 Partin tables

PSA range (ng/mL)	Pathological stage	Biopsy Gleason Score			
		5–6	3 + 4=7	4 + 3 = 7	8–10
Clinical stage T1c (nonpalpable, PSA elevated) (n = 4419)					
0–2.5	Organ confined (n = 226)	93 (91–95)	82 (76–87)	73 (64–80)	77 (65–85)
	Extraprostatic extension (n = 19)	6 (5–8)	14 (10–18)	20 (14–28)	16 (11–24)
	Seminal vesicle (+) (n = 1)	0 (0–1)	2 (0–5)	2 (0–5)	3 (0–8)
	Lymph node (+) (n = 3)	0 (0–1)	2 (0–6)	4 (1–12)	3 (1–12)
2.6–4.0	Organ confined (n = 619)	88 (86–90)	72 (67–76)	61 (54–68)	66 (57–74)
	Extraprostatic extension (n = 92)	11 (10–13)	23 (19–27)	33 (27–39)	26 (19–34)

Table 6.3 Continued

PSA range (ng/mL)	Pathological stage	Biopsy Gleason Score			
		5–6	3 + 4=7	4 + 3 = 7	8–10
	Seminal vesicle (+) (n = 8)	1 (0–1)	4 (2–7)	5 (2–8)	7 (3–13)
	Lymph node (+) (n = 1)	0 (0–0)	1 (0–1)	1 (0–3)	1 (0–3)
4.1–6.0	Organ confined (n = 1266)	**83 (81–85)**	**63 (59–67)**	**51 (45–56)**	**55 (46–64)**
	Extraprostatic extension (n = 297)	16 (14–17)	30 (26–33)	40 (34–45)	32 (25–40)
	Seminal vesicle (+) (n = 37)	1 (1–1)	6 (4–8)	7 (4–10)	10 (6–15)
	Lymph node (+) (n = 12)	0 (0–0)	2 (1–3)	3 (1–6)	3 (1–6)
6.1–10.0	Organ confined (n = 989)	**81 (79–83)**	**59 (54–64)**	**47 (41–53)**	**51 (41–59)**
	Extraprostatic extension (n = 281)	18 (16–19)	32 (27–36)	42 (36–47)	34 (26–42)
	Seminal vesicle (+) (n = 36)	1 (1–2)	8 (6–11)	8 (5–12)	12 (8–19)
	Lymph node (+) (n = 5)	0 (0–0)	1 (1–3)	3 (1–5)	3 (1–5)
>10.0	Organ confined (n = 324)	**70 (66–74)**	**42 (37–48)**	**30 (25–36)**	**34 (26–42)**
	Extraprostatic extension (n = 165)	**27 (23–30)**	**40 (35–45)**	**48 (40–55)**	**39 (31–48)**
	Seminal vesicle (+) (n = 25)	2 (2–3)	12(8–16)	11 (7–17)	17 (10–25)
	Lymph node (+) (n = 13)	1 (0–1)	6 (3–9)	10 (5–17)	9 (4–17)
Clinical stage T2a (palpable < ½ of one lobe) (n = 998)					
0–2.5	Organ confined (n = 156)	**88 (84–90)**	**70 (63–77)**	**58 (48–67)**	**63 (51–74)**
	Extraprostatic extension (n = 18)	**12 (9–15)**	**24 (18–30)**	**32 (24–41)**	**26 (18–36)**
	Seminal vesicle (+) (n = 2)	0 (0–1)	2 (0–6)	3 (0–7)	4 (0–10)
	Lymph node (+) (n = 1)	0 (0–1)	3 (1–9)	7 (1–17)	6 (1–16)

Table 6.3 Continued

PSA range (ng/mL)	Pathological stage	Biopsy Gleason Score			
		5–6	3 + 4=7	4 + 3 = 7	8–10
2.6–4.0	Organ confined (n = 124)	79 (75–82)	57 (51–63)	45 (38–52)	50 (40–59)
	Extraprostatic extension (n = 49)	20 (17–24)	37 (31–42)	48 (40–55)	40 (30–50)
	Seminal vesicle (+) (n = 5)	1 (0–1)	5 (3–9)	5 (3–10)	8 (4–15)
	Lymph node (+) (n = 0)	0 (0–0)	1 (0–2)	2 (0–5)	2 (0–4)
4.1–6.0	Organ confined (n = 171)	71 (67–75)	47 (41–52)	34 (28–41)	39 (31–48)
	Extraprostatic extension (n = 101)	27 (23–31)	44 (39–49)	54 (47–60)	46 (37–54)
	Seminal vesicle (+) (n = 10)	1 (1–2)	7 (4–10)	7 (4–11)	11 (6–17)
	Lymph node (+) (n = 3)	0 (0–1)	2 (1–4)	5 (2–8)	4 (2–9)
6.1–10.0	Organ confined (n = 142)	68 (64–72)	43 (38–48)	31 (26–37)	36 (27–44)
	Extraprostatic extension (n = 99)	29 (26–33)	46 (41–51)	56 (49–62)	47 (37–56)
	Seminal vesicle (+) (n = 12)	2 (1–3)	9 (6–13)	9 (5–14)	13 (8–20)
	Lymph node (+) (n = 6)	0 (0–1)	2 (1–4)	4 (2–8)	4 (1–8)
>10.0	Organ confined (n = 36)	54 (49–60)	28 (23–33)	18 (14–23)	21 (15–28)
	Extraprostatic extension (n = 47)	41 (35–46)	52 (46–59)	57 (48–66)	49 (39–59)
	Seminal vesicle (+) (n = 9)	3 (2–5)	12 (7–18)	11 (6–17)	17 (9–25)
	Lymph node (+) (n = 7)	1 (0–3)	7 (3–14)	13 (6–24)	12 (5–22)

Clinical stage T2b (palpable ≥ ½ of lobe) or T2c (palpable both lobes) (n = 313)

PSA range (ng/mL)	Pathological stage	5–6	3 + 4=7	4 + 3 = 7	8–10
0–2.5	Organ confined (n = 16)	84 (78–89)	59 (47–70)	44 (31–58)	49 (32–65)
	Extraprostatic extension (n = 10)	14 (9–19)	24 (16–33)	29 (19–42)	24 (14–36)

Table 6.3 Continued

PSA range (ng/mL)	Pathological stage	Biopsy Gleason Score			
		5–6	3 + 4=7	4 + 3 = 7	8–10
	Seminal vesicle (+) (n = 0)	1 (0–3)	6 (0–14)	6 (0–14)	8 (0–21)
	Lymph node (+) (n = 0)	1 (0–3)	10(2–25)	19 (4–40)	17 (3–42)
2.6–4.0	Organ confined (n = 28)	74 (68–80)	47 (39–56)	36 (27–45)	39 (28–50)
	Extraprostatic extension (n = 15)	23 (18–29)	37 (28–45)	46 (36–55)	37 (27–48)
	Seminal vesicle (+)(n = 3)	2 (1–5)	13(7–21)	13 (7–22)	19 (9–32)
	Lymph node (+) (n = 2)	0 (0–1)	3 (0–7)	5 (0–14)	4 (0–13)
4.1–6.0	Organ confined (n = 46)	66 (59–72)	36 (29–43)	25 (19–32)	27 (19–37)
	Extraprostatic extension (n = 40)	30 (24–36)	41 (33–47)	47 (38–55)	38 (28–48)
	Seminal vesicle (+)(n = 7)	4 (2–6)	16(10–23)	15 (9–23)	22 (13–33)
	Lymph node (+) (n = 4)	1 (0–2)	7 (3–12)	13 (6–21)	11 (4–23)
6.1–10.0	Organ confined (n = 53)	62 (55–68)	32 (26–38)	22 (17–29)	24 (17–33)
	Extraprostatic extension (n = 28)	32 (26–38)	41 (33–49)	47 (38–56)	38 (29–48)
	Seminal vesicle (+) (n = 15)	5 (3–8)	20 (13–28)	19 (11–28)	27 (16–39)
	Lymph node (+) (n = 5)	1 (0–2)	6 (3–11)	11 (5–19)	10 (3–20)
>10.0	Organ confined (n = 8)	46 (39–53)	18 (13–24)	11 (7–15)	12 (7–18)
	Extraprostatic extension (n = 15)	41 (34–50)	40 (31–51)	40 (30–52)	33 (22–46)
	Seminal vesicle (+) (n = 10)	7 (4–12)	23 (15–33)	19 (10–29)	28 (16–42)
	Lymph node (+) (n = 8)	5 (2–8)	18(9–30)	29(15–44)	26 (12–44)

Reprinted with permission from Makarov DV, Trock BJ, Humphreys EB, et al. (2007). *Urology* 69(6):1095–1101.

Prostate cancer grading

Adenocarcinoma of the prostate is graded using the Gleason system (see Fig. 6.4). Microscopically, adenocarcinoma is graded as a pattern 1 to 5 according to its gland-forming differentiation at relatively low magnification. Cytological features play no part in this grading system.

Since most are multifocal, an allowance is made by adding the two dominant grades to give a sum score between 2 and 10. If only one pattern is observed, the grade is simply doubled. The system is used with needle biopsies, TURP, and radical prostatectomy specimens.

Tertiary Gleason score is sometimes reported on radical prostatectomy specimens and represents the third-most prevalent grade present on the entire surgical specimen and may have prognostic significance if high grade.

Gleason scores 2–4 are considered well differentiated; 5–7 are moderately differentiated; and 8–10 are poorly differentiated. In practice, over 80% of PCs are graded 6 or 7, and, fortunately, only 15% are graded 8–10. Gleason score of less than 6 are uncommon in modern series.

Among expert pathologists, there is good interobserver reproducibility with Gleason scoring. However, scores assigned to needle biopsies are lower than those assigned to the subsequent radical prostatectomy specimen in 30% of cases, while overgrading on needle biopsy is less commonly seen.

The importance of the Gleason score is that it correlates well with prognosis, stage for stage, however the patient is managed. For example, a Gleason 4+4 = 8 adenocarcinoma carries a worse prognosis than a 3+3 = 6 cancer of equivalent stage. Moreover, cancers of the same Gleason score have a worse prognosis if the predominant grade is higher (for example, 4+3 = 7 is worse than 3+4 = 7).

Some men with low-grade tumors develop high-grade tumors after several years. This is most likely due to clonal expansion of high-grade cells rather than to dedifferentiation of low-grade tumor cells. In general, large-volume tumors are more likely to be high-grade than low-volume tumors, but occasionally exceptions are seen.

Finally, caution must be taken when Gleason-scoring prostate tissue that has been subjected to certain interventions, such a hormonal or radiation therapy. It is well recognized that prostate cancer treated with androgen ablation exhibits changes very similar to those seen in Gleason scores 8–10.

It is possible that even treatment of BPH with 5α-reductase inhibitors could adversely affect the Gleason score of cancer present in the gland. Pathologists should be informed of these important aspects of the patient history to provide the most accurate Gleason scores.

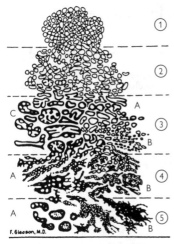

Figure 6.4 A diagrammatic representation of the Gleason grading system for prostate cancer. The grade depends on the structure of the prostatic glands and their relationship to the stromal smooth muscle.

Risk stratification in management of prostate cancer

Prostate cancer treatment options have varying levels of success. A challenge is to choose the most appropriate therapy based on the risk of disease progression with a given treatment and based on an individual's cancer characteristics. It is often useful to assign a relative risk to an individual.

The risk groups were established from literature and are based on known prognostic factors: PSA biopsy Gleason score, and AJCC TNM stage. One typical system described by D'Amico[1] is described below.

This is risk of PSA progression post-therapy and not overall or disease specific-survival.

• *Low risk:* stages T1c and T2a, PSA level of 10 ng/mL or less, and biopsy Gleason score of 6 or less (<25% PSA progression at 5 years post-therapy)
• *Intermediate risk:* PSA levels 10–20 ng/mL or lower, biopsy Gleason score of 7, or clinical stage T2b (25–50% PSA progression at 5 years post-therapy)
• *High risk:* T2c disease or a PSA level >20 ng/mL or a biopsy Gleason score of 8 or more (>50% PSA progression at 5 years post-therapy)

1 D'Amico, et al. (1998). Biochemical outcome after radical prostatectomy, external beam radiation therapy, or interstitial radiation therapy for clinically localized prostate cancer. *JAMA.* 280 (11): 969–974.

General principles of management of localized prostate cancer

When considering treatment options for the man with localized prostate cancer, the following factors should be considered in the discussion:
- Patient's life expectancy and overall health status
- Tumor characteristics, including Gleason score, tumor stage, PSA levels, PSA velocity and PSA doubling times
- Risk stratification
- Outcome tools such as nomograms[1] and Partin tables (p. 208) that give specific likelihood of final pathological stage or specific outcomes based on tumor characteristics and individual treatments (e.g., brachytherapy, radical prostatectomy, etc.)

1 http://www.mskcc.org/mskcc/html/10088.cfm

Management of localized prostate cancer: watchful waiting and active surveillance

More men die with prostate cancer than because of it, as most prostate cancers are slow growing and the majority of men diagnosed are often older with limited life expectancies, often with competing morbidities. This scenario forms the basis for less aggressive approaches to prostate cancer; some men diagnosed with nonmetastatic prostate cancer are offered no initial treatment.

Watchful waiting is based on the premise that some patients will not benefit from definitive treatment of the primary prostate cancer. The decision is made at the time of diagnosis to forgo definitive treatment and to instead provide palliative treatment for local or metastatic progression if and when it occurs.

The risks of developing metastatic disease and of death due to prostate cancer after 10–15 years of watchful waiting can be considered using published data, according to biopsy grade. Table 6.4 summarizes these data.

In contrast, *active surveillance* is based on the concept that some, but not all, patients may derive benefit from treatment of their primary prostate cancer. There are several international trials attempting to answer this question, which will take many years to complete.

The goals of active surveillance are to provide definitive treatment for men with localized cancers that are likely to progress and to reduce the risk of treatment-related complications for men with cancers that are not likely to progress.

Advantages of active surveillance include avoidance of possible side effects and costs of definitive therapy that may be unnecessary, and maintaining quality of life.

Disadvantages include possibly missing an opportunity for cure, the risk of progression and/or metastases, increased anxiety, increased physician visits and tests, and causing subsequent treatment to be more aggressive.

Selection of patients for active surveillance and suggested protocols

There are many different opinions on the best approach to active surveillance. The following represents guidelines from the National Comprehensive Cancer Network (NCCN).[1]

Characteristics of the patient and disease state for whom active surveillance may be considered are the following:
- Low risk prostate cancer (T1–T2a and Gleason 2–6 and PSA <10 ng/mL) regardless of life expectancy
- Intermediate risk prostate cancer T2b–T2c or Gleason 7 or PSA 10–20 ng/mL with <10 year life expectancy

---

1 National Comprehensive Cancer Network (NCCN) Clinical Practice Guidelines in Oncology: Prostate Cancer V.2.2009. Available at: www.nccn.org (registration required).

Surveillance protocol (if life expectancy <10 years follow up may be less frequent) is as follows:
- Patients must have clinically localized disease and be candidates for definitive treatment and choose observation.
- DRE and PSA as often as every 6 months but at least every 12 months
- Repeat prostate needle biopsy within 6 months of diagnosis if initial biopsy was <10 cores
- Needle biopsy may be performed within 18 months if >10 cores obtained initially, then done periodically.

Cancer progression may have occurred if
- Primary Gleason grade 4 or 5 cancer is found on repeat prostate biopsy.
- Prostate cancer is found in a greater number of prostate biopsies or occupies a greater extent of prostate biopsies.
- PSA doubling time is <3 years or PSA velocity is >0.75.
- A repeat prostate biopsy is indicated for signs of disease progression by exam or PSA.

Table 6.4 Natural history of localized prostate cancer managed with no initial treatment

Biopsy grade	% Risk of metastasis (10 years)	% Risk of prostate[1] cancer death (15 years)	Estimated lost years of life
2–4	19	4–7	<1 year
5	42	6–11	4
6	42	18–30	4
7	42	42–70	5
8–10	74	56–87	6–8

1 Albertsen PC, Hanley JA, Gleason DF, et al. (1998). Competing risk analysis of men aged 55 to 74 years at diagnosis managed conservatively for clinically localized prostate cancer. *JAMA* 280:975–980.

Management of localized prostate cancer: radical prostatectomy

Radical (total) prostatectomy (RP) is excision of the entire prostate, including the prostatic urethra, with the seminal vesicles. It may be performed by open retropubic, perineal, laparoscopic, or robotically assisted laparoscopic approaches.

At most U.S. centers, the robotically assisted technique has replaced the laparoscopic approach. The perineal approach does not allow a simultaneous pelvic lymph node dissection and is also not commonly performed in the United States.

Following excision of the prostate, reconstruction of the bladder neck and vesicourethral anastomosis completes the procedure.

RP is indicated for the treatment of men in good health with localized prostate cancer whose life expectancy exceeds 10 years, with curative intent. The indications of radical prostatectomy have been expanded as benefits to the multimodality approach to prostate cancer have become more accepted. As an example, the use of adjuvant radiation therapy following radical prostatectomy with positive surgical margins has allowed more patients with clinical non-organ-confined disease to be offered this surgical option.

Patients with Gleason score 2–4 disease appear to do as well with watchful waiting as with any other treatment. The patient should consider all available treatment options and the complications of RP prior to proceeding.

The surgeon should take part in multidisciplinary team discussion of each case. The most recent AUA guidelines no longer recommend absolute age as a cutoff for recommending treatment options. They recommend using life expectancy and overall health as factors to consider.

Stages in the open retropubic procedure

- The patient is under anesthetic, catheterized, and positioned supine with the middle of the table separated to open up entry to the pelvis.
- Through a lower midline incision, staying extraperitoneal, the retropubic space is opened.
- Obturator fossa lymphadenectomy is recommended for a PSA >10 or Gleason score ≥7. Others consider this to be essential, as many patients will be clinically understaged on the basis of Gleason grading.
- Incisions in the endopelvic fascia on either side allow access to the prostatic apex and membranous urethra.
- Division and hemostatic control of the dorsal vein complex passing under the pubic arch allow access to the membranous urethra, which is divided at the prostatic apex.
- The prostate is mobilized retrogradely from apex to base, taking Denonvilliers fascia on its posterior surface.
- If cavernous nerve sparing is undertaken, the apical and posterior dissection is modified to allow preservation of the neurovascular bundles as they course posterior–laterally between the rectum and prostate.

- Denonvilliers fascia is incised at the prostatic base, allowing access to the vasa (divided) and seminal vesicles (excised).
- The bladder neck is divided, freeing the prostate.
- The bladder neck is reconstructed to the approximate diameter of the membranous urethra.
- A sutured vesicourethral anastomosis is stented by a urethral catheter, typically for 2 weeks.
- The wound is closed, leaving pelvic drains, typically for 48 hours.

The nerve-sparing modification aims to reduce the risk of postoperative erectile dysfunction. The surgeon seeks to minimize injury to the cavernosal nerves passing from the autonomic pelvic plexus on either side in the groove between prostate and rectum, during mobilization of the prostate. This should not be attempted in the presence of palpable disease as it may compromise cancer control. The tips of the seminal vesicles may also be spared in cases with low risk of cancer involvement, potentially reducing bleeding and cavernosal nerve injury.

Stages in the robotically assisted laparoscopic prostatectomy

- The patient is given a general anesthetic and positioned in a low lithotomy position with either Allen stirrups or spreader bars, and an orogastric tube and sterile bladder catheter are placed.
- Through a 1-inch supraumbilical incision, pneumoperitoneum is established up to 15 mmHg with a Veress needle, and 4 to 5 additional working ports (4 total robotic and 1–2 for an assistant) are placed in the lower abdomen and pelvis.
- The patient is placed in a steep Trendelenburg position and the robot is rolled in and docked to the patient.
- The vasa deferentia are dissected posterior to the bladder bilaterally to the level of the seminal vesicles, and these structures are ligated individually, with the vasa divided and the seminal vesicles excised.
- Denonvilliers fascia is incised at the posterior border of the prostate to reveal perirectal fat.
- Anteriorly, bilateral obliterated umbilical ligaments are divided and an inverted U incision is made in the urachus and, using the vasa deferentia as the lateral and posterior border, the bladder is dropped posteriorly to enter the space of Retzius.
- The endopelvic fascia is incised bilaterally to reveal the entire lateral border of the prostate up to the level of the apex, where the puboprostatic ligaments are divided.
- The bladder neck is incised anteriorly to the level of the bladder catheter, which is retracted superiorly so that the bladder neck can be incised posteriorly and the bladder peeled off the prostate.
- The vasa deferentia and seminal vesicles are located and divided, if not done so at the beginning of the procedure, and retracted cephalad and superiorly so that the prostate can be dissected antegrade.

- If cavernous nerve sparing is undertaken, the posterior and apical dissections are modified to allow preservation of the neurovascular bundles as they course posterior–laterally between the rectum and the prostate.
- The dorsal venous complex is ligated and divided, and the distal urethra is divided, freeing the prostate, which is placed in a laparoscopic entrapment bag and moved out of the field.
- Obturator fossa lymphadenectomy is recommended for a PSA >10 or Gleason score ≥7. Others consider this to be essential because many patients will be clinically understaged on the basis of Gleason grading.
- If needed, the bladder neck is reconstructed to approximate the diameter of the membranous urethra.
- A sutured vesicourethral anastomosis is completed over a fresh bladder catheter that is left in for 7–10 days.
- A pelvic drain is placed through one of the working ports under direct vision and left in for approximately 24 hours.
- The robot is rolled away and the specimen is delivered out of the supraumbilical port site, which is increased in size to accommodate the prostate.
- The port sites are all closed.

Postoperative course after radical prostatectomy

Patients are generally hospitalized for 24–48 hours and maintain Foley catheter drainage for 10–14 days. The robotically assisted laparoscopic prostatectomy (RALP) is associated with reduced blood loss and more rapid discharge from the hospital. Currently, there are no convincing data that the long-term functional and oncological outcomes are improved by the less invasive robotically assisted laparoscopic approach.

Complications of radical prostatectomy

General complications

These include those of any major surgery: bleeding requiring reoperation and/or transfusion; infection; thromboembolism; and cardiopulmonary complications or disturbance. These are minimized by attention to hemostasis, prophylactic antimicrobials, pneumatic calf compression, low-dose heparin postoperatively, and early mobilization.

Specific complications—early

Intraoperative obturator nerve, ureteral, or rectal injury (all rare) should be managed immediately if recognized, with end-to-end nerve anastomosis; ureteral reimplantation; or primary three-layer rectal closure with or without a temporary loop colostomy.

Postoperative catheter displacement (rare) is managed with careful replacement using cystoscopic guidance over a wire if there are any concerns over the integrity of the anastamosis. If beyond 3–5 days postoperatively, a urethrogram may reveal no leak and the catheter may not need be replaced.

Postoperative urine or lymphatic leak (distinguished by fluid creatinine concentration) through drains (occasional) is managed by prolonged catheter and wound drainage; lymphatic leaks may require sclerotherapy with tetracycline.

Lymphocele (encapsulated collection of lymphatic fluid) can cause lower extremity swelling or abdominal discomfort. It is unusual with the RALP as the peritoneum is usually opened. Lymphocele can be sclerosed or drained intraperitoneally by a laparoscopic approach.

Specific complications—late

Erectile dysfunction (ED) affects >50% of patients who were potent preoperatively; spontaneous erections may return up to 3 years postoperatively. Men >65 years or with pre-existing ED are more likely to suffer long term.

From 40% to 70% respond to oral PDE5 inhibitors at 6 months, while others require intraurethral or intracavernosal prostaglandin E1 treatments, a vacuum device, or (rarely) a prosthesis. Penile rehabilitation protocols (immediate use of PDE5 inhibitors, vacuum devices, or prostaglandins) may enhance the return of spontaneous erectile function.

Incontinence (stress-type) requiring >1 pad/day affects 5% of patients beyond 6 months and is due to injury of the external urethral sphincter during division and hemostatic control of the dorsal vein complex. The predisposing factors include age >65 years and excessive intraoperative blood loss.

Pelvic floor exercises (Kegel exercises) and the use of biofeedback techniques can help the return of continence. Periurethral bulking injections or implantation of an artificial urinary sphincter are occasionally necessary.

The use of male urethral slings has gained popularity. Incontinence may also develop secondary to bladder neck stenosis or detrusor instability; flow rates, post-void residual measurement, urodynamics, and cystoscopy may help.

Bladder neck stenosis (bladder neck contracture) affects 5–8% of patients and typically occurs 2–6 months postoperatively, rarely becoming a recurrent problem. Predisposing factors include heavy bleeding, postoperative urinary leak, and previous TURP.

Patients complain of new voiding difficulties, and treatment is by endoscopic bladder neck incision with a laser, cold knife, or electrocautery. Occasionally, chronic dilation may be necessary.

Prostate cancer control with radical prostatectomy

While there are no randomized studies comparing RP outcomes to those of radiotherapy, a randomized study comparing RP to watchful waiting has demonstrated a 40% reduction in death due to prostate cancer and a significant reduction in local and metastatic progression in the RP group with a mean follow-up of 8.2 years.[1] High-grade cancers were excluded from this trial, though nonrandomized data suggest that more patients with Gleason 7–10 localized disease survive 10 years following RP than with watchful waiting or radiotherapy.

Excellent long-term results are seen in well-selected patients following RP, particularly those with organ-confined disease and prior lower urinary tract symptoms from bladder outflow obstruction. Serum PSA is usually measured at least 6–12 weeks postoperatively, then every 6 months; it should fall to <0.2 ng/mL.

The 10-year PSA progression rate following RP (usually defined as a serum PSA >0.2 ng/mL) is about 2–30%. Of these, the majority will fail within 3 years of RP. Without additional treatment, the time to development of clinical disease after PSA progression averages 8 years.[2]

A 20-year clinical disease-free survival of 60% is reported.[3] Outcome following radical prostatectomy correlates with Gleason score; preoperative PSA; pathological T stage; and surgical margin status.

Progression-free probabilities are shown in Table 6.5.

Neoadjuvant hormone therapy given 3 or more months prior to RP does not alter the PSA progression rate, despite reducing the incidence of positive surgical margins, and is not routinely used.

Two large studies have demonstrated that adjuvant radiation therapy in the setting of adverse pathology can greatly reduce the rate of PSA progression following radical prostatectomy. SWOG 8794 demonstrated a 50% reduction in PSA recurrence in patients with positive surgical margins who received adjuvant radiation therapy.[4]

Similarly, in EORTC 22911, adjuvant RT improved progression-free survival from 74% to 52.6%.[5] Neither study has yet demonstrated an absolute survival advantage.

1 Holmberg L, et al. (2002). A randomized trial comparing radical prostatectomy with watchful waiting in early prostate cancer. *N Engl J Med* 347:781–789. An update has been published: Bill-Axelson A, Holmberg L, Ruutu M, et al. (2005). Radical prostatectomy versus watchful waiting in early prostate cancer. *N Engl J Med* 352:1977–1984.

2 Pound CR, Partin AW, Eisenberger MA, et al. (1999). Natural history of progression after PSA elevation following radical prostatectomy. *JAMA* 281:1591–1597.

3 Swanson GP, Riggs MW, Earle JD (2002). Long-term follow-up of radical retropubic prostatectomy for prostate cancer. *Eur Urol* 42:212–216.

4 Swanson GP, Hussey MA, Tangen CM, et al. (2007). Predominant treatment failure in postprostatectomy patients is local: analysis of patterns of treatment failure in SWOG 8794. *J Clin Oncol.* 25(16):2225–2229.

5 Bolla M, Van Poppel H, Collette L (2007). Preliminary results for EORTC trial 22911: radical prostatectomy followed by postoperative radiotherapy in prostate cancers with a high risk of progression. *Cancer Radiother* 11(6–7):363–369.

Table 6.5 Progression-free and metastasis-free survival after open retropubic RP without adjuvant therapy, probability (%)

	Progression-free, 5 years	Progression-free, 10 years	Disease-specific, 10 years	Metastasis-free, 10 years
Gleason 2–4	90	88	94	87
Gleason 5–6	84	79	80	68
Gleason 7	60*	56*	80	68
Gleason 8–10	49	—	77	52
PSA <4	91			
PSA 4–9.9	87			
PSA 10–19.9	70			
PSA 20–50	50			
PT1–2		93		
PT3a		76		
PT3b		37		
N†		7		
Margin clear		81		
Margin positive		36+		

* 3+4 = 7 fares better than 4+3 = 7.

† Only 40–50% of patients with a positive surgical margin after RP develop a rising PSA

Management of biochemical relapse post-RP

The definition of PSA recurrence following RP is generally agreed to be a PSA of >0.3 ng/mL and rising. DRE should be performed in case there is a nodule. Biopsy of the vesicourethral anastomosis is not widely practiced unless there is a palpable abnormality.

Studies have shown that MRI and bone scans are rarely helpful in searching for metastatic disease unless the PSA is >7 ng/mL.

Current management options include observation, pelvic radiotherapy, or hormone therapy. A good response to pelvic radiotherapy is likely with the following:

• Positive surgical margins at the time of the RP
• PSA rise is delayed >1 year
• PSA doubles in >10 months
• PSA is <1 ng/mL at the initiation of radiation
• The original disease was low grade and low stage
• The radiation dose exceeds 64 Gy

If the PSA never falls below 0.2 or it rises in the first year with a doubling time of <10 months, the response to pelvic radiotherapy is less effective. It is likely in these circumstances that micrometastatic disease is present, and some form of androgen ablation therapy is usually recommended.

Management of localized prostate cancer: radical external beam radiotherapy (EBRT)

Advances in radiotherapy for localized prostate cancer have included the development of conformal and intensity-modulated techniques to minimize toxicity to the rectum and bladder. EBRT is administered with curative intent, often accompanied by neoadjuvant and adjuvant hormone therapy in high-risk disease.

In general, 2–3 years of hormonal therapy are given for high-risk disease, usually starting before the initiation of radiation therapy. While some data suggest that a shorter course of hormonal therapy (i.e., 6 months) may suffice for intermediate-stage disease, it is not considered standard. There is no role for adding hormonal therapy in low-risk disease.

Hypofractionation (delivery of a total dose of radiation but in a shorter time frame (i.e., 5 days) by use of various stereotactic body radiotherapy (SBRT) platforms has been promoted. Hypofractionation is currently not considered a standard treatment and is under study by groups such as the Radiation Therapy Oncology Group (RTOG).

Proton beam therapy (in contrast to photons used in standard radiation) is a very costly radiation technique that is gaining interest as more centers adopt this technology. The promise is that the side-effect profile may be improved using protons over standard radiation. The role of proton therapy remains to be determined.

Indications

These are clinically localized prostate cancer and life expectancy >5 years. Patients with Gleason score 2–4 disease appear to do as well with watchful waiting as with any other treatment, with 15-year follow-up.

Contraindications

- Severe lower urinary tract symptoms
- Inflammatory bowel disease
- Previous pelvic irradiation

Protocol

EBRT involves a 6- to 7-week course of daily treatments amounting to a dose of 60–72 Gy. Some centers use higher doses of radiation (up to 80 Gy) in an attempt to improve disease control.

Side effects

The use of contemporary radiation techniques that limit the exposure of normal tissues has greatly reduced the complication rates.

- Transient moderate/severe filling-type LUTS (common, rarely permanent)
- Hematuria, significant: 4%
- Moderate to severe gastrointestinal symptoms, bloody diarrhea, pain: 3–32% (common, rarely permanent)

- Erectile dysfunction (ED) gradually develops in 30–50%.
- The risk of a second solid pelvic malignancy is estimated to be 1 in 300, falling to 1 in 70 long-term survivors.

Outcomes of EBRT

Definition of treatment failure

The traditional American Society of Therapeutic Radiation Oncologists (ASTRO) definition is 3 consecutive PSA increases measured 4 months apart for 2 years, thereafter every 6 months. Time to failure is midway through the 3 PSA measurements.

This has been recently updated to the so-called Phoenix definition PSA nadir + 2 ng/mL; the Phoenix definition is now preferred.[1]

Pretreatment prognostic factors

These include PSA, Gleason score, clinical stage, and percentage of positive biopsies.

5-year PSA failure-free survival

- 85% for low risk (T1–2a or PSA <10 ng/mL or Gleason <7)
- 50% for intermediate risk (T2b or PSA 10–20 or Gleason 7)
- 33% for high risk without hormonal therapy (T2c or PSA >20 ng/mL or Gleason 8–10), improved with the use of neoadjuvant and adjuvant hormonal therapy

Treatment of PSA relapse post-EBRT

Hormone therapy, either as monotherapy or with antiandrogens, is currently the mainstay of treatment in this setting. However, local salvage treatment appears attractive, potentially offering another chance of cure if metastases cannot be demonstrated at repeat staging.

Salvage radical prostatectomy is technically demanding and can often be associated with poor outcomes; it appears best suited to younger patients in good health. Other local salvage treatments include *cryotherapy* and *high-intensity focused ultrasound* (HIFU), but outcomes data and access to these treatments are currently limited (see p. 230).

If salvage local treatment is being considered, repeat prostatic biopsies should be performed to demonstrate viable tumor cells. This should be at least 30 months post-EBRT, because fatally damaged cells may survive a few cell divisions.[1]

1 Roach M 3rd, Hanks G, Thames H Jr, Schellhammer P, Shipley WU, Sokol GH, Sandler H (2006). Defining biochemical failure following radiotherapy with or without hormonal therapy in men with clinically localized prostate cancer: recommendations of the RTOG-ASTRO Phoenix Consensus Conference. *Int J Radiat Oncol Biol Phys* 65(4):965–974.

Management of localized prostate cancer: brachytherapy (BT)

This is ultrasound-guided transperineal implantation of radioactive seeds, usually I^{125}, less commonly Pd^{103}, into the prostate. BT is minimally invasive, requires general anesthesia, and delivers up to 150 Gy. It is sometimes augmented by an EBRT boost.

Another approach is to use iridium^{192} wires, known as high-dose radiation (HDR), left for several hours in situ in a series of applications, either before or after EBRT. HDR is not widely available.

Indications for BT as monotherapy

BT is best for low-risk disease: localized T1–2a, Gleason <6, PSA <10 ng/mL prostate cancer, with a life expectancy >5 years.

Indications for BT with EBRT

In the non-protocol setting, patients with intermediate-risk prostate cancer are sometimes treated in combination: T2b–T2c, Gleason 7, PSA 10–20 ng/mL.

Contraindications to BT

These include previous TURP (risk of incontinence); large-volume prostate (>60 mL), which causes difficulty with seed placement; and moderate to severe lower urinary tract symptoms (risk of retention).

High-risk prostate cancer does not do well with BT monotherapy and should not be performed.

Complications

- Perineal hematoma (occasional)
- Lower urinary tract symptoms (common), due to prostatic edema post-implant
- Urinary retention (5–20%)
- Incontinence (5%), if TURP is required to treat urinary retention
- ED affects up to 50% of patients; gradual onset
- Luteinizing hormone–releasing hormone (LHRH) analogue use to reduce prostatic volume prior to treatment is discouraged, as many men develop retention with this approach. α-Blockers are often used to treat LUTS.

Outcomes of BT

PSA rises in the first 3 months post-implant; it subsequently declines. As with EBRT, the ASTRO definition (see p. 227) has been used to define progression:

- 5-year progression-free survival for T1 + 2a, Gleason ≤6, PSA <10 ng/mL is 80–90%
- 5-year progression-free survival for T2c, Gleason >6, PSA >10 ng/mL is 30–50%

- 8-year progression-free survival for T1 + 2a, Gleason <7, PSA <10 ng/mL is 79%
- 12-year progression-free survival for T1 + 2a, Gleason <7, PSA <10 ng/mL is 66%

It is noteworthy that 50% of the patients in these published series had a normal PSA and Gleason score <5; these patients would have done well with watchful waiting. Patients with Gleason 8–10 do poorly after BT.

PSA progression continues steadily several years after treatment.

Outcomes of BT plus EBRT
Five-year progression-free survival is 75–95%.

Comparisons of BT or BT plus EBRT with RP and EBRT alone
- There are no randomized studies.
- In nonrandomized comparisons, an age- and tumor-matched radical prostatectomy series at 8 years yielded a progression-free survival of 98% (compared to 79% with BT).
- Outcome of BT appears inferior to that with EBRT and RP in men with high-risk prostate cancer PSA >10–20 and Gleason score 7–10.

Rising PSA post-BT
Cryotherapy in an option if local recurrence is suspected; repeat staging and biopsy are indicated. Ultrasound images may be compromised in the setting of prior brachytherapy. Salvage prostatectomy can be considered in highly selected patients.

If metastatic disease is suspected or proven, hormone therapy is appropriate.

Management of localized and radiorecurrent prostate cancer: cryotherapy and HIFU

These two minimally invasive treatments for localized prostate cancer are in use in many locations. Proponents claim that they are viable alternatives to radical surgery or radiotherapy and that they are options for salvage treatment of organ-confined recurrent disease following radical radiotherapy.

Furthermore, there is growing interest in "focal therapy," whereby only a portion of the prostate is treated, sparing side effects that may be associated with more aggressive treatments.

Proponents note that of all local therapies, these are the only two that can be repeated if there is a recurrence. Cryotherapy is widely available, whereas HIFU is not yet FDA approved in the United States.

Cryotherapy

A transperineal ultrasound-guided cryoprobe delivers argon or liquid nitrogen at a temperature of $-20°C$ to $-40°C$. When applied in two cycles of freeze–thaw, cellular necrosis occurs. The diameter of the ice ball is monitored using ultrasound; precautions must be taken to protect the urethra, external sphincter, and rectal wall, such as using warming devices.

An anesthetic is required; this is a day-case procedure that can be repeated.

Results

PSA nadir is usually achieved within 3 months; 25–48% of men with localized disease achieve a PSA nadir of <0.1 ng/mL in 3 months, and 96% of men achieve PSA <0.2 ng/mL within 6 months. Positive biopsies are observed in 8–25% of patients after cryotherapy.

Long-term results are promising but appear inferior to other standard therapies and are not endorsed by the AUA in their 2007 treatment guidelines for localized disease.[1]

Complications

These include ED (40–80%); incontinence (4–27%); LUTS due to urethral sloughing; pelvic pain; transient penile numbness; and rectourethral fistula (rare).

In the salvage setting, good short-term PSA responses are reported in 66% of men, at the expense of significant morbidity, including incontinence and urinary retention (70% each).

High-intensity focused ultrasound (HIFU)

HIFU has the potential of selective destruction of tissues at depth without damaging intervening structures. Tissue is heated to the point of

---

1 Gleave M, Klotz L, Taneja SS. (2009). The continued debate: intermittent vs. Continuous hormonal ablation for metastatic prostate cancer. *Urol Oncol.* 27(1):81–86.

coagulative necrosis by high-energy ultrasound transmitted to the prostate using a transrectal device. The tissue temperature is raised locally at this point (over 85°C).

With each firing of the probe, a cigar-shaped volume of damage is produced (a lesion). After one lesion is created, the focus is repositioned by computer guidance to create the next lesion with the same heating process. Lesions are placed side by side to create a continuous volume in which the tissue is necrosed. The rectal wall and the surrounding tissues are undamaged.

An anesthetic is required; this is a day-case procedure that can be repeated. The likelihood of morbidity is increased in the salvage treatment setting. Long-term results are awaited.

Complications
These include ED, urinary retention, stress incontinence, and recto-urethral fistula (rare).

Management of locally advanced nonmetastatic prostate cancer (T3–4 N0M0)

EBRT

EBRT in combination with hormone therapy has consistently demonstrated better outcomes than those with EBRT alone, which is associated with a 15–30% 10-year survival. In a European randomized study[1] the hormone therapy group received LHRH analogues for 3 years starting at the time of EBRT. Their 5-year overall survival was 79% compared to 62% in the group treated with EBRT alone; the 5-year disease-free survival was 85% compared to 48%.

There are potential advantages in starting hormone therapy prior to EBRT as has been performed in other positive studies. The optimal timing and duration of hormone therapy in this setting remain unclear, but most agree that 6 months is inadequate, and 24–36 months should be considered a standard of care in high-risk disease.[1]

Hormone therapy

Hormone therapy alone is another option in elderly patients or those unwilling to consider radiotherapy, but its risk and benefit ratio are not clear. Outside the United States, a nonsteroidal antiandrogen (e.g., bicalutamide 150 mg) regimen is often used.

In the U.S., standard androgen ablation involves orchiectomy or LHRH analogue or antagonist. However, discussion should include the point at which hormone therapy is not a treatment offered with curative intent.

A randomized trial of hormone therapy alone vs. EBRT plus hormone therapy demonstrated that the hormone-only regimen was inferior to the combination treatment.[2]

Watchful waiting or active surveillance

This is also an option for nonmetastatic T3 disease in an elderly asymptomatic man who may wish to avoid side effects of treatment.

Palliative treatment of locally advanced disease

Palliative TURP or medical therapy for LUTS or retention may be necessary. Incontinence can be due to sphincter involvement, though bladder outflow obstruction and instability should be considered: a urinary convene sheath or catheter may be required.

Percutaneous nephrostomies or ureteral stents are occasionally necessary for ureteral obstruction.

---

1 Bolla M, de Reijke TM, Van Tienhoven G, et al. (2009). Duration of androgen suppression in the treatment of prostate cancer. *N Engl J Med* 360(24):2516–2527.
2 Widmark A, Klepp O, Solberg A, et al. (2009). Endocrine treatment, with or without radiotherapy, in locally advanced prostate cancer (SPCG-7/SFUO-3): an open randomised phase III trial. *Lancet* 373(9660):301–308.

Management of advanced prostate cancer: hormone therapy I

Metastatic disease is the cause of nearly all prostate cancer–related deaths. Currently incurable, 5-year survival is 25%; 10% survive <6 months, while <10% survive >10 years. The mainstay of treatment is hormone therapy, with cytotoxic chemotherapy used in cases of castration-resistant prostate cancer.

The concept of hormone therapy was realized in 1941 when Huggins and Hodges reported favorable acid and alkaline phosphatase responses in prostate cancer patients who were castrated or given estrogens.

Hormone dependence of prostate cancer

Of circulating androgen, 95%, mainly testosterone, is produced by the Leydig cells of the testes under the influence of luteinizing hormone (LH). The anterior pituitary synthesizes LH, stimulated by LH-releasing hormone (LHRH) produced by the hypothalamus. The remaining 5% of circulating androgen is synthesized by adrenal cortex from cholesterol.

Testosterone is metabolized to the more potent dihydrotestosterone (DHT), by types 1 and 2 5α-reductase (5AR) enzymes. DHT binds to the androgen receptor, travels to the cell nucleus, and exerts its positive effect on cell growth and division in the androgen-sensitive cell.

All prostate epithelial cells are dependent on androgens and fail to grow or undergo programmed cell death in their absence. Similarly, most previously untreated prostate cancer cells are dependent on androgens.

Androgen deprivation results in a reduction in PSA and clinical improvement in the majority of patients. However, most will still die within 5 years because of the development of androgen-independent growth, a state now commonly referred to as "castration resistant disease." This is considered due to growth of androgen-independent cell clones rather than to a dedifferentiation of previously androgen-dependent cells.

Traditionally, the mean time to disease progression after androgen deprivation is 14 months in men with metastatic disease, although more recent series suggest that this time is actually longer.

Prognostic factors

Predictors of poor hormone therapy response include the following:
- ≥5 metastatic lesions at presentation
- Elevated alkaline phosphatase at presentation
- Anemia at presentation
- Poor performance status at presentation
- Low serum testosterone at presentation
- Failure of bone pain to improve within 3 months of treatment
- Failure of PSA to normalize within 6 months of treatment (a PSA nadir (= lowest value) of <0.1 ng/mL predicts a long-term response)

Management of advanced prostate cancer: hormone therapy II

Mechanisms of androgen deprivation

- **Surgical castration**: bilateral orchiectomy
- **Medical castration**: LHRH agonists, LHRH antagonists, estrogens
- **Antiandrogens** (steroidal or nonsteroidal): androgen receptor blockade at target cell
- **Maximal androgen blockade** (MAB): medical or surgical castration plus antiandrogen

Both forms of castration (*androgen ablation* or *deprivation* are the preferred terms today) have equivalent efficacy, so patients should be given the choice. Estrogens are no longer first-line agents because of the significant cardiovascular morbidity. Antiandrogens alone are less effective in treating metastatic disease, but equivalent for nonmetastatic disease.

MAB has a theoretical advantage over castration in blocking the effects of the adrenal androgens, but significant clinical advantages have not been demonstrated in trial meta-analyses.

5AR inhibitors such as finasteride or dutasteride are not used in the treatment of prostate cancer but appear to have a role in prevention.

Bilateral orchiectomy

This is a simple procedure usually carried out under general anesthesia. Through a midline scrotal incision, both testes may be accessed. The testes are entirely removed or some prefer to incise the tunica albuginea of each testis and the soft tissue content is removed, after which the capsule is closed.

The epidiymes and testicular appendages are preserved; this allows some fullness to remain in the scrotal sac and may psychologically benefit the patient.

Postoperative complications include scrotal hematoma or infection (both rare). Serum testosterone falls within 8 hours to <0.2 nmol/L.

LHRH agonists

Developed in the 1980s, LHRH agonists give patients an alternative to bilateral orchiectomy, with which they are clinically equivalent. They are given by subcutaneous (SC) or intramuscular (IM) injection, as monthly or 3-, 6-, or 12-month depots. Some examples of these peptides include goserelin, triptorelin, histrelin, and leuprolide (see Table 6.6). Nasal forms are available outside the U.S.

If the anterior pituitary is desensitized to the pulsatile release of natural LHRH by the analogue of LHRH, it switches off LH production, although serum testosterone rises in the first 14 days because of a surge of LH. This can result in "tumor flare," manifest in 20% patients with increased symptoms, including catastrophic spinal cord compression. To prevent this, cover with antiandrogens is recommended for a week before and 2 weeks after the first dose of LHRH agonist.

An injectable LHRH antagonist (degarelix) (Table 6.6) rapidly reduces serum testosterone by blockade of the LHRH receptors.

Table 6.6 LHRH agonists and antagonists for primary androgen ablation for prostate cancer

Medications	Class	Administration	Notes
Abarelix (Plenaxis)	LHRH antagonists	Intramuscular injection every 2–4 weeks	Chance of anaphylaxis; no hormonal surge (not available in the U.S. for new patients)
Buserelin (Suprefact)	LHRH agonists	SC: 500 mcg q8h × 7 days then 200 mcg daily; Depot 2-month: 6.3 mg implant every 8 weeks Depot 3-month: 9.45 mg implant every 12 weeks Intranasal: 400 mcg (200 mcg into each nostril) 3 times/day	Not available in the U.S.
Degarelix (Firmagon)	LHRH antagonists	120 mg IM 2 doses initially, maintenance 80 mg IM every month	No hormonal surge. Requires two injections first month
Goserelin (Zoladex 3.6mg and 10.8mg)	LHRH agonist	3.6 mg implant SC every month; 10.8 mg implant SC every 3 months	Subcutaneous absorbable implant
Histrelin implant (Vantas)	LHRH agonists	SC implant 50 mg every 12 months	Remove implant device at reinsertion
Leuprolide (Lupron Depot, Lupron Depot 3 month, Lupron Depot 4 month)	LHRH agonists	7.5 mg IM monthly (depot) 22.5 mg IM every 3 months; 30 mg IM every 4 months	Intramuscular injection
Leuprolide gel (Eligard 7.5 mg, Eligard 22.5 mg, Eligard 30 mg, Eligard 45 mg)	LHRH agonists	7.5 mg SC monthly; 22.5 mg SC every 3 months; 30 mg SC every 4 months; 45 mg SC every 6 months	Formulation requires refrigerated storage
Leuprolide implant (Viadur)	LHRH agonists	SC implant every 12 months (contains 65 mg leuprolide)	Remove implant device at reinsertion. Off market for new patients in 2008
Triptorelin (Trelstar 3.75, 11.25, 22.5)	LHRH agonists	3.75 mg IM monthly 11.15 mg IM every 3 months 22.5 mg IM every 6 months	Intramuscular injection

Side effects of bilateral orchiectomy and LHRH agonists/antagonists
- Loss of sexual interest (libido) and ED
- Hot flushes and sweats can be frequent and troublesome during work or social activity
- Weight gain and obesity
- Gynecomastia
- Anemia
- Cognitive (mood) changes
- Metabolic syndrome (increased blood glucose and lipid profile)
- Osteoporosis and pathological fracture secondary to osteoporosis may occur in patients on long-term treatment.

Antiandrogens
These are administered as tablets. Examples include the nonsteroidal antiandrogens such as bicalutamide (50 mg daily for MAB, in combination with LHRH analogues or orchiectomy; 150 mg daily as monotherapy [not FDA approved in the U.S.]), flutamide, nilutamide, and the steroidal antiandrogen cyproterone acetate.

Bicalutamide monotherapy raises the serum testosterone slightly, so sexual interest and performance are often maintained.

Side effects include frequent gynecomastia, breast tenderness, and occasional liver dysfunction; flutamide can cause GI upset.

At its full dose, cyproterone acetate may cause reversible dyspnea; it may be used at 50 mg bid for treatment of castration-induced hot flushes.

Management of advanced prostate cancer: hormone therapy III

Monitoring treatment

Typically, patients with advanced prostate cancer will have baseline PSA, full blood count, renal and liver function tests, imaging (renal ultrasound or CT), and a bone scan. The PSA is repeated after 3 months, with long-term follow-up every 3–6 months along with periodic serum testosterone to assure castrate levels (< 50 ng/mL).

Liver function is checked every 3 months if antiandrogen monotherapy is used. Renal function should be checked on disease progression, and bone imaging used if clinically indicated.

While PSA is very useful as a marker for response and progression, 5–10% of patients can show clinical progression without PSA rise. This may occur in anaplastic tumors that fail to express PSA.

Advice on exercise, diet, and treatment of erectile dysfunction is often sought by patients during treatment.

Early versus delayed hormone therapy

Traditionally, hormone therapy was reserved for patients with symptomatic metastatic disease. Arguments against early hormone therapy revolve around its side effects and cost. However, studies of patients with locally advanced and metastatic disease have demonstrated slower disease progression and reduced morbidity when treated with androgen deprivation early (i.e., before the onset of symptoms).

Improved survival has also been reported in patients without bone metastases but including node-positive disease, when treated immediately.

Intermittent hormone therapy

The potential advantages of stopping hormone therapy when the disease has remitted, then restarting it when the PSA has risen again, are the reduced side effects and cost. Small series have suggested disease control equivalent to that with continuous hormonal ablation with reduced side effects.[1] However, large randomized trials are lacking and none of the agents is FDA approved for intermittent use.

Regardless, this approach is becoming increasingly popular among clinicians and patients. It can take up to 6 months after stopping treatment for the serum testosterone to recover, hence side effects may persist into off-treatment periods.

Additional therapies

Androgen blockade can cause osteopenia/osteoporosis; bisphosphonate therapy can limit reductions in bone mineral density. Bisphosphonates inhibit osteoclast bone resorption. Patients should receive calcium (1200 mg/d) and vitamin D (800–1000 IU/day) supplements and be encouraged to exercise and stop smoking and drink in moderation.

1 HYPERLINK "/pubmed/19683858" Potential benefits of intermittent androgen suppression therapy in the treatment of prostate cancer: a systematic review of the literature.
Abrahamsson PA. *Eur Urol.* 2010 Jan;57(1):49–59. Epub 2009 Aug 7. Review

With androgen ablation, consider bisphosphonates (e.g., zoledronic acid 4 mg IV yearly or alendronate 70 mg PO/week.) Adjust zoledronic acid on the basis of creatinine level.

Osteonecrosis of the jaw can result from any bisphosphonates, so patients should avoid major dental work while on this treatment.

In castration-resistant prostate cancer, zoledronic acid 4 mg (the most widely studied agent) adjusted to renal function every 3–4 weeks IV to prevent skeletal-related events (SREs). SREs are defined as pathological fracture, spinal compression/vertebral body collapse, radiation or surgery to bone, or change in antineoplastic therapy.

Management of advanced prostate cancer: androgen-independent/ castration-resistant disease

Second-line hormone therapy

When the PSA rises from its lowest (nadir) value, or if symptomatic progression occurs despite a favorable biochemical response to first-line hormone therapy, the disease has entered its *androgen-independent phase*. It is essential to verify that the current androgen ablation regimen is resulting in castrate levels of testosterone (<50 ng/dL), as there are some cases of LHRH analogue therapy that do not develop an adequate response to the ablation therapy.

If the patient is confirmed to be in the castrate testosterone range, further treatment is usually considered. If there is relapse during androgen ablation, up to 25% of patients respond by adding an antiandrogen (e.g., bicalutamide 50 mg daily) to establish maximal androgen blockade (MAB). The addition of an antiandrogen will result in PSA declines of 50% in 15–54% of patients (median duration 4–6 months).

If MAB was used from initiation of hormone therapy, withdrawal of the antiandrogen paradoxically elicits a favorable PSA response in 5–25% of patients; unfortunately this "anti-androgen withdrawal phenomenon" is rarely durable.

A further rise in PSA may require other hormonal manipulations such as the use of ketoconazole or the addition of estrogens. No secondary hormonal manipulation has been shown to extend survival in any trial.

The prognostic factors for survival with androgen-independent disease are identical to the factors predicting response to hormone therapy (see p. 233), plus time from initiation of hormone therapy to initiation of chemotherapy and visceral metastasis status.

Cytotoxic chemotherapy

Systemic chemotherapy is offered to appropriate patients with androgen-independent metastatic disease and disease progression. LHRH agonists are continued during therapy to prevent escape from androgen blockade.

Currently FDA-approved agents include docetaxel, mitoxantrone, and estramustine. Estramustine has limited utility due to cardiovascular and thromboembolic toxicity. Mitoxantrone at a dose of 12 mg/m^2 with prednisone 5 mg PO bid every 3 weeks palliates bone pain in 30%. Improved survival was not seen when mitoxantrone with prednisone was compared to prednisone alone.

Two major trials (TAX 327/SWOG 99–16) showed that docetaxel 60–70 mg/m^2 every 3 weeks with estramustine 280 mg PO tid for 5 days or docetaxel 75 mg/m^2 every 3 weeks with prednisone had a 20–24 % improvement in survival compared to mitoxantrone 12–14 mg/m^2 and prednisone. Palliation of bone pain was superior in those treated with docetaxel compared with those treated with mitoxantrone (TAX 327 study). Many consider docetaxel to be the current standard of care in this setting.

Clinical trials are under way to evaluate docetaxel combined with other agents (e.g., targeting angiogenesis [bevacizumab], and bone-targeted agents [atrasentan].) There is no standard therapy for patients who fail docetaxel; mitoxantrone in this setting has PSA decline rates of 50%, in 10%–20% of men treated.

Clinical trials are evaluating novel immunotherapeutic, cytotoxic, and antiangiogenic agents. In men with prostate cancer exhibiting neuroendocrine features, androgen blockade should be initiated along with immediate chemotherapy using cisplatin/etoposide or carboplatin/etoposide or a docetaxel-based regimen.

Newer agents for castration-resistant prostate caner

Abiraterone acetate is an inhibitor of the enzyme CYP17 that is critical to the generation of androgens and estrogens. It is 10 times more potent than ketoconazole in this activity and has shown promise in castration-resistant prostate cancer (CRPC).

ZD4054 is an endothelin receptor antagonist that appears to extend survival in men with CRPC and is in phase III trials. A variety of agents in late-stage clinical testing rely on immune modulation of the prostate cancer cell. Sipuleucel-T (Provenge, Dendreon Seattle, WA) was approved by the FDA in 2010. A patient's own ex vivo processed dendritic cells expressing a key tumor antigen (prostate acid phosphatase), are reinfused for 3 cycles. In patients with minimally symptomatic, castrate resistant metastatic prostate a statistically significant survival extension of at least 4 months at an overall survival of about 20 months has been shown[1].

1 Bot, Adrian (2010) The Landmark Approval of Provenge®, What It Means to Immunology and "In This Issue": The Complex Relation Between Vaccines and Autoimmunity International Reviews of Immunology Vol. 29, No. 3, 235–238.

Palliative management of prostate cancer

Involvement of the acute pain team, palliative care physicians, and nurses is often necessary in the terminal phase of the illness to optimize quality of life.

Pain

Pain is undoubtedly the most debilitating symptom of advanced prostate cancer. The pathogenesis of this pain is poorly understood, but there is known to be increased osteoclastic and osteoblastic activity. Table 6.7 categorizes the pain syndromes and their management.

Radiation can be given for palliation of painful bony metastases rather than for curative intent (typical treatment 300 cGy in 10 divided doses). Strontium-89 and samarium-153 can palliate bone pain and are most useful for diffuse metastasis, but they can have an adverse effect on platelets in particular.

Spinal cord compression (see p. 457)

Lower urinary tract symptoms/urinary retention

A TURP may be required for bladder outflow obstruction (BOO) or retention. Instrumentation can be difficult if there is a bulky fixed prostate cancer. The bladder may be contracted due to disease involvement, causing misery even after relief of BOO. This may respond to anticholinergic therapy.

A long-term urethral or suprapubic catheter may be required for difficult voiding symptoms or recurrent retention.

Ureteral obstruction (see p. 456)

This is a urological oncological emergency. Locally advanced prostate cancer and bladder cancer may cause bilateral ureteral obstruction. The patient presents with symptoms and signs of renal failure or is anuric without a palpable bladder. Renal ultrasound will demonstrate bilateral hydronephrosis and an empty bladder.

After treating any life-threatening metabolic abnormalities such as hyperkalemia, the treatment options include bilateral percutaneous nephrostomies or ureteral stents. Insertion of retrograde ureteral stents in this scenario is often unsuccessful because tumor on the trigone obscures the location of the ureteral orifices.

Antegrade ureteral stenting following placement of nephrostomies is usually successful.

Unilateral ureteral obstruction

This is occasionally observed at presentation or on progression. If asymptomatic, this may be managed conservatively provided there is a normal contralateral kidney.

Anemia, thrombocytopenia, and coagulopathy

For some patients, hemoglobin levels drop rapidly and they become symptomatic on a regular basis. Some of this drop may be due to the androgen ablation. In more advanced disease, bone marrow replacement is the cause. This tends to be normochromic and normocytic and often occurs without other symptoms and with normal renal function.

Such patients require regular transfusions. Platelet transfusions are rarely required for bleeding.

Terminal patients may develop a clinical picture similar to disseminated intravascular coagulation (DIC) leading to problematic hematuria.

Table 6.7 Pain syndromes and their management

Pain type	Initial management	Other options
Focal bone pain	Medical: simple, NSAIDs, opiates Single-shot radiotherapy, 800 cGy (75% respond up to 6 months)	Surgical fixation of pathological fracture or extensive lytic metastasis
Diffuse bone pain	Medical: NSAIDs, opiates Multishot radiotherapy or radiopharmaceutical (e.g., Strontium[89])	Steroids; bisphosphonates; chemotherapy
Epidural metastasis and cord compression	See p. 457	
Plexopathies (rare—caused by direct tumor extension)	Medical: NSAIDs, opiates Radiotherapy; nerve blocks	Tricyclics; anticonvulsants
Other pain syndromes: skull/cranial nerve, liver, rectum/perineum	Radiotherapy Medical: NSAIDs, opiates, steroids	Intrathecal chemotherapy for meningeal involvement

Prostate cancer: prevention; complementary and alternative therapies

As many as 27% of men in their third decade have histological prostate cancer, even though the disease is rarely detected clinically <50 years of age. Further, a likely premalignant lesion (high-grade PIN) has been identified. This suggests there may be opportunity for preventative strategies.

Dietary intervention

There are many epidemiological and laboratory data supporting dietary interventions, though randomized prospective trials are awaited.

High-fat diets, particularly those rich in saturated fat and omega-6 fatty acids, are linked to increased risk of prostate cancer diagnosis.

Soy products contain phytoestrogens including the isoflavone genistein. Genistein is a natural inhibitor of tyrosine kinase receptors and inhibits prostate cancer cell lines. Chinese Americans have a 24-fold risk of developing prostate cancer compared to that of native Chinese, perhaps because of a difference in their respective diets.

Lycopene, present in cooked tomatoes and tomato products, is thought to reduce risk of prostate cancer progression and inhibit cell lines.

Vitamins A (retinoids) and D both inhibit growth of prostate cell lines, and vitamin D receptor polymorphisms appear to predispose certain individuals to prostate cancer.

The SELECT Trial is the largest cancer prevention trial to date that studied the effect of selenium and vitamin E, alone and in combination, on reducing the risk of prostate cancer. Preliminary data suggested that these agents might be effective. Unfortunately, the trial did not demonstrate an advantage for these agents; there was an early suggestion of an increased health risk with these agents.[1]

Studies from the UK, Europe, and the United States have shown that 25–40% of prostate cancer patients are taking some form of complementary therapy, most without informing their doctor. These can occasionally be harmful: for example, a Chinese herb mixture called PC-SPES, now withdrawn, frequently caused thromboembolism to contamination with estrogenic compounds that likely accounted for some of its reported activity.

Smoking has been shown in population studies to be significantly associated not with prostate cancer diagnosis but with fatal prostate cancer. No definite link exists between alcohol consumption, vasectomy, or sexual activity and prostate cancer.

Studies have suggested an increased risk associated with early sexual activity and a reduced risk associated with frequent masturbation, but these require substantiation.

---

1 Lippman SM, Klein EA, Goodman PJ, .et al. (2009). Effect of selenium and vitamin E on risk of prostate cancer and other cancers: the Selenium and Vitamin E Cancer Prevention Trial (SELECT). *JAMA* 301(1):39–51.

Chemoprevention with antiandrogens

Given that prostate cancer is believed to start as an androgen-dependent disease, interest in its prevention has also focused on antiandrogens. While nonsteroidal antiandrogens would have unacceptable side effects and cost, the 5-α reductase inhibitors could be feasible chemoprevention agents as they are already used for the treatment of symptomatic BPH.

The Prostate Cancer Prevention Trial (PCPT) recruited 18,000 men who had no clinical or biochemical evidence of prostate cancer. They were randomized to placebo or finasteride 5 mg daily for up to 7 years. The men were offered biopsy if they developed a rising PSA or an abnormality on DRE, or at end of study.

Prostate cancer was detected in 24% and 18% of participants in placebo and finasteride arms, respectively, a 25% reduction in prostate cancer. However, Gleason 7+ cancers were significantly more frequent in the finasteride arm. This increase in high-grade cancer has been ascribed to sampling artifact due to the reduction in the size of the prostate.

The REDUCE trial in over 8000 men used the 5-α reductase inhibitor dutasteride in a placebo-controlled trial to attempt to reduce the risk of prostate cancer in a group of high-risk men (i.e., previous negative biopsy). Follow-up biopsy was performed at 2 and 4 years and for cause (i.e., rising PSA, new prostate nodule). The study demonstrated a 23% reduction in cancer with improvements in BPH-related outcomes. There was no suggestion of increased Gleason score cancers.

A 2008 joint recommendation of the American Society of Clinical Oncology (ASCO) and the American Urological Association states that healthy men who have a prostate-specific antigen score of 3.0 or lower, have no signs of prostate cancer, and plan to be screened regularly for the disease should discuss with their physician whether to take 5-α reductase inhibitors to decrease their risk of developing prostate cancer.[2]

2 Kramer BS, et al. (2009). Use of 5-α-reductase inhibitors for prostate cancer chemoprevention: American Society of Clinical Oncology/American Urological Association 2008 Clinical Practice Guideline. *J Urol* 181:1642–1657.

Bladder cancer: epidemiology and etiology

Bladder cancer is the second-most common urological malignancy, accounting for 70,980 total cases in men and women with 14,330 total deaths in the United States. This represents 2.3% of all cancer deaths. The majority of patients have localized curable or controllable disease.

Risk factors

- **Men** are 2.5 times more likely than women to develop the disease and die from it. The reasons for this are unclear but may be associated with greater urine residuals or toxic exposure.
- **Age** increases risk; it is most commonly diagnosed in the eighth decade and is rare in those <50 years of age.
- **Race:** Black people have a lower incidence than that of White people, but inexplicably they appear to carry a poorer prognosis.
- **Environmental carcinogens**, found in urine, are the major cause of bladder cancer.
- **Chronic inflammation** of bladder mucosa: bladder stones, long-term catheters, and the ova of *Schistosoma haematobium* (bilharziasis) are implicated in development of squamous cell carcinoma of the bladder.
- **Smoking** is the major cause of bladder cancer in the developed world. Cigarette smoke contains the carcinogens 4-aminobiphenyl (4-ABP) and 2-naphthylamine (see Fig. 6.5). Slow hepatic acetylation (detoxification) of 4-ABP by N-acetyltransferase and glutathione S-transferase M1 (GST M1), or induction of the cytochrome p-450 1A2 demethylating enzyme, appears to increase urinary carcinogenic exposure of the urothelium. Smokers have a 2- to 5-fold risk compared to that of non-smokers of developing bladder cancer and subsequent recurrences. Estimates suggest that 30–50% of bladder cancer is caused by smoking. There is a slow (20-year) reduction in risk following cessation of smoking. Passive exposure to cigarette smoke is also implicated.
- **Occupational exposure** to carcinogens, in particular aromatic hydrocarbons like aniline (see Fig. 6.5), is a recognized cause of bladder cancer. See Box 6.3 for examples of at-risk occupations. A latent period of 25–45 years exists between exposure and carcinogenesis.
- **Drugs:** phenacetin and cyclophosphamide
- **Pelvic radiotherapy** for other malignancies such as prostate, rectal or cervical cancer

No evidence for a hereditary genetic etiology exists, though many somatic genetic abnormalities have been identified. The most common cytogenetic abnormality is loss of chromosomes 9p, 9q, 11p 13q, and 17q.

Activation or amplification of oncogenes (*p21 ras, c-myc, c-jun, erbB-2*), inactivation of tumor suppressor genes (*p53* mutations appear to worsen survival after treatment, retinoblastoma, *p16* cyclin-dependent kinse inhibitor), and increased expression of angiogenic factors (e.g., vascular endothelial growth factor [VEGF]) are reported in transitional cell carcinomas.

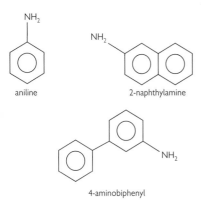

aniline

2-naphthylamine

4-aminobiphenyl

Figure 6.5 Carcinogens known to increase risk of bladder cancer.

Box 6.3 Occupations associated with urothelial carcinoma

- Drivers exposed to diesel exhaust
- Dye manufacture
- Fine chemical manufacture (e.g., auramine)
- Hairdressers
- Leather workers
- Painters
- Plumbers
- Rope and textile manufacture
- Rubber manufacture (e.g., tires or electric cable)

Bladder cancer: pathology and staging

Benign tumors of the bladder, including inverted papilloma and nephrogenic adenoma, are uncommon. The vast majority of primary bladder cancers are malignant and epithelial in origin:

- >90% are transitional cell carcinoma (TCC); *urothelial carcinoma* (UC) is now the preferred term.
- 1–7% are squamous cell carcinoma (SCC).
- 75% are SCC in areas where schistosomiasis is endemic.
- 2% are adenocarcinoma
- Rarities include pheochromocytoma, melanoma, lymphoma, and sarcoma arising within the bladder muscle.
- Secondary bladder cancers are mostly metastatic adenocarcinoma from gut, prostate, kidney, or ovary.

Tumor spread

- **Direct** tumor growth to involve the detrusor, the ureteral orifices, prostate, urethra, uterus, vagina, perivesical fat, bowel, or pelvic side walls.
- **Implantation** into wounds/percutaneous catheter tracts
- **Lymphatic** infiltration of the iliac and para-aortic nodes
- **Hematogenous**, most commonly to liver (38%), lung (36%), adrenal gland (21%), and bone (27%). Any other organ may be involved.

Histological grading

Grading is divided into well, moderately, and poorly differentiated (abbreviated to G1, G2, and G3, respectively).

Staging

Staging is by the TNM (2002) classification (see Fig. 6.6 and Table 6.8). All rely on physical examination and imaging (prefixed c), the pathological classification (prefixed p) corresponding to the TNM categories.

Urothelial carcinoma (transitional cell carcinoma)

UC may be single or multifocal. Because 5% of patients will have a synchronous upper tract UC and metachronous recurrences may develop after several years, the urothelial field-change theory of polyclonality is favored over the theory of tumor monoclonality with implantation (seeding).

Primary UC is considered clinically as superficial or muscle invasive: 70% of tumors are papillary, usually G1 or G2, exhibiting at least 7 transitional cell layers covering a fibrovascular core (normal transitional epithelium has ≤5 cell layers). Papillary UC is most often superficial, confined to the bladder mucosa (Ta) or submucosa (T1). 10% of patients subsequently develop muscle-invasive or metastatic disease.

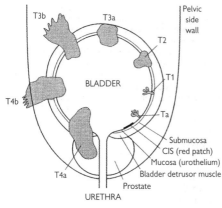

Figure 6.6 Diagrammatic representation of T staging of bladder urothelial cell carcinoma. Reprinted with permission from Brewster S, Cranston D, Noble J, Reynard J (2001) *Urology: A Handbook for Medical Students*. Informa Healthcare, p. 97.

Table 6.8 2002 TNM staging of bladder carcinoma

Tx	Primary tumor cannot be assessed
T0	No evidence of primary tumor
Ta	Noninvasive papillary carcinoma
Tis	Carcinoma in situ
T1	Tumor invades subepithelial connective tissue
T2	Tumor invades muscularis propria (detrusor): T2a inner half; T2b outer half
T3	Tumor invades beyond muscularis propria into perivesical fat: T3a = microscopic; T3b = macroscopic (extravesical mass)
T4a	Tumor invades any of prostate, uterus, vagina, bowel
T4b	Tumor invades pelvic or abdominal wall
Nx	Regional (iliac and para-aortic) lymph nodes cannot be assessed
N0	No regional lymph node metastasis
N1	Metastasis in a single lymph node <2 cm in greatest dimension
N2	Metastasis in a single lymph node 2–5 cm or multiple nodes <5 cm
N3	Metastasis in a single lymph node or multiple nodes >5 cm in greatest dimension
Mx	Distant metastasis cannot be assessed
M0	No distant metastasis
M1	Distant metastasis present

However, a subset of superficial UC, G3T1 tumors, are more aggressive, with 40% subsequently upstaging. 10% of UC have mixed papillary and solid morphology and 10% are solid. These are usually G3, half of which are muscle invasive at presentation.

Ten percent of UC is flat carcinoma in situ (CIS). This is poorly differentiated carcinoma, but confined to the epithelium and associated with an intact basement membrane. Half of CIS lesions occur in isolation; the remainder occur in association with muscle-invasive UC.

CIS usually appears as a flat, red, velvety patch on the bladder mucosa; 15–40% of such lesions are CIS, the remainder being focal cystitis of varying etiology. The cells are poorly cohesive, up to 100% of patients with CIS exhibiting positive urine cytology, in contrast to much lower yields (17–72%) with G1/2 papillary UC.

From 40% to 83% of untreated CIS lesions will progress to muscle-invasive UC, making CIS the most aggressive form of superficial UC. 5% of patients with G1/2 UC and at least 20% with G3 UC (including CIS) have vascular or lymphatic spread.

Metastatic node disease is found in 0% Tis, 6% Ta, 10% T1, 18% T2 and T3a, and 25–33% T3b and T4 UC.

Papillary urothelial neoplasm of low malignant potential (PUNLMP)
The World Health Organization (WHO) defines PUNLMP as a papillary urothelial tumor that resembles an exophytic urothelial papilloma but shows increased cellular proliferation exceeding the thickness of normal urothelium. They are typically small (1–2 cm) and have little, if any, cytological atypia.

Treatment and follow-up are the same as for low-grade noninvasive urothelial carcinoma.

Squamous cell carcinoma (SCC)
SCC is usually solid or ulcerative and muscle invasive at presentation. SCC accounts for only 2–5% of bladder cancers in North America and Europe. SCC in the bladder is associated with chronic inflammation (bladder calculi, indwelling catheters) and urothelial squamous metaplasia, rather than CIS.

Bilharzial SCC is the most common form of bladder cancer in East Africa and the Middle East and is related to infection with *Schistosoma hematobium*. In Egypt, 80% of SCC cases are induced by the ova of *Schistosoma hematobium*.

Non-bilharzial SCC is the second-most common form of bladder cancer in North America and Europe. 5% of paraplegics with long-term catheters develop SCC. Smoking is also a risk factor for SCC.

The prognosis is better for bilharzial SCC than for non-bilharzial disease, probably because it tends to be lower grade and metastases are less common in these patients.

Adenocarcinoma

Adenocarcinoma is rare, is usually solid/ulcerative and high grade, and carries a poor prognosis. It is frequently advanced at initial presentation (muscle invasive or metastatic). One-third of cases originate in the urachus, the remnant of the allantois, located deep to the bladder mucosa in the dome of the bladder.

Adenocarcinoma is a long-term (10–20+ year) complication of bladder exstrophy and bowel implantation into the urinary tract, particularly bladder substitutions and ileal conduits after cystectomy. There is association with cystitis glandularis, rather than CIS.

Secondary adenocarcinoma of the bladder may arise as discussed earlier.

Bladder cancer: presentation

Symptoms

The most common presenting symptom (85% of cases) is painless total hematuria. This may be initial or terminal if the lesion is at the bladder neck or in the prostatic urethra. 34% of patients >50 years of age and 10% under age 50 with macroscopic hematuria have bladder cancer. History of smoking or occupational exposure should raise suspicion for UC in the setting of hematuria.

Asymptomatic microscopic hematuria is found on routine urine stick-testing. Up to 16% of females and 4% of males have dipstick hematuria: <5% of these patients are <50 years of age, while 7–13% of those >50 years will have a malignancy.

Pain is unusual, even if the patient has obstructed upper tracts, since the obstruction and renal deterioration arise gradually. Pain may be caused by locally advanced (T4 disease).

Filling-type lower urinary tract symptoms, such as urgency or suprapubic pain occur. There is almost always microscopic or macroscopic hematuria. This so-called malignant cystitis is typical in patients with CIS.

Recurrent urinary tract infections and pneumaturia due to malignant colovesical fistula are also found. However, this is less common than benign causes such as diverticular and Crohn disease.

More advanced cases may present with lower limb swelling due to lymphatic/venous obstruction, bone pain, weight loss, anorexia, confusion, and anuria (renal failure due to bilateral ureteral obstruction).

Urachal adenocarcinomas may present with a blood or mucus umbilical discharge or a deep subumbilical mass (rare).

Signs

As most patients have superficial localized disease, signs are generally absent. General examination may reveal pallor, indicating anemia due to chronic renal impairment or blood loss in more advanced disease. Abdominal examination may reveal a suprapubic mass in the case of locally advanced disease.

Digital rectal examination may reveal a mass above or involving the prostate. A pelvic exam in females should also be performed. Although the likelihood of diagnosing bladder cancer in patients <50 years of age is low, all patients with these presenting features should be investigated.

Bladder cancer: diagnosis and staging

After a urinary tract infection has been excluded or treated, all patients with microscopic or macroscopic hematuria require investigation of their upper tracts, bladder, and urethra. Usually, renal imaging and flexible cystoscopy with local anesthetic are first-line investigations.

CT urography (CTU) before and after IV contrast is becoming the first-line radiological investigation of hematuria. It is faster and more sensitive than ultrasound or IVP in the detection of renal (parenchymal and urothelial) and ureteral tumors.

CTU also detects some bladder tumors, but may overcall bladder wall hypertrophy as tumor and will miss flat CIS and urethral pathology. CTU cannot replace cystoscopy. If there is hydronephrosis in association with a bladder tumor, it is likely that the tumor is causing the obstruction to the distal ureter caused by muscle-invasive disease.

False-negative cytology is frequent (40–70%) in patients with papillary UC. Overall, routine urine cytology has 50% sensitivity but a high 96% specificity and is most reliable with high-grade UC and CIS. False-positive cytology can occur from infection, inflammation, instrumentation, and chemotherapy.

Fluorescent in situ hybridization (FISH) (sensitivity 77%, specificity 98%) and other tests such as NMP-22 (sensitivity 56%, specificity 85%) may be helpful in the evaluation.

If all investigations are normal, consideration should be given to "medical" causes of hematuria, such as glomerulonephritis or IGA nephropathy. In patients with persisting microscopic hematuria, especially those with associated proteinuria or hypertension, nephrology consultation should be considered.

Transurethral resection of bladder tumor (TURBT)

TURBT usually provides definitive histological diagnosis (see p. 248). This is usually undertaken under general or spinal anesthesia. Bimanual examination is mandatory before and after bladder tumor resection in order to assess size, position, and mobility.

The pathologist should report on the tumor type, grade, and stage. In particular, the presence or absence of muscularis propria should be noted, since its absence will preclude reliable T staging. Suspicious areas are biopsied separately and consideration given to random biopsies to evaluate for CIS.

The prostatic urethra is biopsied if radical reconstructive surgery such as orthotopic neobladder is under consideration. Care should be taken in resecting tumors at the dome, since intraperitoneal bladder perforation may occur, especially in women with thin-walled bladders.

Mitomycin C, given as a single dose within 24 hours of TURBT (40 mg in 40 mL of saline or sterile water), can reduce tumor recurrence but is contraindicated with bladder perforation.

Staging investigations

These are usually reserved for patients with biopsy-proven muscle-invasive bladder cancer unless clinically indicated, since superficial UC and CIS disease are rarely associated with metastases.

- **Pelvic CT or MRI** may demonstrate extravesical tumor extension or pelvic lymphadenopathy, reported if >5–8 mm in maximal diameter.
- **Chest X-ray**
- **Isotope bone scan** (positive in 5–15% of patients with muscle-invasive UC) is obtained in cases being considered for radical treatment.
- **Staging lymphadenectomy** (open or laparoscopic) may be indicated in the presence of CT-detected pelvic lymphadenopathy if radical treatment is under consideration. However, this is most often performed at the time of radical cystectomy.

Management of superficial UC: transurethral resection of bladder tumor (TURBT)

The diagnostic role of TURBT is discussed on p. 254. Therapeutically, a visually complete tumor resection is adequate treatment for 70% of newly presenting patients with Ta/T1 superficial disease. The remaining 30% of patients experience early recurrence, 15% with upstaging. Because of this, it is proposed that all new patients receive adjuvant treatment (see below).

Complications are uncommon and include bleeding, sepsis, bladder perforation, incomplete resection, and urethral stricture. Alternatively, transurethral laser ablation is less likely to cause bleeding, but histological sampling would be inadequate.

Follow-up after TURBT

Most urologists perform review cystoscopy at 3 months. If this demonstrates recurrence, 70% of cases will further recur. If no recurrence is evident, only 20% will further recur. If the bladder is clear at follow-up, further cystoscopies are performed at 6 months and thereafter annually until the patient is no longer fit to undergo treatment.

There is no accepted protocol for upper tract surveillance in patients with a history of bladder UC, although some urologists recommend IVP every 2 years.

Transurethral fulguration (electrosurgical or laser)

This procedure is accepted more quickly and is less morbid for ablating very small, superficial papillary recurrences.

Patients with G3T1 UC and CIS are at significantly higher risk of recurrence and 40% are upstaged. Also, some patients experience persistent symptomatic multifocal G1/2, Ta/1 recurrent UC, which requires frequent follow-up procedures. In these circumstances, adjuvant treatment is indicated (see p. 258).

Patients with high-grade (G3) disease whose biopsy material does not contain muscularis propria should be re-resected early (within a few weeks) since the possibility of muscle invasion has not been excluded. Table 6.9 summarizes the management of bladder cancer, stage by stage.

Table 6.9 Summary of management of bladder cancer

Histology	Risk of recurrence post-TURBT	Risk of stage progression	Further treatment	Urological follow-up
G1/2, Ta/1 UC	30%	10–15%	Consider peri-operative single-dose intravesical mitomycin C chemotherapy	Review cystoscopies, commencing 3 months
Persistent multifocal recurrent G1/2, Ta/1	70%+	10–15%	Intravesical chemotherapy, 6-week doses	Follow-up cystoscopies, commencing 3 months
G3, T1 UC	80%	40%	Intravesical BCG, 6-week doses	Follow-up cystoscopies, commencing 6–12 weeks
CIS (also called severe urothelial dysplasia)	80%	40%	Intravesical BCG, 6-week doses, then maintenance	Cystoscopies + biopsy and cytology, commencing 3 months
pT2/3, N0, M0 UC, SCC, or adeno-carcinoma	Usually TUR is incomplete	N/A	Radical cystectomy, radiotherapy with chemotherapy ("bladder preservation," or palliative TURBT (if unfit for radical procedure)	Cystoscopies if bladder is preserved; urethral washings for cytology
T4 or metastatic UC, SCC, or adeno-carcinoma	Usually TUR is incomplete	N/A	Systemic chemotherapy; multidisciplinary team; symptom palliation	Palliative treatment for local bladder symptoms

Management of superficial UC: adjuvant intravesical chemotherapy and BCG

Adjuvant intravesical chemotherapy

Depending on patient and tumor characteristics, a number of patients may benefit from some form of intravesical therapy.[1] Intravesical chemotherapy (e.g., mitomycin C [MMC] 40 mg in 50 mL saline) is used for G1–2, Ta or T1 tumors, and recurrent multifocal UC. MMC is an antibiotic chemotherapeutic agent that inhibits DNA synthesis. In experimental studies, it may cause regression of small papillary UC, so it should be cytotoxic for microscopic residual disease post-TURBT.

It significantly reduces the likelihood of tumor recurrence compared to that with TURBT alone, but has never been shown to prevent progression to muscle invasion and has no impact on survival. It is used either as a single dose within 24 hours of first TURBT, or weekly for 6 weeks commencing up to 2 weeks post-TURBT.

It is administered by urethral catheter and held in the bladder for 1 hour. Thiotepa is no longer used in most centers for superficial UC.

Other potential agents include doxorubicin and gemcitabine.

Toxicity of MMC

Fifteen percent of patients report transient filling-type LUTS; occasionally, dermatitis develops on the external genitalia or palms of the hands, so treatment must be stopped. Systemic toxicity is rare with MMC given the large size of the molecule and low rate of systemic absorption.

Adjuvant intravesical BCG

Bacille Calmette–Guérin (BCG) is an attenuated strain of *Mycobacterium bovis*. It acts as an immune stimulant, up-regulating cytokines such as IL-6 and IL-8 in the bladder wall.

BCG is given as a 6-week course for G3T1 UC and for CIS, starting at least 2 weeks post-TURBT. It is administered via a urethral catheter, 80 mg in 50 mL saline, and retained in the bladder for 1 hour. BCG should never be given sooner than 10 days after tumor resection.

BCG produces complete responses in 60–70% of patients, compared with TURBT alone. 30% do not respond, and 30% of responders relapse within 5 years. It is more effective than MMC for adjuvant treatment of G1/2,Ta/1 UC, but is not often used (except as second-line treatment occasionally) because of the additional toxicity. Two studies have suggested that BCG may delay tumor progression to muscle invasion.

Though less expensive and more effective, BCG is potentially more toxic than intravesical chemotherapy, causing irritative symptoms in nearly all patients and low-grade fever with myalgia in 25%.

---

1 AUA Guideline for the management of nonmuscle invasive bladder cancer: Stages Ta, T1 and TIS: 2007 Update available at: www.auanet.org/content/guidelines-and-quality-care/clinical-guidelines/main-reports/bladcan07. Accessed August 2009.

BCG infection (BCGosis), especially if BCG is administered in a setting of recent surgery or traumatic catheterization, can be seen in a small percentage of patients. They develop a high, persistent fever, requiring antituberculous therapy for up to 6 months with isoniazid and pyridoxine, or standard triple therapy (rifampicin, isoniazid, and ethambutol) in critically ill patients. Granulomatous prostatitis and epididymo-orchitis are rare complications.

Contraindications to intravesical BCG
- Immunosuppressed patients
- Pregnant or lactating women
- Patients with hematological malignancy
- After a traumatic catheterization
- Active UTI

Cystoscopy done too early after BCG can produce alarming-looking effects because of the generalized inflammatory response. Follow-up cystoscopy and biopsy 3 months after BCG may still reveal chronic granulomatous inflammation.

Maintenance BCG (e.g., treatment every 3 months and then every 6 months for 3 years after the initial 6-week course or monthly regimen) demonstrated a benefit for superficial UC, excluding CIS, compared with a single 6-week course.

Maintenance may be associated with a higher risk of side effects.

Recurrent G3T1 UC or CIS
A second course of BCG could be offered; 50% of patients will respond. Otherwise, proceed without delay to radical cystectomy. The latter has a cure rate of 90%.

Muscle-invasive bladder cancer: surgical management of localized (pT2/3a) disease

This is a dangerous disease; untreated 5-year survival is 3%. In the absence of prospective randomized trials comparing the surgical and nonsurgical treatments, the options for a patient with newly diagnosed confined muscle-invasive bladder cancer are as follows.

Bladder preservation

- Radical transurethral resection of bladder tumor (TURBT) plus systemic chemotherapy, mostly done in setting of clinical trial at present or in patients clearly unfit for radical cystectomy. With hydronephrosis, bladder preservation relative contraindication.
- Palliative TURBT palliative radiotherapy (RT): for elderly/unfit patients
- Partial cystectomy in highly selected patients without evidence of CIS
- TURBT plus definitive RT (see p. 264): poor options for SCC and adenocarcinoma as they are seldom radiosensitive

Radical cystectomy with:

- Ileal conduit urinary diversion
- Continent urinary diversion (orthotopic neoblader or catherizable stoma)
- Neoadjuvant chemotherapy: some evidence of benefit (see p. 264)
- Neoadjuvant RT: no evidence of benefit

Partial cystectomy

A good option for well-selected patients with small solitary disease located near the dome, and for urachal carcinoma. Morbidity is less than with radical cystectomy.

The surgical specimen should be covered with perivesical fat, with a 1.5 cm margin of macroscopically normal bladder around the tumor. There should be no biopsy evidence of CIS elsewhere in the bladder.

The bladder must be closed without tension and catheterized for 7–10 days to allow healing. Subsequent review cystoscopies ensure no tumor recurrence.

Radical cystectomy with urinary diversion

This is the most effective primary treatment for muscle-invasive UC, SCC, and adenocarcinoma, and can be used as salvage treatment if bladder preservation has failed. It is also a treatment for G3T1 UC and CIS, refractory to BCG.

However, this is a major undertaking for the patient and surgeon, requiring support from cancer specialist nurse, stoma therapist, or continence advisor.

The procedure

Some centers are exploring laparoscopic radical cystectomy with urinary diversion. However, it is not currently considered the standard of care. Standard open surgical radical cystectomy is described.

Through a midline abdominal transperitoneal approach, the entire bladder is excised along with perivesical vascular pedicles, fat, and urachus, plus the prostate or anterior vaginal wall. The anterior urethra is not excised unless there is prior biopsy evidence of tumor at the female bladder neck or prostatic urethra (when recurrence occurs in 37%).

The ureters are divided close to the bladder, ensuring their disease-free status by frozen-section histology if necessary, and anastomosed into the chosen urinary diversion (see p. 266).

A bilateral pelvic lymphadenectomy is undertaken at the time. The extent and completeness of the lymphadenectomy can have important therapeutic implications.

Node burden (>8 positive) and node density, the ratio of involved nodes to total lymph nodes (>20%) has worse prognosis

Major complications

Affect 25% of cystectomy patients. These include perioperative death (1%), re-operation (10%), bleeding, thromboembolism, sepsis, wound infection/dehiscence (10%), intestinal obstruction or prolonged ileus (10%), cardiopulmonary morbidity, and rectal injury (4%).

Erectile dysfunction is likely in men after cystectomy due to cavernosal nerve injury.

The complications of urinary diversion are discussed on p. 266.

Postoperative care

Monitoring in the intensive care unit for 24 hours is considered standard at most centers.

Daily clinical evaluation, including inspection of the wound (and stoma if present), plus monitoring of blood count and creatinine/electrolytes, is mandatory. Broad-spectrum antimicrobial prophylaxis and thromboembolic prophylaxis with TED stockings, pneumatic calf compression, and subcutaneous heparin are standard.

Assisted ambulation after 24 hours is ideal. Chest physiotherapy and adequate analgesia is especially important in smokers and patients with chest comorbidity. Oral intake is restricted until bowel sounds are present; some patients may require parenteral nutrition in the presence of gastrointestinal complications.

Drains are usually placed in the pelvis or near the ureterodiversion anastomosis. Ureteral catheters passing from the renal pelves through the diversion and exiting percutaneously or through the stoma are used. If a continent diversion is performed, a catheter draining the diversion will be exiting urethrally or suprapubically.

Most patients are hospitalized 7–10 days.

Salvage radical cystectomy is technically a more difficult and slightly more morbid procedure. Relatively few patients who have failed primary RT and chemotherapy are suitable for this second chance of a cure.

Efficacy of radical cystectomy 5-year survival rates are as follows:

- Stage T1/CIS   +90%
- Stages T2, T3a   63–88%
- Stage T3b   37–61%
- Stage T4a (into prostate)   10%
- Stage TxN1–2   30%
- Salvage T0   70%
- Salvage T1   50%
- Salvage T2, 3a   25%

Muscle-invasive bladder cancer: radical and palliative radiotherapy

Radical external beam radiotherapy (RT)

This is a good option for treating muscle-invasive (pT2/3/4) UC in patients who are not healthy or unwilling to undergo cystectomy. The 5-year survival rates are inferior to those of surgery, but the bladder is preserved and the complications are less significant.

Typically, a total dose of 70 Gy is administered in 30 fractions over 6 weeks. Higher-grade tumors tend to do less well, perhaps because of the undetected presence of disease outside the field of irradiation. Beyond this, prediction of radiotherapy response remains difficult, relying on follow-up cystoscopy and biopsy. CIS, SCC, and adenocarcinoma are poorly sensitive to radiotherapy.

Neoadjuvant or adjuvant cisplatin-based combination chemotherapy with RT is used in locally advanced (pT3b/4) disease (see p. 264) and is more commonly performed than RT monotherapy.

Complications

These occur in 70% of patients; they are self-limiting in 90% of cases. Complications include radiation cystitis (LUTS and dysuria) and proctitis (diarrhea and rectal bleeding). These effects usually last only a few months.

Refractory radiation cystitis and hematuria may rarely require measures such as intravesical alum, formalin, hyperbaric oxygen, iliac artery embolization, or even palliative cystectomy.

Efficacy of RT monotherapy

5-year survival rates are as follows:

- Stage T1   35%
- Stage T2   40%
- Stage T3a   35%
- Stage T3b, T4   20%
- Stage TxN1–2   7%

If disease persists or recurs, salvage cystectomy may still be successful in appropriately selected patients; 5-year survival rates are 30–50%.

Otherwise, cytotoxic chemotherapy (see p. 265) and palliative measures may be considered.

Palliative treatment

This includes radiotherapy for metastatic bone pain (30 Gy) or to palliate symptomatic local tumor (40–50 Gy). Intractable hematuria may be controlled by intravesical formalin or alum, hyperbaric oxygen, bilateral internal iliac artery embolization or ligation, or palliative cystectomy.

Ureteral obstruction may be relieved by percutaneous nephrostomy and antegrade stenting (see p. 456). Involvement of a palliative care team can be very helpful to the patient and family.

Muscle-invasive bladder cancer: management of locally advanced and metastatic disease

Locally advanced bladder cancer (pT3b/4)

Many patients treated with primary cystectomy or radiotherapy (RT) with curative intent succumb to metastatic disease due to incomplete tumor excision or micrometastases.

At this stage, 5-year survival is only 5–10%. There is interest in augmenting primary treatment in an effort to improve outcomes.

Neoadjuvant RT

Randomized studies have suggested improvements in local control using RT prior to cystectomy, but no survival benefit has been demonstrated.

Adjuvant RT

The rationale for post-cystectomy RT is that patients with proven residual or nodal disease may benefit from locoregional treatment. However, it leads to unacceptably high morbidity and has no demonstrable advantages. Post-treatment bowel obstruction occurs 4.5 times more commonly in RT patients.

Adjuvant cystectomy

Two studies have demonstrated an improvement in local control and a survival advantage when treating locally advanced disease with cystectomy after RT, compared to RT alone. However, this treatment strategy is associated with increased morbidity of surgery in this setting.

Neoadjuvant chemotherapy

Neoadjuvant chemotherapy with methotrexate, vinblastine, adriamycin, and cisplatin (MVAC) should be considered in all patients with muscle-invasive (T2–4a) disease. A randomized trial comparing the median survival among patients assigned to cystectomy alone was 46 months, compared with 77 months among patients assigned to 3 cycles of MVAC combined with cystectomy. Similar findings have been demonstrated using CMV chemotherapy.

For patients with localized disease, pathological complete response (P0) after chemotherapy results in a relapse-free survival at 5 years of 85%. For patients who do not have a complete response to therapy, patients treated with MVAC chemotherapy prior to cystectomy have similar survival rates to those with cystectomy alone.

Adjuvant chemotherapy

The rationale for post-cystectomy chemotherapy is that patients with proven residual or nodal disease may benefit from systemic treatment. Patients with T3–4a, or N+ disease are at high risk for relapse following radical cystectomy.

Adjuvant MVAC or gemcitabine/cisplatin can be considered, although there are no trials demonstrating a survival advantage for adjuvant therapy. Clinical trial enrollment should be encouraged.

Neoadjuvant or adjuvant chemotherapy with RT

The recent meta-analysis also showed a 5% survival advantage with the use of cisplatin-based combination chemotherapy when RT was used as definitive treatment. This may be offered to patients suspected of having locally advanced disease after clinical examination and staging imaging.

Metastatic bladder cancer

Systemic chemotherapy

This modality is routine for patients with unresectable, diffusely metastatic measurable disease. Complete responses are rare with single agents. When chemotherapeutic agents are combined, however, complete responses are observed.

The most active agents include cisplatin, taxanes (docetaxel, paclitaxel), gemcitabine, and cisplatin. Clinical trials have established the MVAC combination as the standard of care.[1] This multidrug treatment has been found to be superior to single-agent cisplatin, the combination of docetaxel and cisplatin, and the multidrug regimen CISCA. The median survival of patients treated with MVAC for metastatic disease is 14.2–16.1 months. Using MVAC, 20% of patients develop neutropenia and 3% die of sepsis.

Trials comparing gemcitabine combined with cisplatin to MVAC found similar survival rates. Gemcitabine/cisplatin-treated patients have significantly less neutropenia and fewer hospitalization days for treating infection. Gemcitabine/cisplatin is currently considered an alternative standard of care to MVAC.

Second-line therapy for patients who fail either gemcitabine cisplatin or MVAC is limited. Median time to progression is approximately 3 months, and median survival ranges between 6 and 9 months. Single-agent therapy is used over combination treatment since there are fewer toxicities.

Radiotherapy

Roles for RT include palliation of metastatic pain and spinal cord compression.

Surgery

There is no surgical role in treatment of extravesical metastatic disease. However, some publications suggest that surgical resection of metastatic lesions that have responded to chemotherapy can result in durable responses.

1 Sternberg CN (2007). Chemotherapy for bladder cancer: treatment guidelines for neoadjuvant chemotherapy, bladder preservation, adjuvant chemotherapy, and metastatic cancer. *Urology* 69(1 Suppl):62.

Bladder cancer: urinary diversion after cystectomy

Ureterosigmoidostomy

This is the oldest form of urinary diversion, whereby the ureters drain into the sigmoid colon, either in its native form or following its detubularization and reconstruction into a pouch (Mainz II). This diversion requires no appliance (stoma bag, catheter) so remains popular in developing countries.

In recreating a cloaca, the patient may be prone to upper UTI with the risk of long-term renal deterioration, metabolic hyperchloremic acidosis, and loose, frequent stools. The low-pressure and capacious Mainz II pouch reduces these complications.

There is a long-term risk of colon cancer with this type of diversion and it is not popular in the United States.

Ileal conduit

This was developed in 1950 and remains the most popular form of urinary diversion. A 15 cm segment of of subterminal ileum is isolated on its mesentery, the ureters are anastomosed to the proximal end, and the distal end is brought out in the right lower quadrant as a stoma. The ileum is anastomosed to gain enteral continuity (ileoileostomy).

Complications
- Prolonged ileus
- Urinary leak
- Enteral leak
- Pyelonephritis
- Ureteroileal stricture
- Stoma problems—skin irritation, stenosis, and parastomal hernia

Patients require stoma therapy support and some find difficulty in adjusting their lifestyle to cope with a stoma bag. Metabolic complications are uncommon.

In post-RT salvage patients, a jejunal or colonic conduit is used because of concerns about the healing of radiation-damaged ileum. The conduit may be brought out in the upper abdomen. Patients require careful electrolyte monitoring due to sodium loss and hyperkalemia.

Continent diversion

The advantage of such a diversion is the absence of an external collection device. A neobladder (pouch) is fashioned from 60–70 cm of detubularized ileum or right hemicolon. The ureters drain into the neobladder, usually through an anti-reflux submucosal tunnel. This may be drained by the patient via a catheterizable stoma, such as the appendix or uterine tube (the Mitrofanoff principle) brought out in the right iliac fossa.

Alternatively, the neobladder may be anastomosed to the patient's urethra so that natural voiding can be established. Patients void by relaxing their external sphincter and performing a Valsalva maneuver.

This orthotopic neobladder should require no catheter, unless the pouch is too large and fails to empty adequately. In this case, the patient must be prepared to perform intermittent self-catheterization. Initially, bladder irrigations once or twice a day are necessary because of mucous production that gradually diminishes with time.

Popular ileal pouches include those of Studer (Fig. 6.7), Camey II, and Kock; ileocecal pouches include the Indiana and Mainz I. The choice of pouch often comes down to the surgeon's preference; they all carry similar complication risks.

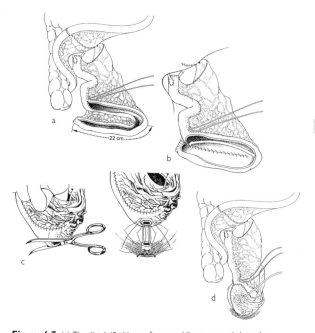

Figure 6.7 (a) The distal 40–44 cm of resected ileum opened along the antimesenteric border with scissors. Spatulated ureters are anastomosed end to side with 4–0 running suture on either side of proximal end of afferent tubular ileal limb. Ureters are stented. (b) The two medial borders of the U-shaped, opened, distal ileal segment are oversewn with a single-layer seromuscular continuous suture. The bottom of the U is folded between the two ends of the U. (c) Before complete closure of the reservoir, an 8–10 mm hole is cut into the most caudal part of the reservoir (**left**). Six sutures are placed between the seromuscular layer of the anastomotic area of the reservoir and the membranous urethra (**right**). An 18 Fr urethral catheter is inserted. (d) Before complete closure of the pouch, a cystostomy tube is inserted and brought out suprapubically adjacent to the wound. Reprinted with permission from Studer UE, Danuser H, Hochreiter W, et al. (1996). *World J Urol* 14(1):29–39.

Previously irradiated bowel can be cautiously used to form pouches, though complications are more likely. In orthotopic neobladders, incontinence is more common in men than in women, and women have a higher likelihood of being in retention and requiring long-term intermittent catheterization.

Complications relating to continent diversions and neobladders
- Urinary leakage and peritonitis
- Pelvic abscess
- Stone formation
- Catheterizing difficulties and stomal stenosis
- Urinary incontinence and nocturnal enuresis
- Pouch-ureteral reflux and UTI
- Uretero-pouch anastomotic stricture
- Late neobladder rupture

Metabolic abnormalities
These include early fluid and electrolyte imbalances. Later, urinary electrolyte absorption may cause hyperchloremic acidosis, and loss of the distal small bowel (distal 15 cm of ileum) may result in vitamin B_{12} deficiency. Metabolic acidosis is less likely in patients with normal renal function; treatment is with sodium bicarbonate and potassium citrate.

Annual B_{12} and CBC monitoring should be undertaken, with supplementation if necessary.

Adenocarcinoma
Adenocarcinoma may develop (5%) in diversions that involve a segment of colon. While more likely with ureterosigmoidostomy with constant contact of feces with the urinary stream, the cause is the carcinogenic bacterial metabolism of urinary nitrosamines.

This tends to occur near the inflow of urine. It is therefore advisable to perform annual visual surveillance of colon urinary diversions after 10 years. If the urethra is in situ, as with orthotopic neobladder, annual urethroscopy and cytology are suggested.

Transitional cell carcinoma (UC) of the renal pelvis and ureter

UC accounts for 90% of upper urinary tract tumors, the remainder being benign inverted papilloma, fibroepithelial polyp, squamous cell carcinoma (associated with longstanding calculus disease), adenocarcinoma (rare), and various rare nonurothelial tumors, including sarcoma.

- Renal pelvic UC is uncommon, accounting for 10% of renal tumors and 4% of all UC.
- Ureteral UC is rare, accounting for only 1% of all newly presenting UC. Half are multifocal; 75% are located distally; while only 3% are located in the proximal ureter.

Risk factors are similar to those for UC in the bladder (see p. 246).

- **Males** are affected three times more than females.
- Incidence increases with **age**.
- **Smoking** confers a two-fold risk, and there are various occupational causes.

UC does not have a genetic hereditary form, although there is a high incidence of upper tract UC in families from some villages in Balkan countries (Balkan nephropathy) that remains unexplained.

Pathology and staging

The tumor usually has a papillary structure, but occasionally it is solid. It is bilateral in 2–4%. It arises within the renal pelvis, less frequently in one of the calyces or ureter. Histologically, features of UC are present, described below. Staging is by the TNM classification. Spread is by

- Direct extension, including into the renal vein and vena cava
- Lymphatic spread to para-aortic, paracaval, and pelvic nodes
- Blood-borne spread, most commonly to liver, lung, and bone

Presentation

- Painless hematuria (80%)
- Flank pain (30%), often caused by clots passing down the ureter ("clot colic")
- Associated with synchronous bladder UC (4%)
- At follow-up, ~50% of patients will develop a metachronous bladder UC and 2% will develop contralateral upper tract UC

Investigations

Diagnosis is usually made on urine cytology and IVP or CTU, respectively, revealing malignant cells and a filling defect in the renal pelvis or ureter. If doubt exists, selective ureteral urine cytology, retrograde pyeloureterography, or flexible ureteroscopy are indicated.

If ultrasound and cystoscopy are normal during the investigation of hematuria, an IVP or CT is recommended. Staging imaging is obtained by contrast-enhanced abdominal CT, chest X-ray, and, occasionally, isotope bone scan.

Staging is by the TNM (2002) classification (see Table 6.10) following histological confirmation of the diagnosis. All cases rely on physical examination and imaging, the pathological classification corresponding to the TNM categories See Box 6.4 for corresponding 5-year survival rates.

Treatment and prognosis

Nephroureterectomy

If staging indicates nonmetastatic disease in the presence of a normal contralateral kidney, the gold-standard treatment with curative intent is nephroureterectomy, open or laparoscopic.

The open approach uses either a long transperitoneal midline incision or separate flank and iliac fossa incisions. The entire ureter is taken with a cuff of bladder, because of the 50% incidence of subsequent ureteral stump recurrence. Follow-up should include annual cystoscopy and IVP or CTU to detect metachronous UC development.

Table 6.10 TNM staging of carcinomas of the renal pelvis and ureter

Tx	Primary tumor cannot be assessed
T0	No evidence of primary tumor
Ta	Noninvasive papillary carcinoma
Tis	Carcinoma in situ
T1	Tumor invades subepithelial connective tissue
T2	Tumor invades muscularis propria
T3	Tumor invades beyond muscularis propria into perinephric or periureteral fat or renal parenchyma
T4	Tumor invades adjacent organs or through kidney into perinephric fat
Nx	Regional (para-aortic) lymph nodes cannot be assessed
N0	No regional lymph node metastasis
N1	Metastasis in a single lymph node <2 cm
N2	Metastasis in a single lymph node 2–5 cm or multiple nodes <5 cm
N3	Metastasis in a single lymph or multiple nodes >5 cm
Mx	Distant metastasis cannot be assessed
M0	No distant metastasis
M1	Distant metastasis present

Box 6.4 5-year survival

• Organ-confined disease	T1,2	60–100%
• Locally advanced	T3,4	20–50%
• Node-positive disease	N+	15%
• Pulmonary, bone metastases	M+	10%

Multiple techniques for laparoscopic management of the distal ureter have been described, including pure laparoscopic, endoscopic through the bladder, and open resection of the distal ureter after laparoscopic dissection of the kidney and ureter.

Percutaneous/ureteroscopic resection/ablation

For patients with a single functioning kidney or bilateral disease, or those who are unfit, percutaneous or ureteroscopic resection or ablation of the tumor are the minimally invasive options. Topical chemotherapy (e.g., mitomycin C) may subsequently be instilled through the nephrostomy or ureteral catheters. This nephron-sparing approach is less likely to be curative than definitive surgery.

Systemic combination chemotherapy for unresectable or metastatic disease using cyclophosphamide, methotrexate, and vincristine is associated with a 30% total or partial response at the expense of moderate toxicity.

Palliative surgery or arterial embolization may be necessary for troublesome hematuria.

Radiotherapy is generally ineffective.

Radiological assessment of renal masses

Abdominal ultrasound

This is considered by many to be the first-line investigation for a patient with flank pain or a suspected renal mass. The size resolution for renal masses is 1.5 cm, exhibiting variable echo patterns.

Ultrasound may also detect renal cysts, most of which are simple: smooth-walled, round or oval, without internal echoes and complete transmission with a strong acoustic shadow posteriorly. If the cyst has a solid intracystic element, septations, or an irregular or calcified wall, further imaging with CT is indicated.

CT scan

If a renal mass is detected, a thin-slice CT scan before and after contrast is the most important investigation. In general, any solid-enhancing renal mass is considered a renal carcinoma until proven otherwise. Even relatively avascular renal carcinomas enhance by 10–25 Hounsfield units.[1]

Occasionally, an isodense but enhancing area of kidney is demonstrated ("pseudotumor") and may correspond to a harmless hypertrophied cortical column (of Bertin) or a dysmorphic renal segment. CT may mislead with respect to liver invasion (rare) because of "partial volume effect"; real-time ultrasound is more accurate. Lymphadenopathy >2 cm is highly indicative of metastases, but occasionally can be inflammatory or due to another process such as lymphoma.

Bosniak developed a radiological classification of renal cysts (Table 6.11).[2] The classification is based on homogeneity and complexity of cystic fluid, presence or absence of septations, calcifications, or solid components; and the density of cystic fluid is determined by Hounsfield units. Hounsfield units are a measure of X-ray attenuation applied to CT scanning: –1000 units equate with air, 0 units equate with water, and +1000 equate with bone.

MRI with gadolinium contrast may be used for imaging the inferior vena cava or renal vein (MRV), locally advanced disease, or renal insufficiency, or for patients allergic to iodinated contrast. Renal arteriography is seldom used in the diagnostic setting but may be helpful to delineate the number and position of renal arteries in preparation for nephron-sparing surgery or surgery for horseshoe kidneys.

Nephrogenic systemic fibrosis (NSF) is a scleroderma-like skin disease that affects patients with renal insufficiency. There is a strong association with the development of NSF and exposure to gadolinium contrast agents used in performing MRI. Therefore, in patients with GFRs <30 mL/min/1.73 m^2, these agents should not be used.

Fine needle aspiration/needle biopsy

Ultrasound or CT-guided fine needle aspiration (FNA) or needle biopsy in the investigation of renal masses is of limited value because of the better accuracy of modern cross-sectional imaging, false-negative biopsy results

1 Barbaric ZL. (1994). Principles of Genitourinary Radiology. 2nd Edn. Thieme Medical Publishers: New York.
2 Israel GM, Bosniak MA (2005). An update of the Bosniak renal cyst classification system. *Urology* 66(3):484–488.

(5–15%), and risks of hemorrhage (5%) and tumor spillage (rare). FNA is useful for aspiration of renal abscess or an infected cyst, or to diagnose suspected lymphoma or metastatic lesions.

Table 6.12 provides a practical radiological classification of renal masses.

Table 6.11 Bosniak renal cyst classification system based on CT findings

I	Benign simple cysts; thin wall without septa, calcifications, or solid components, water density and no contrast enhancement. No further imaging is needed.
II	Benign cysts with a few thin septa; the wall or septa may contain fine calcification and sharp margins; they are non-enhancing, and usually <3 cm.
IIF	Well marginated and may have thin septa or minimal smooth thickening of the septa or wall, which may contain calcification that may also be thick and nodular; no contrast enhancement. Includes totally intrarenal non-enhancing lesions > 3 cm. These require follow-up (designated by the *F* designation).
III	Indeterminate cysts with thickened irregular or smooth walls or septa; enhancement present. 40–60% are malignant (cystic renal cell carcinoma and multiloculated cystic renal cell carcinoma). Other class III lesions are benign and include hemorrhagic cysts, infected cysts, and multiloculated cystic nephroma. Surgery is recommended, although additional imaging by MRI or with biopsy is supported by some clinicians.
IV	Risk of malignancy is 85–100%. Characteristics of category III cysts plus they contain contrast-enhancing soft-tissue components that are adjacent to and independent of the wall or septum. Surgery is recommended.

Table 6.12 Classification of renal masses by radiographic appearance

Simple cyst	Complex cyst	Fatty mass	Others (excluding very rare lesions)
Cyst	Renal carcinoma	Angiomyo-lipoma	Renal cell carcinoma
Multiple cysts	Cystic nephroma	Lipoma	Metastasis
Parapelvic cyst	Hemorrhagic cyst	Liposarcoma	Lymphoma
Calyceal diverticulum	Metastasis; Wilms tumor		Sarcoma Abscess
	Infected cyst		Tuberculosis
	Lymphoma		Oncocytoma
	Tuberculosis		Xanthogranulomatous pyelonephritis
	Renal artery aneurysm		Pheochromocytoma (adrenal)
	Arteriovenous malformation		Wilms tumor (p. 328)
	Hydrocalyx		Transitional cell carcinoma

Benign renal masses

The most common (70%) are simple cysts, present in >50% of >50-year-olds. Rarely symptomatic, treatment by aspiration or laparoscopic unroofing is seldom considered.

Most benign renal tumors are rare; the two most clinically important are oncocytoma and angiomyolipoma. Solid masses <2.0 cm are benign in up to 30% of cases, therefore a period of observation is reasonable as many of these may not grow, especially in older or debilitated patients.

Oncocytoma

This is uncommon, accounting for 3–7% of renal tumors. Males are twice as commonly affected as females. They occur simultaneously with renal cell carcinoma in 7–32% of cases.

Pathology

Oncocytomas are spherical, capsulated, and brown/tan in color, with a mean size of 4–6 cm. Half contain a central scar. They may be multifocal and bilateral (4–13%) and 10–20% extend into perinephric fat.

Histologically, they comprise aggregates of eosinophilic cells, packed with mitochondria. Mitoses are rare and they are considered benign, not known to metastasize.

It is often difficult to distinguish oncocytoma from chromophobe RCC. There is often loss of the Y chromosome.

Presentation

Oncocytomas often (83%) present as an incidental finding, or with flank pain or hematuria.

Investigations

Oncocytoma cannot often be distinguished radiologically from RCCs; it may coexist with RCC. Rarely, they exhibit a spoke-wheel pattern on CT scanning, caused by a stellate central scar. Percutaneous biopsy is not recommended since it often leads to continuing uncertainty about the diagnosis.

Treatment

Partial nephrectomy (open or laparoscopic) is indicated whenever technically feasible, based on lesion size and location. Radical nephrectomy is rarely indicated unless the lesion is very large and partial nephrectomy is not possible or diagnosis is uncertain. Ablation is used in selected cases.

No aggressive follow-up is usually necessary.

Angiomyolipoma (AML)

Eighty percent of these benign clonal neoplasms (hamartomas) occur sporadically, mostly in middle-aged females. 20% are in association with tuberous sclerosis (TS)—an autosomal dominant syndrome characterized by mental retardation, epilepsy, adenoma sebaceum, and other hamartomas.

Half of TS patients develop AMLs. The mean age is 30 years, and 66% of patients are female. Frequently, AMLs are multifocal and bilateral.

Pathology

AML is composed of blood vessels, smooth muscle, and fat. They are always considered benign, although extrarenal AMLs have been reported in venous system and hilar lymph nodes. Macroscopically, it looks like a well-circumscribed lump of fat. Solitary AMLs are more frequently found in the right kidney.

HMB-45 is a monoclonal antibody against a melanoma-associated antigen seen in AML and can differentiate cases from other renal cortical neoplasms.

Presentation

AMLs frequently present as incidental findings (>50%) on ultrasound or CT scans. They may present with flank pain, palpable mass, or painless hematuria. Massive and life-threatening retroperitoneal bleeding occurs in up to 10% of cases (Wunderlich syndrome).

Pregnant women appear to be at an increased risk for hemorrhage.

Investigations

Ultrasound reflects from fat, hence it has a characteristic bright echo pattern. This does not cast an acoustic shadow beyond, helping to distinguish an AML from a calculus. CT shows fatty tumor as low-density (Hounsfield units <10) in 86% of AMLs. If the proportion of fat is low, a definite diagnosis cannot be made.

Measurement of the diameter is relevant to treatment. On MRI, adipose tissue has high signal intensity on T_1-weighted images and lower on T_2-weighted images

Treatment

In studies, 52–82% of patients with AML >4 cm are symptomatic compared with only 23% with smaller tumors. Therefore, asymptomatic AMLs can be followed with serial ultrasound if <4 cm, while those bleeding or >4 cm should be treated surgically or by embolization.

Emergency nephrectomy or selective renal artery embolization may be life saving. In patients with TS, in whom multiple bilateral lesions are present, conservative treatment should be attempted.

Renal cell carcinoma: epidemiology and etiology

Renal cell carcinoma (RCC)—also known as hypernephroma (since it was erroneously believed to originate in the adrenal gland), clear cell carcinoma, and Grawitz tumor—is an adenocarcinoma. It is the most common of renal tumors, accounting for 85% of renal malignancies and 2% of all cancer deaths.

In the United States, 57,760 patients were diagnosed in 2009 and 12,980 patients died of RCC. RCC is the considered the most lethal of all urological tumors, approximately 40% of patients dying of the condition. Incidence has increased since the 1980s, when imaging such as ultrasound and CT scanning became more commonplace to investigate nonspecific abdominal symptoms.

The size of the masses has also decreased with time as more and more masses are discovered incidentally. It occurs in sporadic (common) and hereditary (rare) forms.

Etiology

Males are affected twice as commonly as females. Peak incidence of sporadic RCC is the sixth to eighth decade.

Environmental

Studies have shown associations with the following:

- Analgesic phenacetin use
- Asbestos exposure
- Family history in a first- or second-degree relative (relative risk of 2.9)
- Hypertension (1.4- to 2-fold risk)
- Low socioeconomic status
- Obesity
- Renal failure and dialysis (30-fold risk)
- Smoking cigarettes, pipe, or cigars (1.4- to 2.3-fold increased risk smoking cessation can reduce the relative risk by 20–50%)
- Tobacco chewing
- Urban dwelling

Nutrition is considered important: Asian migrants to Western countries are at increased risk of RCC; vitamins A, C, E, and fruit and vegetable consumption are protective.

Anatomical risk factors include polycystic and horseshoe kidneys.

Genetics

Clear cell renal cell carcinoma

This is associated with deletion of chromosome 3p and/or mutations of the VHL gene.

Von Hippel–Lindau (VHL) syndrome

Half of individuals with this autosomal dominant syndrome, characterized by pheochromocytoma, renal and pancreatic cysts, and cerebellar hemangioblastoma, develop RCC, often bilateral and multifocal. Patients typically present in third, fourth, or fifth decades.

VHL syndrome occurs from loss of both copies of a tumor suppressor gene at chromosome 3p25–26; this and other genes on 3p are also implicated in causing the common sporadic form of RCC.

Inactivation of the VHL gene leads to effects on gene transcription, including dysregulation of hypoxia inducible factor 1 (HIF-1), an intracellular protein that plays an important role in the cellular response to hypoxia and starvation. This results in up-regulation of vascular endothelial growth factor (VEGF), the most prominent angiogenic factor in RCC, which is why some RCCs are highly vascular.

Chromophobe RCC is a result of loss of chromosome 17.

Non-hereditary papillary RCC is linked with changes in both chromosome 7 and 17.

Hereditary papillary RCC (HPRCC)
HPRCC arises from mutation and activation of the met proto-oncogene on chromosome 7p34 and has an autosomal dominant familial component. c-MET encodes the receptor tyrosine kinase for hepatocyte growth factor, which regulates epithelial proliferation and differentiation in a wide variety of organs, including the normal kidney.

Birt-Hogg-Dubé (BHD) syndrome
This is a rare, autosomal dominant disorder caused by germ-line mutations in the BHD (FLCN) gene within the chromosomal band 17p11.2 and encodes for a tumor-suppressor protein, folliculin. BHD syndrome is characterized by the cutaneous triad of fibrofolliculomas (hamartoma of the hair follicle), trichodiscomas, and skin tags, along with a propensity for renal tumors.

The renal tumors are often chromophobe RCC or oncocytoma or hybrids of these tumors. A substantial number of patients will develop clear cell tumors as well. These tumors are more likely to be multiple and bilateral.

Renal cell carcinoma: pathology, staging, and prognosis

RCC is adenocarcinoma of the renal cortex, believed to arise from proximal convoluted tubule. It is usually tan colored and solid; 7–20% are multifocal, 10–20% contain calcification, and 10–25% contain cysts or are predominantly cystic. Smaller lesions are rarely grossly infiltrative. They are usually circumscribed by a pseudocapsule of compressed tissue.

Spread
- By direct extension to adrenal gland (7.5% in tumors >5 cm), through the renal capsule, into the renal vein (5% at presentation), inferior vena cava (IVC), right atrium
- By lymphatics to hilar and para-aortic lymph nodes
- Hematogenous to lung (75%), bone (20%), liver (18%), and brain (8%).

Histological classification of RCC
- **Conventional** (70–80%): arise from the proximal tubule; highly vascular; cells clear (glycogen, cholesterol) or granular (eosinophilic cytoplasm, mitochondria)
- **Papillary** (10–15%): papillary, tubular, and solid variants; 40% multifocal; small incidental tumors could equate with Bell's legendary "benign adenoma"
- **Chromophobe** (5%): arises from the cortical portion of the collecting duct; possess a perinuclear halo of microvesicles
- **Collecting duct (Bellini)**: rare; young patients; poor prognosis
- **Medullary cell**: rare; arises from calyceal epithelium; young, Black, sickle-cell sufferers; poor prognosis

The term *sarcomatoid* is used to describe an infiltrative, poorly differentiated variant of any type.

Genetic changes associated with RCC are described on p. 278. RCC is an unusually immunogenic tumor. Reports of spontaneous regression, prolonged stabilization, and complete responses to immunotherapy support this. RCC is also unusually vascular, overexpressing angiogenic factors, principally VEGF but also basic FGF and TGF-α.

Grading is by the Fuhrman system (1 = well-differentiated; 2 = moderately differentiated; 3 and 4 = poorly differentiated) based on nuclear size, outline, and nucleoli.

Staging is by the TNM (2002) classification following histological confirmation of the diagnosis (see Fig. 6.8 and Table 6.13). All cases rely on physical examination and imaging; the pathological classification (prefixed *p*) corresponds to the TNM categories. Staging is the most important prognostic indicator for RCC (see Box 6.5). Fuhrman grade and histological subtypes are also important.

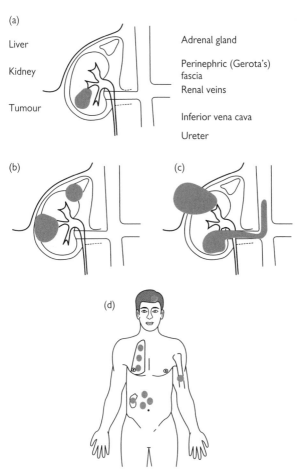

Figure 6.8 Renal cell carcinoma staging. (a) Primary tumor is limited to kidney (T1/T2). T1a is <4 cm and T1b is >4 cm but not >7 cm. T2 is >7 cm. (b) Primary tumor invades perinephric tissue but not beyond perinephric fascia or invades adrenal gland (T3a). (c) Primary tumor extends into renal veins or IVC below the diaphragm (T3b); above the diaphragm into right atrium or invades wall of vena cava (T3c); or outside perinephric fascia (e.g., into liver, bowel, or posterior abdominal wall) (T4). (d) N and M staging: involves multiple para-aortic or paracaval nodes; pulmonary, bone, or brain metastases (T1–4N2M1).

Box 6.5 Prognosis—5-year survival

• Organ-confined	T1a	90–100%
	T1b	80–90%
	T2	70–80%
• Capsular transgression/adrenal	T3a	60–70%
• Renal vein or IVC thrombus	T3b/c	50–80% (25% with IVC wall invasion)
• Visceral/lymph node involvement	T4 or N+	5–30%
• Distant metastasis	M+	5–100%

Nomograms have been developed to predict risk of recurrence

Reprinted with permission from Kattan MW, Reuter V, Motzer RJ, Katz J, Russo P. (2001). *J Urol* 166(1): 63–67.

Table 6.13 TNM staging of RCC

Tx	Primary tumor cannot be assessed
T0	No evidence of primary tumor
T1	Tumor <7 cm, limited to the kidney
T1a	Tumor is 4 cm or less, limited to kidney
T1b	Tumor >4 cm but <7 cm, limited to kidney
T2	Tumor >7 cm, limited to the kidney
T3	Tumor extends outside the kidney, but not beyond Gerota's (perinephric) fascia
T3a	Tumor invades adrenal gland or perinephric fat
T3b	Tumor grossly extends into renal vein or subdiaphragmatic IVC
T3c	Tumor grossly extends into supradiaphragmatic IVC or heart; invades wall of vena cava
T4	Tumor invades beyond Gerota's fascia
Nx	Regional (para-aortic) lymph nodes cannot be assessed
N0	No regional lymph node metastasis
N1	Metastasis in a single regional node
N2	Metastasis in 2 or more regional nodes
Mx	Distant metastasis cannot be assessed
M0	No distant metastasis
M1	Distant metastasis present

Renal cell carcinoma: presentation and investigations

More than 50% of RCCs are now detected incidentally on abdominal imaging carried out to investigate vague or unrelated symptoms. Thus, the stage at diagnosis of RCC is lower than it was because of widespread use of imaging modalities.

Presentation

Of the symptomatic RCCs diagnosed, 50% of patients present with hematuria, 40% with flank pain, 30% of patients notice a mass, and 25% have symptoms or signs of metastatic disease (night sweats, fever, fatigue, weight loss, hemoptysis).

Less than 10% patients exhibit the classic triad of hematuria, flank pain, and mass. Less common presenting features include acute varicocele due to obstruction of the testicular vein by tumor within the left renal vein (5%) and lower limb edema due to venous obstruction.

Paraneoplastic syndromes due to ectopic hormone secretion by the tumor occur in 10–40% of patients; these may be associated with any disease stage (Table 6.14).

Investigations

- Radiological evaluation of hematuria, flank pain, and renal masses is described on p. 5.
- Needle biopsy of renal masses is not recommended, since the result may be misleading and complications include hemorrhage and seeding of the biopsy tract.
- Urine cytology and culture should be normal.
- Full blood count may reveal polycythemia or anemia.
- Serum creatinine and electrolytes, calcium, and liver function tests are essential.

When RCC is diagnosed radiologically, staging chest CT and bone scan (if clinically indicated) will follow. Any suggestion of renal vein or IVC involvement on CT may be further investigated with MRI.

Angiography may be helpful in planning partial nephrectomy or surgery for horseshoe kidneys. Contralateral kidney function is assessed by uptake and excretion of CT contrast and the serum creatinine. If doubt persists, an isotope renogram is obtained.

Table 6.14 Paraneoplastic syndromes

Syndrome associated with RCC	Cause
Anemia	Hematuria, chronic disease
Polycythemia	Ectopic secretion of erythropoietin
Hypertension (25%)	Ectopic secretion of renin, renal artery compression, or AV fistula
Hypoglycemia	Ectopic secretion of insulin
Cushing	Ectopic secretion of ACTH
Hypercalcemia (10–20%)	Ectopic secretion of parathyroid hormone–like substance
Gynecomastia, amenorrhea, reduced libido, baldness	Ectopic secretion of gonadotrophins
Stauffer syndrome: hepatic dysfunction (increased liver function testing), fever, anorexia	Unknown; resolves in 60–70% of patients post-nephrectomy

Renal cell carcinoma: active surveillance

Surveillance of localized renal tumors is now performed more often in carefully selected patients. For incidental stage T1 renal masses, prolonged follow-up will be necessary, similar to that for low-risk prostate cancer. There are no currently established protocols.

Active surveillance is a reasonable option for patients with limited life expectancy or for those who are unfit for or do not desire intervention, especially those with T1a renal masses (<4 cm). These masses grow slowly growth and very infrequently progress to metastasis.[1]

The patient should be counseled about the small risk of cancer progression, possible loss of window of opportunity for nephron-sparing surgery, lack of curative salvage therapies if metastases develop, limitations of renal mass biopsy, and deficiencies of the current literature.

1 AUA Guideline for Management of the Clinical Stage 1 Renal Mass (2009). Available at: www. auanet.org/content/guidelines

Renal cell carcinoma: surgical treatment I

Surgery is the mainstay of treatment for RCC. Increases in diagnosis of smaller early-stage RCC and the concept of cytoreductive surgery for advanced disease has affected surgical treatment strategies of the disease, while the absolute reduction in mortality remains elusive.

Localized disease—radical nephrectomy

Open approach

This remains the gold-standard curative treatment of localized RCC, however, properly performed laparoscopic techniques are becoming the "new" standard at many centers. The aim is to excise the kidney with the perinephris (Gerota fascia), perhaps with ipsilateral adrenal gland (for tumors >5 cm, upper pole tumors, or with evidence of adrenal invasion) and regional nodes (controversial), removing all tumor with adequate surgical margins.

Surgical approach is usually transperitoneal (subcostal, midline), which provides good access to hilar and major vessels, or thoracoabdominal (for very large or T3c tumors). Smaller masses can be approached retroperitoneally through a flank incision.

Following renal mobilization, the ureter is divided. Ligation and division of the renal artery or arteries should ideally take place prior to ligation as well as division of the renal vein to prevent vascular swelling of the kidney. If present, excision of hilar or para-aortic or paracaval lymph nodes will improve pathological tumor staging (for adequate TNM classification at least 8 nodes are necessary, but nodes may not be easily identified).

Complications include mortality up to 2% from bleeding or embolism of tumor thrombus; and bowel, pancreatic, splenic, or pleural injury.

Laparoscopic approach

Well accepted for treating benign disease, this approach is becoming commonplace for larger renal masses as experience increases. Masses of up to 10–12 cm can usually be removed by this approach, with larger masses requiring advanced skills.

Approaches are either transperitoneal or retroperitoneal, using straight laparoscopic technique or hand-assisted laparoscopic technique.

The specimen should be removed whole in a bag through the hand port or similar-sized (7–8 cm) lower abdominal incision; morcellation interferes with complete pathologic evaluation.

Advantages over open surgery include less pain, reduced hospital stay, and quicker return to normal activity.

Morbidity is reported in 8–38% of cases, including pulmonary embolism. Long-term (10-year) results demonstrate similar outcomes for both laparoscopic and open techniques.

Localized disease—partial nephrectomy

Nephron-sparing surgery is the best option for multifocal, bilateral tumors, particularly if the patient has VHL syndrome or single functioning kidney when the prospect of renal replacement therapy looms. It has become acceptable to treat small (<4 cm) tumors, even with a normal contralateral kidney, unless the tumor is close to the pelvicaliceal or hilar vessels. Arteriography or three-dimensional CT/MRI reconstructions are helpful to the surgeon.

Open transperitoneal or flank approaches are used; laparoscopic partial nephrectomy is now standard at most U.S. centers. The renal artery is clamped and, if the procedure is expected to last >30 minutes, the kidney packed with crushed ice for open procedures. "Enucleation" of masses <4 cm with a rim of normal tissue is also acceptable.

Results of partial nephrectomy performed laparoscopically are comparable to those with open surgery and should be considered for patients with small peripheral lesions who otherwise meet the criteria for open partial nephrectomy.

Specific complications include failure of complete excision of the tumor(s) leading to local recurrence in up to 10% of cases, and urinary leak from the collecting system.

Postoperative follow-up

The aim is to detect local or distant recurrence (incidence is 7% for T1N0M0, 20% for T2N0M0, and 40% for T3N0M0) to permit additional treatment if indicated. After partial nephrectomy, concern will also focus on recurrence in the remnant kidney.

There is no consensus regarding the optimal regimen; typically, it includes stage-dependent 6-month clinical assessment and annual CT imaging of chest and abdomen for 3–10 years.

Localized disease—tumor ablation therapy

Given the relatively benign nature and progression of the small renal mass, the increase in detection of these smaller lesions of the kidney and the improvements in technological ablative therapies have become more frequently employed. These technologies include thermal ablation by heating (radiofrequency ablation, or RFA) and cryotherapy and may be accomplished by open, laparoscopic, or percutaneous approaches.

According to the AUA 2009 guidelines,[1] "ongoing concerns include increased local recurrence rates when compared to surgical excision, controversy about radiographic parameters of success and difficulty with surgical salvage if required. Nevertheless, even in their current iteration, cryoablation and RFA represent valid treatment alternatives for many older patients or those with substantial comorbidities, presuming judicious patient selection and thorough patient counseling."

In series reviewed to date, cryoablation is associated with a lower rate of incomplete ablation (4.8%) than RFA (14.2%).

Technologies that employ novel techniques (HIFU, radiosurgical ablation ["Cyberknife", others]) and microwave and laser interstitial therapy remain investigational.

---

1 AUA Guidelines for Management of the Clinical Stage 1 Renal Mass. (2009). AUAnet.org.

Renal cell carcinoma: surgical treatment II

Localized RCC—lymphadenectomy

Lymph node involvement in RCC is a poor prognostic factor. Incidence ranges from 6% in T1–2 tumors, 46% in T3a, to 62–66% in higher-stage disease.

Lymphadenectomy at the time of nephrectomy may add prognostic information, especially if there is obvious lymphadenopathy, but therapeutic benefit remains unclear. Formal lymphadenectomy adds time and increases blood loss, while nodes are clear in about 95% of cases.

Localized RCC—treatment of local recurrence

Though uncommon, if there is local recurrence in the renal bed after radical nephrectomy, surgical excision remains the preferred treatment choice, provided there are no signs of distant disease. Local recurrence is more common after partial nephrectomy, where it can be treated by a further partial or total nephrectomy.

While radiation therapy can palliate distant metastasis, it is not considered to be effective in local recurrences.

Locally advanced RCC

Disease involving the IVC right atrium, liver, bowel, or posterior abdominal wall demands special surgical skills. In appropriate patients, an aggressive surgical approach involving a multidisciplinary surgical team to achieve negative margins appears to provide survival benefit.

Adjuvant treatment

Early studies suggested a role for preoperative RT, though recent studies have failed to show a survival benefit for either pre- or postoperative RT. It may retard growth of residual tumor after nephrectomy, but toxicity is high.

Randomized trials of adjuvant immunotherapy vs. observation alone and the use of the new tyrosine kinase inhibitors are ongoing for patients with large tumors, positive nodes, surgical margins, and venous invasion.

Metastatic RCC

Nephrectomy has long been indicated for palliation of symptoms (pain, hematuria) in patients with metastatic RCC (if inoperable, arterial embolization can be helpful).

A recent study demonstrated a median survival benefit of 10 months for patients with good performance status treated with cytoreductive nephrectomy prior to immunotherapy (interferon α-2B) and has further expanded the indications for surgery in RCC.[1]

Resection of solitary metastases is an option after nephrectomy and can extend survival.

1 Flanigan RC et al. (2001). Nephrectomy followed by interferon alfa-2b compared with interferon alfa-2b alone for metastatic renal-cell cancer. *N Engl J Med.* 345(23):1655–1659.

Renal cell carcinoma: management of metastatic disease

Surgery

Approximately 25–30%of patients with RCC exhibit metastatic disease at presentation; 20–30% progress subsequently to this stage following nephrectomy.

Metastatic RCC is defined as tumor spread to one regional lymph node <2 cm (N1), or more than a single regional lymph node (N2). Distant metastatic sites (M1) include lung, liver, bone subcutaneous sites, and central nervous system. The prognosis is poor, so despite the rare possibility of spontaneous metastatic regression following nephrectomy, it was not usually undertaken except to relieve local symptoms of pain or hematuria.

The case for nephrectomy in metastatic RCC has reopened, as discussed on p. 290. Metastasectomy may be of benefit to the 1.5–3% of patients who develop a solitary metastasis (particularly in lung, adrenal, or brain) following nephrectomy.

Hormone therapy and cytoxic chemotherapy have little role in RCC.

Radiotherapy is useful for palliation of metastatic lesions in bone and brain, and in combination with surgery for spinal cord compression.

Immunotherapy

Responses are more likely in patients with good performance status, prior nephrectomy, and small-volume metastatic burden.

IL-2 (Aldesleukin)

IL-2 is the only agent shown to produce complete and durable responses in 6–8% of patients, with partial responses in 10–15%. A typical high-dose (bolus) is 600,000–720,000 IU/kg IV q8h for 5 days. It is usually given as several cycles.

Significant toxicity includes fever, chills, nausea, vomiting, hypotension, arrhythmias, and metabolic acidosis. Low-dose IL-2 is an alternative regimen to reduce toxicity.

Varying regimens are reported, generally 10% of a high-dose regimen administered as an outpatient.

Interferon A-2b

This offers a complete response of 1% and a partial-response rate of 10–15%. Varying regimens are described.

The SWOG Intergroup regimen for interferon α-2b is induction of 1.25 million IU m^2 to 5 million IU m^2 over 3 days and continued at 5 million IU m^2 Monday, Wednesday, and Friday until progression.

The dose is modified on the basis of toxicity, which can include hematological and hepatic symptoms, diarrhea, anorexia, and hypotension.

Molecular targeted therapies

The model for molecular targeted therapy in urology is highlighted by the development of new targeted therapies based on the molecular biology of RCC.[1]

- Sunitinib targets VEGF receptor tyrosine kinase and other pathways and is FDA approved for treatment of metastatic clear cell carcinoma. In RCC, a 30% partial-response rate is noted, with a 6-month improvement in progression-free survival, although, no complete responses are reported. The dose is 50 mg PO qd × 4 weeks of a 6-week cycle (4 weeks on, 2 weeks off). Noteworthy are reports of microangiopathic hemolytic anemia (MAHA) when used with bevacizumab.
- Sorafenib targets multiple tryosine kinases (VEGF receptor PDGF) receptor, fibroblast growth factor receptor-1 [FGFR-1], others). It is FDA approved for metastatic clear cell RCC at a dose of 400 mg PO bid.
- Temsirolimus is FDA approved for first-line therapy in poor-risk patients and offers approximately a 3-month improvement in survival. It is a parenteral rapamycin analogue that inhibits mTOR kinase given at a dose 25 mg IV weekly (premedicate with diphenhydramine 25–50 mg IV).
- Everolimus is approved for advanced RCC after failure of sunitinib or sorafenib. It is an mTOR (mammalian target of rapamycin) inhibitor dosed at 10 mg PO daily.
- Bevacizumab is a VEGF inhibitor given at 10 mg/kg IV every 2 weeks. It is not currently FDA approved for RCC.

Palliative care

Medications such as megestrol acetate (40–320 mg/day divided dose) or steroids (e.g., dexamethasone 4 mg daily) improve appetite and mental state, but are unlikely to have an impact on tumor growth.

The involvement of multidisciplinary uro-oncology, palliative, and primary care teams is essential to support these patients and their relatives.

1 Basso M, Cassano A, Barone C (2010). A survey of therapy for advanced renal cell carcinoma. *Urol Oncol*. 28(2):121–133.

Testicular cancer: epidemiology and etiology

Incidence and mortality

Primary testicular cancer (TC) is the most common solid cancer in men ages 20–45 years; it is rare below age 15 years and above 60 years. Constituting 1–2% of all male cancers, the lifetime risk of developing testicular cancer is 1 in 500. It is also considered the most curable cancer.

There were 8400 U.S. cases in 2009 but only 380 deaths. It is apparently increasing in incidence; it is reported to affect 7 per 100,000 men.

Public health campaigns encouraging testicular self-examination (TSE) for young men are ongoing in countries such as England.

Epidemiology and etiology

- *Age:* the most commonly affected age group is 20–45 years, with germ cell tumors; teratomas are more common at ages 20–35, while seminoma is more common at ages 35–45 years. Rarely, infants and boys below age 10 years develop yolk sac tumors, and 50% of men >60 years with TC have lymphoma.
- *Race:* White people are three times more likely to develop TC than are Black people in the United States.
- *Cryptorchidism:* 10% of TC cases occur in undescended testes: the risk increases by 3–14 times compared to men with normally descended testes. Ultrastructural changes are present in these testes by age 3 years, although earlier orchidopexy does not completely eliminate the risk of developing TC. 5–10% of patients with a cryptorchid testis develop malignancy in the normally descended contralateral testis.
- *Intratubular germ cell neoplasia (IGCN)* is synonymous with carcinoma in situ, although the disease arises from malignant change in spermatogonia. 50% of cases develop invasive germ cell TC within 5 years. The population incidence is 0.8%. Risk factors include cryptorchidism, extragonadal germ cell tumor, previous or contralateral TC (5%), atrophic contralateral testis, 45XO karyotype, and infertility.
- *Human immunodeficiency virus (HIV)* patients infected with the HIV virus are developing seminoma more frequently than expected.
- *Genetic factors* appear to play a role, given that first-degree relatives are at higher risk, but a defined familial inheritance pattern is not apparent.
- *Maternal estrogen ingestion* during pregnancy increases the risk of cryptorchidism and TC in the male offspring.

Trauma and viral-induced atrophy have not been convincingly implicated as risk factors for TC.

Bilateral testicular cancer occurs in 1–2% of cases.

Testicular cancer: clinical presentation

Symptoms

Most patients present with a scrotal lump, usually painless or slightly aching. Delay in presentation is not uncommon, particularly in those with metastatic disease. This may be due to patient factors (fear, self-neglect, ignorance, denial) or earlier misdiagnosis.

Occasionally (5%), acute scrotal pain may occur, due to intratumoral hemorrhage, causing diagnostic confusion.

The lump may have been noted by the patient, sometimes after minor trauma, or by his partner. In 10%, symptoms suggestive of advanced disease include weight loss, lumps in the neck, cough, and bone pain.

Signs

Examination of the genitalia should be carried out in a warm room with the patient relaxed. Observation may reveal asymmetry or slight scrotal skin discoloration. Using careful bimanual palpation, the normal side is first examined, followed by the abnormal side. This will reveal a hard, non-tender, irregular, non-transilluminable mass in the testis or replacing the testis.

Care should be taken to assess the epididymis, spermatic cord, and overlying scrotal wall, which may be normal or involved in 10–15% of cases. Rarely, a reactive hydrocele may be present if the tunica albuginea has been breached.

General examination may reveal cachexia, supraclavicular lymphadenopathy, left-sided neck mass, chest signs, hepatomegaly, lower limb edema, or abdominal mass—all suggestive of metastatic disease.

Gynecomastia is seen in <5% of patients with TC and is due to endocrine manifestations of some tumors.

Differential diagnosis

The majority of scrotal masses are benign; however, no risks should be taken. Every patient who is concerned should be seen, examined, and if any doubt persists, investigated further.

There is often a delay in diagnosis of testicular cancer either because of denial by the patient or delayed diagnosis by the physician, who may ascribe the mass to an infectious cause and initially treat with antibiotics.

Box 6.6 provides a comprehensive listing of scrotal and testicular masses in adults and children.

Investigations

Scrotal ultrasound

This is an extension of the physical examination and will confirm that the palpable lesion is within the testis, distorting its normally regular outline and internal echo pattern. Any hypoechoic area within the tunica albuginea should be regarded with suspicion. It may distinguish a primary from a secondary hydrocele.

Box 6.6 Differential diagnosis of testicular and scrotal masses in adults and children

Adult or pediatric painful mass
- Epididymitis/orchitis; bacterial, STD, mumps, tuberculosis
- Incarcerated/strangulated hernia
- Testicular trauma: usually blunt; contusion, rupture; usually associated hematocele
- Torsion (testicle, testicular or epididymal appendage)
- Tumor (pain infrequent unless traumatized or rapidly growing; see below)

Adult painless mass
- Adenomatoid tumor of testis or epididymis
- Adrenal rest tumors
- Adenocarcinoma of the rete testis
- Chylocele: usually associated with filariasis
- Fibrous pseudotumor of the tunica albuginea
- Hydrocele, primary or due to trauma, torsion, tumor, epididymitis; hydrocele of the cord
- Lipoma of the cord
- Mesothelioma of tunica vaginalis
- Polyorchidism
- Paratesticular sarcomas: rhabdomyosarcoma, fibrosarcoma, leiomyosarcoma, liposarcoma
- Scrotal edema (insect bite, nephrotic syndrome, acute idiopathic scrotal edema)
- Scrotal wall: sebaceous and inclusion cysts, idiopathic calcinosis, fat necrosis, malignancy
- Sperm granuloma following vasectomy
- Spermatocele (epididymal cyst)
- Testicular cysts (simple, tunica albuginea, epidermoid)
- Testicular tumor
  - Germ cell tumors (95% of testicular malignancies): seminoma, embryonal cell carcinoma, choriocarcinoma, yolk sac carcinoma teratoma (1–5%), teratocarcinoma
  - Gonadal stromal tumors: Leydig, Sertoli cell, granulosa cell tumor
  - Metastatic tumors: prostate, lung, and gastrointestinal tract; rare kidney, malignant melanoma, pancreas, bladder and thyroid
  - Mixed germ cell and stromal tumor (gonadoblastoma)
  - Angioma, fibroma, leiomyoma, hamartoma, carcinoid, mesothelioma, and neurofibroma
  - Malignant fibrous histiocytoma (most common soft tissue sarcoma in late adult life)
  - Leukemia or lymphoma
- Varicocele

Pediatric painless mass
- Similar to adult list; most/more common: hydrocele, hernia, variocele, testicular teratoma, adrenal rest tumor, rhabdomyosarcoma

Reproduced from Carver BS, Sheinfeld J (2010). Testis cancer, general. Gomella LG (Ed.), *5 Minute Urology Consult*, 2nd ed. Philadelphia LWW.

Ultrasound may also be used to identify impalpable lesions as small as 1–2 mm—an occult primary tumor in a patient presenting with systemic symptoms and signs or an incidental finding.

Image contralateral testis as 2% of patients will have bilateral testicular cancers.

Abdominal and chest CT scans are usually obtained for staging purposes if the diagnosis of TC is confirmed, usually following radical orchiectomy.

Serum tumor markers are measured prior to any treatment of a confirmed testicular mass (p. 298).

Treatment

All patients with a testicular mass should be evaluated for testicular cancer. Studies have shown that 18–33% of patients with testicular cancer were initially treated for epididymitis, resulting in a delay in diagnosis.

Radical orchiectomy

Radical orchiectomy should be performed for diagnosis and treatment of the primary tumor. This involves excision of the testis, epididymis, and cord, with their coverings, through a groin incision. The cord is clamped, transfixed, and divided near the internal inguinal ring before the testis is manipulated into the wound, preventing inadvertent metastasis.

A silicone prosthesis may be inserted at the time of the procedure or at a later date. This treatment is curative in up to 80% of patients. Sperm cryopreservation should be offered to patients without a normal contralateral testis.

Contralateral testis biopsy should be considered in patients at high risk for IGCN (see pp. 294, 308).

Testicular cancer: serum markers

Germ cell tumors may express and secrete into the bloodstream relatively specific and readily measurable proteins. These tumor markers (with the exception of PLAP) are useful in diagnosis, staging, prognostication (see p. 303), and monitoring of response to treatment (see p. 304).

Currently, testicular cancer is the only malignancy to incorporate serum markers into the staging system.

Oncofetal proteins

α-Fetoprotein (AFP)

AFP is expressed by trophoblastic elements within 50–70% of teratomas and yolk sac tumors. With respect to seminoma, the presence of elevated serum AFP strongly suggests a non-seminomatous element.

Serum half-life is 3–5 days; normal is <10 ng/mL. It can be elevated.

Human chorionic gonadotrophin, β subunit (β-hCG)

B-hCG is expressed syncytiotrophoblastic elements of choriocarcinomas (100%), teratomas (40%), and seminomas (10%). Serum half-life is 24–36 hours. Assays measure the β subunit with the normal <5 mIU/mL.

When used together, 90% of patients with advanced disease have elevation of one or both markers; it is less among patients with low-stage tumors.

Cellular enzymes

Lactate dehydrogenase (LDH)

LDH is a ubiquitous enzyme, elevated in serum for various causes and is therefore less specific. It is elevated in 10–20% of seminomas, correlating with tumor burden, and is most useful in monitoring treatment response in advanced seminoma.

Other markers with limited current clinical use include PLAP, CD30, and GGTP.

Clinical use

These markers are measured at presentation, 1–2 weeks after radical orchiectomy, and during follow-up to assess response to treatment and residual disease.

Normal markers prior to orchiectomy do not exclude metastatic disease. Normalization of markers post-orchiectomy cannot be equated with absence of disease, and persistent elevations of markers post- orchiectomy may occur with liver dysfunction and hypogonadotrophism, but usually indicate metastatic disease.

Testicular cancer: pathology and staging

Ninety percent of testicular tumors are malignant germ cell tumors (GCT), split into seminomatous and non-seminomatous (NS) GCTs for clinical purposes. Seminoma, the most common germ cell tumor, appears pale and homogeneous. NSGCTs are heterogeneous and sometimes contain bizarre tissues such as cartilage or hair.

Metastases to the testis are rare, notably from the prostate (35%), lung (19%), colon (9%), and kidney (7%). Table 6.15 shows the WHO histo-pathological classification of testicular tumors.

The right testis is affected slightly more commonly than the left; synchronous bilateral TC occurs in 2% of cases. TC spreads by local extension into the epididymis, spermatic cord, and, rarely, the scrotal wall.

Lymphatic spread occurs via the testicular vessels, initially to the para-aortic nodes. Involvement of the epididymis, spermatic cord, or scrotum may lead to pelvic and inguinal node metastasis.

Blood-borne metastasis to the lungs, liver, and bones is more likely once the disease has breached the tunica albuginea.

TC is staged using various classifications, most recently the TNM (2002) system (see Fig. 6.9 and Table 6.16). Here, T stage is pathological, N stage involves imaging, and M stage involves physical examination, imaging, and biochemical investigations. An additional S category is appended for serum tumor markers (see p. 305).

Table 6.15 WHO histopathological classification of testicular tumors

Germ cell tumors (90%)

Seminoma (48%)
- Spermatocytic, classical, and anaplastic subtypes

Non-seminomatous GCT (42%)
- Teratoma
  - Differentiated/mature
  - Intermediate/immature
  - Undifferentiated/malignant
- Yolk sac tumor
- Choriocarcinoma
- Mixed NSGCT

Mixed GCT (10%)

Other tumors (7%)
- Epidermoid cyst (benign)
- Adenomatoid tumor
- Adenocarcinoma of the rete testis
- Carcinoid
- Lymphoma (5%)
- Metastatic, from another site (1%)

Sex cord stromal tumors (3%) (10% malignant)
- Leydig cell
- Sertoli cell
- Mixed or unclassified

Mixed germ cell/sex cord tumors (rare)

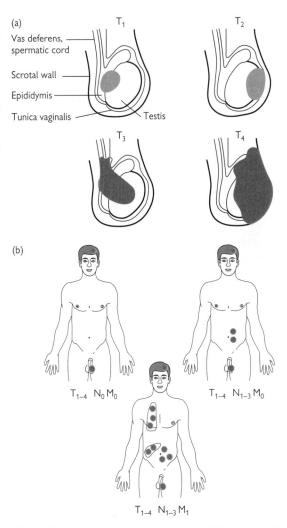

Figure 6.9 Pathological staging of testicular cancer. (a) Primary tumors T1–T4. If radical orchiectomy has not been used, T_x is used. (b) Node/metastasis: para-aortic lymphadenopathy, measured in long axis on CT scan (upper figures); supraclavicular lymphadenopathy and/or pulmonary metastases—M1a, other distant metastases (e.g., liver, brain)—M1b (lower figure).

Table 6.16 TNM staging of testicular germ cell tumors. S staging is presented on p. 305

Tx	The primary tumor has not been assessed (no radical orchiectomy)
T0	No evidence of primary tumor
Tis	Intratubular germ cell neoplasia (carcinoma in situ)
T1	Tumor limited to testis and epididymis without vascular invasion; may invade tunica albuginea but not tunica vaginalis
T2	Tumor limited to testis and epididymis with vascular/lymphatic invasion, or tumor involving tunica vaginalis
T3	Tumor invades spermatic cord with or without vascular invasion
T4	Tumor invades scrotum with or without vascular invasion
Nx	Regional lymph nodes cannot be assessed
N0	No regional lymph node metastasis
N1	Metastasis with a lymph node ≤2 cm or multiple lymph nodes, none >2 cm
N2	Metastasis with a lymph node size 2–5 cm or multiple lymph nodes, collected size 2–5 cm
N3	Metastasis with a lymph node mass >5 cm
Mx	Distant metastasis cannot be assessed
M0	No distant metastasis
M1a	Nonregional lymph node or pulmonary metastasis
M1b	Distant metastasis other than to nonregional lymph node or lungs

Testicular cancer: prognostic staging system for metastatic germ cell cancer

The International Germ Cell Cancer Collaborative Group (IGCCCG) has devised a prognostic factor–based staging system for metastatic germ cell cancer that includes good- and intermediate-prognosis seminoma and good-, intermediate-, and poor-prognosis non-seminomatous germ cell tumors (NSGCT) (Table 6.17).

See p. 299 for discussion on testicular tumor markers, including S staging (p. 305). Primary therapy of testicular cancer is based on the following:
- Histology (seminoma vs. NSGCT)
- Clinical TNM stage.
- International Germ Cell Cancer Collaborative Group (IGCCCG) classification (good, intermediate, or poor risk)

Table 6.17 IGCCCG staging system for metastatic germ cell cancer

	Seminoma	NSGCT
Good	90% of patients	56% of patients
5-year progression-free survival	86%	92%
All factors listed present:	Any primary site; *no* nonpulmonary visceral metastases; normal AFP; any hCG or LDH	Testis or retroperitoneal primary site; *no* nonpulmonary visceral metastases; AFP <1000 ng/mL; hCG <5000 mIU/L; and LDH <1.5 normal upper limit (S1)
Intermediate	10% of patients	28% of patients
5-year progression-free survival	73%	80%
All factors listed present:	Any primary site; nonpulmonary visceral metastases present; normal AFP; Any hCG or LDH	Testis or retroperitoneal primary site; no nonpulmonary visceral metastases; AFP 1000–9999 ng/mL or hCG 5000–49999 mIU/L; LDH 1.5–10 normal upper limit (S2)
Poor		16% of patients
5-year progression-free survival	No patients classified as poor prognosis	48%
All factors listed present:		Mediastinal primary; nonpulmonary visceral metastases present; AFP >10,000 ng/mL or hCG >50,000 mIU/L; LDH >10 normal upper limit (S3)

Testicular cancer: management of non-seminomatous germ cell tumors (NSGCT)

Following radical orchiectomy and formal staging, the patient may require a retroperitoneal lymph node dissection (RPLND). Joint management involves urology and medical oncology in most cases of NSCGT.

In the presence of elevated AFP, a seminoma would be managed as for teratoma. Combination chemotherapy, introduced in the 1980s, revolutionized the treatment of metastatic testicular teratoma, which was hitherto virtually untreatable.

The IGCCCG prognostic staging is often used in treatment planning at some centers. General treatment options following radical orchiectomy and staging for NSCGT are outlined here (see Table 6.18 for stage grouping).

Stage I

- Surveillance is appropriate for reliable patients with no risk factors. It has a 25–30% relapse rate.
- Requires close follow-up with imaging (CT, CXR), tumor markers, and physical examination
- RPLND: modified unilateral template/nerve-sparing. Up to 70–75% will be pathologically negative (pN0).
- RPLND offers cure in 95% with negative nodes and may cure low-volume nodal disease. Only 5% will relapse.
- Chemotherapy with two cycles of bleomycin, etoposide, cisplatin (BEP) yields 95% survival.

Stage IIa/IIb

Controversy exists regarding the most effective treatment regimen. Options include RPNLD with modified bilateral template, RPNLD + adjuvant chemotherapy, or primary chemotherapy.

- RPNLD and no tumor found: observe
- RPNLD and positive nodes: two cycles of adjuvant chemotherapy
- RPNLD and high-volume disease or residual tumor left behind: three cycles adjuvant chemotherapy

Stage IIC or III

- Chemotherapy is the initial treatment, with either 3 or 4 cycles depending on risk. Complete responses are frequently observed.
- Partial responses with residual retroperitoneal masses undergo full bilateral RPNLD (nerve-sparing, if applicable). Follow-up is based on pathological findings:
  - Residual masses: fibrosis in 40%, teratoma in 40%, and viable malignancy in 20%
  - Malignancy present and post-resection tumor markers elevated or tumor left behind: use salvage chemotherapy
  - Malignancy present and post-resection tumor markers normal and no tumor left behind: 2 cycles of chemotherapy can be given
  - Teratoma/fibrosis only: observation only

Table 6.18 Simplified stage grouping for testis cancer, including S stage

Simplified stage groupings in testis cancer				
Stage 0	Tis	N0	M0	S0
Stage IA	T1	N0	M0	S0
Stage IB	T2–4	N0	M0	S0
Stage IS	T any	N0	M0	S 1–3
Stage IIA	T any	N1	M0	S 0/1
Stage IIB	T any	N2	M0	S 0/1
Stage IIC	T any	N3	M0	S 0/1
Stage IIIA	T any	N any	M 1a	S 0/1
Stage IIIB	T any	N any	M 0/1a	S2
Stage IIIC	T any	N any	M 0/1a	S3
	T any	N any	M1b	S any

a, nonregional nodes or pulmonary metastasis; b, other distant metastasis.

	LDH	hCG mIU/mL	AFP ng/mL
S0	Normal	Normal	Normal
S1	<1.5 ULN	<5000	<1000
S2	1.6–10 ULN	5100–50,000	1100–10,000
S3	>10.1 ULN	>50,100	>10,100

ULN, upper limit of normal.

- With no response to primary chemotherapy, consider salvage chemotherapy (ifosfamide, vinblastine, cisplatin), or salvage bone marrow transplant.

Chemotherapy

Regardless of histology, patients with advanced germ cell tumors (cIIB–cIII) and those with elevated tumor markers following radical orchiectomy (cIS) are treated initially with platinum-based chemotherapy based on IGCCCG risk stratification.

Good risk

Use BEP regimen every 21 days × 3 cycles
- Bleomycin 30 U IV weekly
- Etoposide 100 mg/m² IV × 5 days
- Cisplatin 20 mg/m² IV × 5 days

Or EP regimen every 21 day × 4 cycles
- Etoposide 100 mg/m² IV × 5 days
- Cisplatin 20 mg/m² IV × 5 days

Intermediate- or high-risk disease

Use 4 cycles BEP every 21 days (as above), or the following given every 21 days x 4 cycles:

- Etoposide 75 mg/m^2 IV x 5 days
- Ifosfamide 1.2 g/m^2 IV x 5 days
- Cisplatin 20 mg/m^2 IV x 5 days

Chemotherapy complications

- Bleomycin: pulmonary toxicity causing pulmonary fibrosis that can be life threatening
- Cisplatin: nephrotoxicity, ototoxicity, peripheral neuropathy
- Etoposide (VP16): hematological toxicity, alopecia, vascular toxicity, metabolic syndrome
- Ifosfamide: hemorrhagic cystitis (can be reduced by the use of MESNA)
- Secondary malignancy: leukemias, lymphomas, skin malignancies
- Infertility: 50% will have normal sperm counts 2 years after chemotherapy, 25% will remain azoospermic (many patients with testicular cancer will have abnormal semen parameters before radical orchiectomy)

Surveillance and follow-up after treatment

Surveillance for low-risk disease requires the following. Patients who undergo definitive therapy can have less aggressive follow-up the first 2 years, but follow-up is also to 10 years. The risk of relapse is highest in the first 2 years.

- Year 1: monthly clinic visit with serum markers and chest X-ray, abdominal CT months 3, 6, 9, and 12
- Year 2: bi-monthly clinic visit with serum markers and chest X-ray, abdominal CT month 24
- Years 3, 4, and 5: 3-monthly clinic visit with serum markers and chest X-ray
- Annual clinic visit with serum markers and chest X-ray thereafter to 10 years

RPLND

RPLND is the gold-standard staging investigation following radical orchiectomy. In the United States, it is the preferred approach for patients at high risk for retroperitoneal relapse (predominant embryonal carcinoma, lymphovascular invasion, or extension into the tunica or scrotum) if serum tumor markers have normalized. In the UK, RPLND is used only to remove or debulk residual mass post-chemotherapy.

Retroperitoneal lymphadenopathy is usually the first and only evidence of extragonadal metastasis of teratoma. For low-stage disease, a modified nerve-sparing template is used.

Open RPLND is the standard, with laparoscopic techniques applied at some centers. It is a technically challenging procedure that requires significant expertise.

Left-sided testicular tumor

The limits of dissection include the left common iliac artery medially and inferiorly up to the aortic bifurcation. Dissection continues along the aorta to the inferior mesenteric artery (IMA), and above the IMA, the dissection is carried out to the lateral edge of the inferior vena cava. The superior limit of the dissection is the renal vessels bilaterally. The ureter and gonadal vessels are the limit laterally.

The spermatic cord stump (marked by a nonabsorbable suture at the time of radical orchiectomy) is included in the specimen.

Right-sided testicular tumor

The limits of dissection include the right common iliac artery medially and inferiorly up to bifurcation of the aorta. Dissection continues along the aorta up to the IMA. Superior to the IMA, the dissection is carried out to the left ureter. Superior limit is the renal hilum bilaterally. On the right side, lateral limit is the ureter and the gonadal vessels.

The stump of the spermatic cord is included in the specimen.

Post-chemotherapy RPLND

Post-chemotherapy RPLND and resection of residual masses involves a complete bilateral resection including the supra hilar nodes. In the setting of post-chemotherapy RPLND, 40% will have teratoma, and 10–15% will have viable germ cell tumor.

RPLND complications

There is <1% mortality. Perioperative morbidity is 5–25% (atelectasis, ileus, lymphocele, pancreatitis, chylous ascites). Late bowel obstruction also occurs (1–2%). Ejaculatory dysfunction, when present, can be markedly decreased with nerve-sparing templates.

Testicular cancer: management of seminoma, IGCN, and lymphoma

Of all seminomas, 75% are confined to the testis at presentation and are cured by radical orchiectomy; 10–15% of patients harbor regional node metastasis, and 5–10% have more advanced disease.

Treatment and follow-up depend largely on disease stage similar to the stratification of NSGCT (p. 304). RPLND is not used for seminoma. Unlike NSCGT, radiation therapy is a therapeutic modality in seminoma.

Subdiaphragmatic radiation is the traditional method: 35 Gy to the para-aortic and ipsilateral iliac lymph nodes following radical orchiectomy using a "hockey stick" template. Newer radiation techniques limit radiation to the paraortic region with contralateral testicular shielding.

Generally, radiation doses in the adjuvant setting are in the range of 25 Gy, with 35 Gy used for more bulky disease.

Prophylactic mediastinal radiation therapy has been abandoned (cardiovascular side effects, failure to significantly improve outcomes, and interference with ability to administer salvage chemotherapy).

Stage I
- Radical orchiectomy and adjuvant radiation therapy in low-stage disease is the most common treatment.
- Close surveillance with imaging and serial tumor markers instead of radiation therapy for low-stage seminoma is gaining acceptance.

Stage IIA
- Non-bulky retroperitoneal nodes: RT 35 Gy or chemotherapy

Stage IIB/IIC
- Bulky lymphadenopathy (>5–7 cm nodes) or visceral metastasis with standard NSCGT: platinum-based chemotherapy (BEP/EP) (see p. 305)

Stage III
- Chemotherapy; with brain metastasis, brain radiation therapy +/ excision

Cure rate
All stages have at least a 90% cure rate:
- Stage I is 98–100%.
- Stage II (B1/B2 non-bulky) is 98–100%.
- Stage II (B3 bulky) and stage III have a >90% complete response to chemotherapy and an 86% durable response rate to chemotherapy.

Management of intratubular germ cell neoplasia (IGCN)
- Observation or orchiectomy for unilateral disease.
- Radiotherapy for unilateral disease in the presence of a contralateral tumor
- Radiotherapy for bilateral disease, to preserve Sertoli cells
- Frozen sperm storage must be offered.

Management of testicular lymphoma

This may be a primary disease or a manifestation of disseminated nodal lymphoma. The median age of incidence is 60 years, but has been reported in children.

One-quarter of patients present with systemic symptoms; 10% have bilateral testicular tumors. These patients have a poorer prognosis following radical orchiectomy and chemotherapy, while those with localized disease may enjoy long-term survival.

Penile neoplasia: benign, viral-related, and premalignant lesions

Benign tumors and lesions (see Table 6.19)

Noncutaneous
- Congenital and acquired inclusion cysts
- Retention cysts
- Syringomas (sweat gland tumors)
- Neurilemoma
- Angioma, lipoma
- Iatrogenic pseudotumor following injections
- Pyogenic granuloma following injections

Cutaneous
- Pearly penile papules (normal in 15% of postpubertal males)
- Zoon balanitis (shiny, erythematous plaque on glans or prepuce)
- Lichen planus (flat-topped violaceous papule)

Viral-related lesions

Condyloma acuminatum

This is also known as genital warts, related to human papillomavirus (HPV) infection. There are soft, usually multiple benign lesions on the glans, prepuce, and shaft; they may occur elsewhere on genitalia or perineum.

A biopsy is worthwhile prior to topical treatment with podophyllin. 5% have urethral involvement, which may require diathermy.

HPV infection (particularly types 16 and 18) is potentially carcinogenic and condylomata have been associated with penile SCC (this is distinct from the premalignant *giant condyloma acuminatum;* see below).

Bowenoid papulosis

This condition resembles carcinoma in situ, but with a benign course. Multiple papules appear on the penile skin, or a flat glanular lesion. These should be biopsied. HPV is the suspected cause.

Kaposi sarcoma

This reticuloendothelial tumor has become the second-most common malignant penile tumor. It presents as a raised, painful, bleeding violaceous papule or as a bluish ulcer with local edema. It is slow growing, solitary, or diffuse. It occurs in immunocompromised men, particularly in gay men with HIV/AIDS. Urethral obstruction may occur.

Treatment is palliative, with intralesional chemotherapy, laser, cryoablation, or radiotherapy.

Premalignant cutaneous lesions

Some histologically benign lesions are recognized to have malignant potential or occur in close association with SCC of the penis. A chronic red or pale lesion on the glans or prepuce is a cause for concern. Note should be made of its color, size, and surface features. Early follow-up after use of steroid, antibacterial, or antifungal creams is recommended. If persistent, biopsy is advised.

Table 6.19 Benign penile tumors and lesions

Disease (organism/ cause)	Characteristics	Therapy
Behçet disease (autoimmune; ? genetic)	Syndrome of oral and genital ulcers, and uveitis; lesions are painful; rule out STDs	Symptomatic against inflammation; If severe, use steroids, immunosuppressants, interferon
Chancroid (Haemophilus ducreyi)	Painful, purulent ulcer, single or multiple, tender suppurative inguinal nodes	Azithromycin or ceftriaxone as a single dose
Erythema multiforme (hypersensitivity to chemicals, drugs, or infection common)	Red target lesions 1–2 cm; with severe form (Steven-Johnson syndrome) blisters and epidermal necrolysis	Discontinue cause, local supportive care
Fixed drug eruption (immune reaction to medication)	Solitary, inflammatory and occasionally bullous; recurrent same site with exposure to medication; post-inflammatory hyperpigmentation common	Stop medication (antibiotics are most common cause)
Genital herpes (herpes simplex virus types 1 and 2)	Multiple painful vesicles with tender nodes	Acyclovir, valacyclovir, famciclovir orally in acute, suppressive, or prodromal therapy
Genital warts/ condylomata acuminata (HPV types 6 and 11)	Non-tender wart-like papillary lesions, sometimes friable, no adenopathy	Surgical ablation, podophyllin
Granuloma inguinale/ donovanosis (Calymmatobacterium granulomatis)	Painless, progressive beefy red ulcers, infrequent adenopathy	Doxycycline or TMP-SMX
Lichen planus (? viral or chemical)	Whitish annular lesion on the glans penis, often itchy papular rash in other parts of body	Usually resolves spontaneously, topical steroids if symptomatic
Lichen sclerosis et atrophicus, penile lesion called balanitis xerotica obliterans or BXO (? autoimmune, infectious, or genetic)	Well-circumscribed white patches on glans/prepuce, thin epidermis ulcer prone that scars and contract; secondary meatal stenosis and phimosis; itching and burning common	High-dose topical steroids or circumcision

Table 6.19 Continued

Disease (organism/ cause)	Characteristics	Therapy
Lymphogranuloma venereum (Chlamydia trachomatis)	Small, painless vesicle or papule progresses to an ulcer Painful matted nodes, fistula common	Doxycycline; azithromycin or erythromycin alternative
Molluscum contagiosum (A pox virus)	Smooth, round, pearly papules, 2–5 mm	Surgical ablation
Pearly penile papules (? viral)	Usually uncircumcised, painless 1–2 mm papules with variable color (translucent/white/yellow) usually around corona an dorsum of penis	Usually not clinically important; ablation if bothersome
Sclerosing lymphangitis (Local trauma)	Asymptomatic subcutaneous cordlike swellings along the dorsal shaft of the penis or around the coronal sulcus; may be edema of glans and coronal sulcus.	Traumatic in origin, self- limited; avoid vigorous sexual activity
Syphilis, primary (Treponema pallidum)	Painless, indurated, with a clean base, usually singular lesion; tender inguinal nodes	Benzthiazide penicillin G (2.4 million units IM) single dose
Zoon balanitis (? Mycobacterium smegmatis)	Found in uncircumcised only, on prepuce or glans, usually painless, solitary shiny lesion with reddish or orange tint; can be to 2 cm, occasionally erosive	Circumcision curative

- **Cutaneous horn:** rare, solid skin overgrowth; extreme hyperkeratosis, the base may be malignant. Treatment is wide local excision.
- **Pseudoepitheliomatous micaceous** and **keratotic balanitis:** unusual hyperkeratotic growths on the glans. They require excision, histological examination, and follow-up, as they may recur.
- **Balanitis xerotica obliterans** (BXO): also known as lichen sclerosus et atrophicus, this is a common sclerosing condition of glans and prepuce. It occurs at all ages and most commonly presents as non-retractile foreskin (phimosis). The meatus and fossa navicularis may be affected, causing obstructed and spraying voiding. The histological diagnosis is usually made after circumcision, with epithelial atrophy, loss of rete pegs, and collagenization of the dermis. BXO occurs in association

with penile SCC, but most pathologists would regard the lesion as benign unless epithelial dysplasia is present.

- **Leukoplakia:** solitary or multiple whitish glanular plaques that usually involve the meatus. Treatment is excision and histology. Leukoplakia is associated with in situ SCC; follow-up is required.
- **Erythroplasia of Queyrat:** also known as carcinoma in situ of the glans, prepuce, or penile shaft. A red, velvety, circumscribed painless lesion occurs, though it may ulcerate, resulting in discharge and pain. Treatment is excision biopsy if possible; radiotherapy, laser ablation, or topical 5-fluorouracil may be required. Histology reveals hyperplastic mucosal cells with malignant features.
- **Bowen disease:** this is carcinoma in situ of the remainder of the keratinizing genital or perineal skin. Treatment is wide local excision, laser, or cryoablation.
- **Buschke–Löwenstein tumor:** also known as *verrucous carcinoma* or *giant condyloma acuminatum*, this is an aggressive locally invasive tumor of the glans. Metastasis is rare, but wide excision is necessary to distinguish it from SCC. Urethral erosion and fistulation may occur.

Penile cancer: epidemiology, risk factors, and pathology

Squamous cell carcinoma (SCC) is the most common penile cancer, accounting for 95% of penile malignancies. Others include Kaposi sarcoma (see p. 310) and, rarely, basal cell carcinoma, melanoma, sarcoma, and Paget disease. Metastases to the penis are occasionally seen from the bladder, prostate, rectum, and other primary sites.

Incidence and etiology of SCC

Penile cancer is rare, representing 1% of male cancers. The incidence appears to be decreasing, occurring mostly in elderly men. In 2009, 1290 cases were reported, with 300 deaths.

Risk factors for SCC

- **Age:** penile cancer incidence rises during the sixth decade and peaks in the eighth decade. It is unusual <40 years of age, but has been rarely reported in children.
- **Premalignant lesions:** 42% of patients with penile SCC are reported to have had a pre-existing penile lesion (see p. 310).
- **A prepuce** (foreskin): penile cancer is rare in men circumcised at a young age. Smegma that forms from desquamated epithelial cells is thought to be a primary instigating factor in penile cancer; good hygiene and circumcision limit smegma accumulation.
- **Geography:** Highest incidence worldwide is in Brazil. It is virtually non-existent in Israel.
- **Human papilloma virus (HPV)** genital wart infection, especially with types 16, 18, and 21.
- **Multiple sex partners**
- **Smoking and tobacco products**

Pathology and staging of penile SCC

Believed to be preceded by carcinoma in situ, SCC starts as a slow-growing papillary, flat or ulcerative lesion on the glans (48%), prepuce (21%), glans and prepuce (9%), coronal sulcus (6%), or shaft (2%). The remainder are indeterminate. It grows locally beneath the foreskin before invading the corpora cavernosa, urethra, and, eventually, the perineum, pelvis, and prostate.

Metastasis is initially to the superficial then deep inguinal and, subsequently, iliac and obturator lymph nodes. Skin necrosis, ulceration, and infection of the inguinal lymph nodes may lead to sepsis or hemorrhage from the femoral vessels. Blood-borne metastasis to lungs and liver is rare (1–10% of cases).

Histologically, SCC exhibits keratinization, epithelial pearl formation, and mitoses. Staging is by the TNM system (see Fig. 6.10 and Table 6.20). Grading scale is as follows: low (75%), intermediate (15%), or high (10%); grading correlates with prognosis, as does presence of vascular invasion.

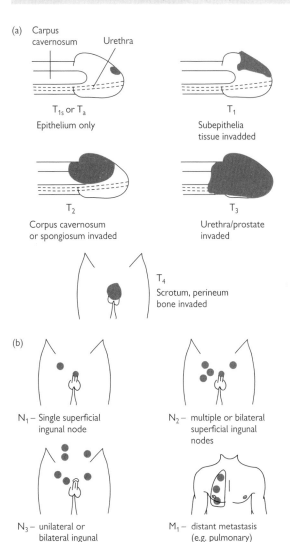

(a) Carpus cavernosum   Urethra

T_{1s} or T_a
Epithelium only

T_1
Subepithelia
tissue invadded

T_2
Corpus cavernosum
or spongiosum invaded

T_3
Urethra/prostate
invaded

T_4
Scrotum, perineum
bone invaded

(b)

N_1 – Single superficial
ingunal node

N_2 – multiple or bilateral
superficial ingunal
nodes

N_3 – unilateral or
bilateral inguinal
or intra-pelvic nodes

M_1 – distant metastasis
(e.g. pulmonary)

Figure 6.10 Pathological staging of penile cancer. (a) T stage: primary tumor;
(b) N and M stages.

Table 6.20 TNM staging of penile carcinoma

Tx	Primary tumor cannot be assessed
T0	No evidence of primary tumor
Tis	Carcinoma in situ
Ta	Noninvasive verrucous carcinoma
T1	Tumor invades subepithelial connective tissue
T2	Tumor invades corpus cavernosum or spongiosum
T3	Tumor invades urethra or prostate
T4	Tumor invades other structures
Nx	Regional nodes cannot be assessed
N0	No regional lymph node metastases
N1	Single superficial inguinal lymph node metastasis
N2	Multiple or bilateral superficial inguinal lymph node metastases
N3	Metastases in deep inguinal or pelvic lymph nodes, unilateral or bilateral
Mx	Distant metastasis cannot be assessed
M0	No distant metastasis
M1	Distant metastasis

SCCs are graded using the Broder classification system:
- Grade I: well differentiated, keratinization, prominent intercellular bridges, keratin pearls
- Grade II to III: greater nuclear atypia, increased mitotic activity, decreased keratin pearls
- Grade IV: cells deeply invasive, marked nuclear pleomorphism, nuclear mitoses, necrosis, lymphatic and perineural invasion, no keratin pearls

Squamous cell carcinoma of the penis: clinical management

Presentation

A hard, painless lump on the glans penis is the most common presentation. About 15–50% of patients delay presentation for >1 year because of embarrassment, personal neglect, fear, or ignorance. A bloody discharge may be confused with hematuria. Rarely, a groin mass or urinary retention are presenting symptoms.

Examination reveals a solid, non-tender mass or ulcer beneath or involving the foreskin. There is usually evidence of local infection. In more advanced disease, the prepuce, glans, shaft, scrotum, and even perineum are replaced by tumor.

The inguinal lymph nodes are examined. They may be enlarged, fixed, or even ulcerate overlying skin.

Investigations

A biopsy is indicated. Chest radiology, pelvic CT scan, serum calcium, and liver function tests are usually obtained.

Treatment

The management of penile cancer should take place in regional or supra-regional centers that can provide multidisciplinary surgical and oncological expertise.

Primary tumor

The first-line treatment of penile cancer, regardless of the inguinal node status, is surgery (see Box 6.7 for 5-year survival rates).

Circumcision is appropriate for preputial lesions, but local recurrence is observed in 22–50%.

Penis-preserving wide excision of glanular lesions with skin graft glanular reconstruction may be suitable for smaller G1–2 Ta–1 tumors, giving good cosmetic and functional results.

Alternatives to surgery include laser or cryoablation, radiotherapy or brachytherapy, photodynamic therapy, or topical 5-fluorouracil. Mohs cutaneous surgery has been used with mixed results.

For G3T1 and more advanced tumors, partial or total penile amputation is required, depending on the extent of the tumor. Partial amputation is preferable, provided a 2 cm margin of palpably normal shaft can be obtained. The patient must be prepared for poor cosmetic and functional results: inability to have sexual intercourse and need to sit to void urine. Local recurrence occurs in 10% if the excision margin is positive.

Total amputation involves excision of the scrotum and its contents, with formation of a perineal urethrostomy. The most common complication is urethral meatal stenosis.

Radiotherapy remains an alternative, but disadvantages include radio-resistance, leading to reported recurrence rates of 30–60%; and tissue necrosis and damage leading to urethral stricture, fistula, and pain. Patients with M1 disease are offered palliative surgery.

Lymphadenopathy

Six weeks of broad-spectrum antimicrobials (e.g., Augmentin or cephalosporin) are given after the primary tumor has been removed. Nodes become clinically nonpalpable in 50% of patients, who may then be followed up.

For those with persistent inguinal lymphadenopathy, in the absence of demonstrable pelvic or metastatic disease, bilateral inguinal lymphadenectomy should be considered, since 5-year survival is 80%. Even if lymphadenopathy is unilateral, >50% will have contralateral metastases. However, this is major surgery with a high morbidity, including lymphedema, thromboembolism, wound breakdown, and flap complications, so it is not suitable for elderly or unfit men.

Fine needle aspiration cytology is not recommended since a negative result will not alter treatment.

Radiotherapy and chemotherapy

Radiotherapy and chemotherapy are alternative or adjuvant treatments for metastatic nodal disease in unfit, elderly, or inoperable patients; 5-year survival is 25%. There is not a standard chemotherapy. Rarely, potential active agents include 5-FU, bleomycin, methotrexate, and cisplatin.

Rarely, lymphadenopathy ulcerates the skin, may encase the femoral vessels, and invade the deeper musculature. In these circumstances, collaboration with plastic and vascular surgeons is necessary if surgery is considered appropriate.

Prophylactic lymphadenectomy

This is currently practiced in the United States for tumors exhibiting vascular invasion, are high grade, or stages T2–4. It is argued that the risk of metastatic disease with palpably normal groins is >20% and delayed lymphadenectomy could reduce the chance of cure. From 20% to 30% of patients with inguinal metastases will also have pelvic node involvement.

Lymph node sampling (either sentinel node biopsy or modified inguinal dissection) may be offered for patients with palpably normal inguinal nodes and T2 or above lesion to avoid the morbidity of formal inguinal lymphadenectomy.

Distant metastatic disease

This is treated using single-agent systemic chemotherapy: cisplatin, bleomycin, or methotrexate. Responses are partial and short-lived in 20–60% of patients. Experience with combination chemotherapy is increasing.

Box 6.7 5-year survival

- Node-negative SCC, after surgery   65–90%
- Inguinal node metastases   30%
- Metastatic SCC   <10%

Carcinoma of the scrotum

Originally described in Victorian chimney sweeps, by Percival Pott, it was the first cancer to be associated with an occupation. A rare disease in men <50 years of age, chronic exposure of the scrotal skin to soot, tar, or oil is the cause.

A squamous cell carcinoma, it presents as a painless lump or ulcer, often purulent, on the anterior or posterior (therefore not obvious if the patient is lying or sitting) scrotal wall. Inguinal lymphadenopathy may suggest metastasis or reaction to infection.

Treatment of a mass or ulcer on the scrotum is wide local excision with a 2 cm margin of skin and dartos. Antimicrobials are administered for 6 weeks if there is lymphadenopathy, then the groin areas are re-evaluated.

Inguinal lymphadenectomy, with adjuvant chemotherapy, is considered if lymphadenopathy persists. Supraclavicular lymphadenopathy, hematogenous visceral, and bony metastasis are rare and carry a poor prognosis.

Tumors of the testicular adnexa

Epithelial tumors arising from the epididymis and paratesticular tissues are rare; they are mostly of mesenchymal origin.

Adenomatoid tumors

These small, solid tumors arise in the epididymis or on the surface of the tunica albuginea. They usually present without change for several years. There are benign vacuolated epithelial and stromal cells.

The origin is unknown. Treatment is local excision.

Cystadenoma of the epididymis

This is a benign epithelial hyperplasia that occurs in young adults. It is often asymptomatic. One-third of cases are bilateral and associated with VHL syndrome.

Mesothelioma

This presents as a firm, painless, scrotal mass associated with hydrocele, which gradually enlarges. It occurs in any age group, with 15% being metastatic to inguinal nodes.

It is treated with orchiectomy and follow-up.

Paratesticular tumors

Rhabdomyosarcoma

A scrotal mass presents in the first or second decade in the spermatic cord and compresses the testis and epididymis. Lymphatic spread is to the para-aortic nodes.

Treatment is multimodal radical orchiectomy with radiotherapy and chemotherapy, with 5-year survival of 75%.

Leiomyoma/sarcoma

This presents as a scrotal mass at age 40–70 years in the spermatic cord. 30% of cases are malignant, 70% are benign; there is hematogenous distant spread.

Treatment is wide excision or radical orchiectomy.

Liposarcoma

This is a spermatic cord tumor. Radical orchiectomy with high ligation of spermatic cord, similar to surgical management of testicular tumors, is the treatment. Wide local excision may be required to ensure complete tumor removal.

Radiation therapy may be required in cases of incomplete resection leaving residual tumor or extensive local disease.

Urethral cancer

Primary urethral cancer is rare, occurring in elderly patients. It is 4 times more common in women than in men.

Risk factors

Urethral stricture and sexually transmitted disease are implicated. Direct spread from tumor in the bladder or prostate is more common.

Pathology and staging

Seventy-five percent of cases are SCC, occurring in the anterior urethra; 15% are UC, occurring in the posterior/prostatic urethra; 8% are adeno-carcinoma; and the remainder include sarcoma and melanoma.

Urethral cancer metastasizes to the pelvic lymph nodes from the posterior urethra and to the inguinal nodes from the anterior urethra in 50% of patients.

Staging is by the TNM system (see Table 6.21) following histological confirmation of the diagnosis.

Presentation

This is often late; many patients have metastatic disease at presentation
• Painless hematuria; initial, terminal, or a bloody urethral discharge
• Voiding-type LUTS (less common)
• Perineal pain (less common)
• Periurethral abscess or urethrocutaneous fistula (rare)
• Past history of sexually transmitted or stricture disease
• Examination may reveal a hard, palpable mass at the female urethral meatus or along the course of the male anterior urethra. Inguinal lymphadenopathy, chest signs, and hepatomegaly may suggest metastatic disease.

Differential diagnosis

In men
• Urethral stricture
• Perineal abscess
• Metastatic disease involving the corpora cavernosa
• Urethrocutaneous fistula (secondary to benign stricture disease)

In women
• Urethral caruncle
• Urethral cyst
• Urethral diverticulum
• Urethral wart (condylomata acuminata)
• Urethral prolapse
• Urethral vein thrombosis
• Periurethral abscess

Investigations

Cystourethroscopy, biopsy, and bimanual examination under anesthesia will obtain a diagnosis and local clinical staging. Chest radiography and abdominopelvic CT scan will enable distant staging.

Table 6.21 TNM staging of urethral carcinoma

Tx	Primary tumor cannot be assessed
T0	No evidence of primary tumor
Urethra (male and female)	
Ta	Noninvasive papillary carcinoma
Tis	Carcinoma in situ
T1	Tumor invades subepithelial connective tissue
T2	Tumor invades corpus spongiosum, prostate, or periurethral muscle
T3	Tumor invades corpus cavernosum, prostatic capsule, vagina, or bladder neck
T4	Tumor invades adjacent organs including bladder
Transitional cell carcinoma of the prostatic urethra	
Tis	Carcinoma in situ, prostatic urethra (pu) or prostatic ducts (pd)
T1	Tumor invades subepithelial connective tissue
T2	Tumor invades prostatic stroma, corpus spongiosum, or periurethral muscle
T3	Tumor invades through prostatic capsule, corpus cavernosum, or bladder neck
T4	Tumor invades adjacent organs including bladder
Nx	Regional (deep inguinal and pelvic) lymph nodes cannot be assessed
N0	No regional lymph node metastasis
N1	Metastasis in a single lymph node <2 cm in greatest dimension
N2	Metastasis in a single lymph node >2 cm in greatest dimension
Mx	Distant metastasis cannot be assessed
M0	No distant metastasis
M1	Distant metastasis present

Treatment

For localized anterior urethral cancer, radical surgery or radiotherapy are the options. Results are better with anterior urethral disease (see Box 6.8). Male patients would require perineal urethrostomy. Postoperative incontinence due to disruption of the external sphincter mechanism is minimal unless the bladder neck is involved, but the patient would need to sit to void.

For posterior/prostatic urethral cancer, cystoprostatourethrectomy should be considered for men in good overall health, while anterior pelvic exenteration (excision of the pelvic lymph nodes, bladder, urethra, uterus, ovaries, and part of the vagina) should be considered for women.

In the absence of distant metastases, inguinal lymphadenectomy is performed if nodes are palpable, since 80% contain metastatic tumor.

For locally advanced disease, a combination of preoperative radiotherapy and surgery is recommended.

For metastatic disease, chemotherapy is the only option with regimens of systemic cisplatin, bleomycin, and methotrexate or 5-fluorouracil and methotrexate in addition to surgical resection in the treatment of metastatic urethral SCC.

Staging

Staging is by the TNM (2002) classification following histological confirmation of the diagnosis (see Table 6.21). All cases rely on physical examination and imaging, the pathological classification (prefixed p) corresponding to the TNM categories.

Box 6.8 5-year survival
- Surgery: anterior urethra   50%
- Surgery: posterior urethra   15%
- Radiotherapy   34%
- Radiotherapy and surgery   55%

Retroperitoneal fibrosis

Retroperitoneal fibrosis (RPF) was first described by the French urologist Albarran at the beginning of the 20th century. The condition is also known as Ormond disease.

Benign causes

Idiopathic RPF comprises two-thirds of benign cases. A fibrous plaque extends laterally and downward from the renal arteries, encasing the aorta, inferior vena cava, and ureters, but rarely extends into the pelvis. The central portion of the plaque consists of woody scar tissue, while the growing margins have the histological appearance of chronic inflammation. It may be associated with the following:

- Mediastinal, mesenteric, or bile-duct fibrosis
- Drugs, including methysergide, β-blockers, haloperidol, amphetamines, and LSD
- Chronic urinary infections including TB and syphilis
- Inflammatory conditions such as Crohn's disease or sarcoidosis
- Abdominal aortic aneurysm (AAA), intra-arterial stents, and angioplasty may induce idiopathic fibrosis due to periaortitis, hemorrhage, or an immune response to insoluble lipoprotein.

Malignant causes

- Lymphoma is the most common cause; RPF is also sometimes due to sarcoma.
- Metastatic or locally infiltrative carcinoma of the breast, stomach, pancreas, colon, bladder, prostate and carcinoid tumors
- Radiotherapy may cause RPF, although this is rare today with more precise field localization.
- Chemotherapy, especially following treatment of metastatic testicular tumors, may leave fibrous masses encasing the ureters. These may or may not contain residual tumor.

Presentation

Idiopathic RPF classically occurs in the fifth or sixth decade of life.

Men are affected twice as commonly as women. In the early stage, symptoms are relatively nonspecific, including loss of appetite and weight, low-grade fever, sweating, and malaise. Lower limb swelling may develop. Dull, non-colicky abdominal or back pain is described in up to 90% of patients. Later, the major complication of the disease develops: bilateral ureteral obstruction causing anuria and renal failure.

Examination may reveal hypertension in up to 60% of patients and an underlying cause such as an AAA.

Investigations

Inflammatory serum markers are elevated in idiopathic RPF (60–90% elevated ESR). Pyuria or bacteriuria is common.

Ultrasound will demonstrate uni- or bilateral hydronephrosis.

CT, IVP, or retrograde ureterography will reveal tapering medial displacement of the ureters with proximal dilatation and will exclude calculus disease. Up to one-third of patients will have a nonfunctioning kidney at the time of presentation due to long-standing obstruction.

CT-guided fine needle or laparoscopic biopsy of the mass may confirm the presence of malignant disease, but a negative result does not exclude malignancy.

Management

Emergency management of a patient presenting with established renal failure requires relief of the obstruction by percutaneous nephrostomy or ureteral stenting. Fluid and electrolyte losses need to be replaced following relief of bilateral ureteral obstruction and postobstructive diuresis. Assess with daily weighing and measurement of blood pressure lying and standing.

Steroids may decrease the edema often associated with RPF and may help reduce the obstruction. If used, they are usually discontinued when inflammatory markers (such as ESR or CRP) return to normal. The anti-estrogen tamoxifen and cyclophosphamide have been used successfully in some patients but are not considered the standard of care.

Surgical ureterolysis with omental wrap is often necessary to free and insulate the ureters from the encasing fibrous tissue. This can be accomplished by the open, laparoscopic or hand-assisted laparoscopic approaches. Biopsies are taken to exclude malignancy. If malignancy is noted, treatment is directed at the cause.

Monitor patient for recurrent disease with serum creatinine and ultrasound every 3–6 months for 5 years.

Wilms tumor and neuroblastoma

Wilms tumor

This is a rare childhood tumor, affecting 1 in 10,000 children. It represents 80% of all genitourinary tumors affecting children under age 15 years. Males and females are equally affected, with 20% being familial and 5% bilateral. Three-quarters of cases present under the age of 5 years. It is rarely reported in adults.

Pathology and staging

Wilms tumor is a soft, pale gray tumor resembling brain tissue. It contains blastema and epithelial and connective tissue components. It is thought to arise from nephrogenic rests in the kidney.

Mutation or deletion of both copies (alleles) of the chromosome 11p WT-1 tumor suppressor gene results in tumorigenesis. The familial disease exhibits autosomal dominant inheritance but is recessive at the cellular level. Affected family members harbor a germ-line WT-1 mutation, conferring susceptibility. One further hit is required, while two hits are required to cause the sporadic disease. This explains why hereditary Wilms tumors tend to develop multifocally and at a slightly younger age than sporadic counterparts.

Tumor staging relates to the relationship of the tumor to the renal capsule, excision margins, and local lymph nodes at nephrectomy, as well as the presence of soft tissue (typically lung) or bone metastases. Histology determines treatment approaches and relates to final outcome:

- Favorable histology in 95% of cases
- Unfavorable (5%) cases: nuclear enlargement (>3-fold), hyperchromasia, abnormal mitoses
- Anaplasia is an unfavorable marker of chemoresistance.

Presentation

Ninety percent of patients have a mass; 33% complain of abdominal or flank pain; 30–50% develop hematuria; 50% are hypertensive; and 15% exhibit other anomalies such as hemihypertrophy, aniridia, and cryptorchidism. It can be a component of Denys–Drash, WAGR (Wilms tumor, Aniridia, Genital anomalies, mental Retardation), Beckwith–Wiedemann, and other uncommon syndromes.

Investigations

The first-line investigation for a child with an abdominal mass or hematuria is ultrasound, which will reveal a renal tumor. Further diagnostic imaging and staging are obtained by CT, including the chest, to evaluate for metastasis.

Percutaneous biopsy is not recommended.

Treatment and prognosis

Children with renal tumors should be managed by a specialist pediatric oncology center. Staging nephrectomy, with or without preoperative or postoperative chemotherapy, remains the mainstay of treatment. NWTSG (National Wilms Tumor Study Group) recommends surgical diagnosis and staging, followed by adjuvant treatment.

In European countries SIOP (International Society of Pediatric Oncology) treatment involves preoperative chemotherapy followed by surgery. The chemotherapy most frequently used is actinomycin D, vincristine, and doxorubicin.

Survival is generally good, at >90% overall, ranging from 55% to 97% according to stage and histology. The unfavorable histology is present in a small percentage but accounts for >50% of deaths. Radiation therapy is used selectively for advance disease or for anaplasia.

Neuroblastoma

This is the most common extracranial solid tumor of childhood, with 80% diagnosed in children <4 years old. The tumor is of neural crest origin; 50% occur in the adrenal gland and most of the remaining cases arise along the sympathetic trunks.

Chromosome 1p deletion is found in 25–35% of tumors. An allelic loss of 11p occurs in up to 45%. Familiar forms are rare (<1%) but 20% of these are autosomal dominant.

Presentation

Systemic symptoms and signs are common: fever, abdominal pain/distension, mass, weight loss, anemia, and bone pain. Retro-orbital metastases may cause proptosis.

Imaging and staging

Use ultrasound initially; CT of chest and abdomen. Calcification in tumor helps distinguish neuroblastoma from Wilms tumor. MIBG scans are very sensitive for detection of neuroblastomas.

- Stage 1   Tumor confined to organ of origin and grossly complete excision
- Stage 2   Unilateral tumor with residual disease post-resection or lymphadenopathy
- Stage 3   Tumor crossing midline or contralateral nodes
- Stage 4   Metastatic disease beyond regional nodes; survival 6%
- Stage 4S   Unilateral tumor with metastasis limited to liver, skin, or bone marrow; survival 77%

Treatment and prognosis

Treatment involves surgical excision; radiotherapy; and combination chemotherapy, possibly with autologous bone marrow transplantation. Stage 4S tumors may resolve with little or no treatment.

Prognosis is poor except for stage 1 and 4S disease.

Miscellaneous urological diseases of the kidney

Cystic renal disease: simple cysts 332
Cystic renal disease: calyceal diverticulum 334
Cystic renal disease: medullary sponge kidney (MSK) 336
Acquired renal cystic disease (ARCD) 338
Autosomal dominant (adult) polycystic kidney disease
    (ADPKD) 340
Vesicoureteric reflux (VUR) in adults 342
Ureteropelvic junction (UPJ) obstruction in adults 346
Anomalies of renal ascent and fusion: horseshoe kidney, pelvic
    kidney, malrotation 348
Renal duplications 352

Cystic renal disease: simple cysts

Simple cysts are single or multiple renal masses ranging from a few to many centimeters in diameter that do not communicate with any part of the nephron or the renal pelvis. They are mainly confined to the renal cortex, are filled with clear fluid, and contain a membrane composed of a single layer of flattened cuboidal epithelium. They can be unilateral or bilateral and often affect the lower pole of the kidney.

In comparison, *parapelvic cysts* are simple parenchymal cysts located adjacent to the renal pelvis or hilum.

The prevalence of simple cysts increases with age. The precise prevalence depends on the method of diagnosis. On CT, 20% of adults have renal cysts by age 40 years and 30% by the age of 60. At postmortem, 50% of subjects aged >50 have simple cysts. Most reports show no gender predilection.

Cysts do not usually increase in size with age, but may increase in number.

Etiology

Both congenital and acquired causes have been suggested. Chronic dialysis is associated with the formation of new simple cysts.

Presentation

Simple cysts are most commonly diagnosed following a renal ultrasound or CT (less commonly after IVP) done for other purposes, and, as such, they represent an incidental finding. Very large cysts may present as an abdominal mass or cause dull flank or back pain.

The great majority of simple renal cysts are asymptomatic. Acute, severe flank pain may follow bleeding into a cyst (causing sudden distension of the wall).

Rupture (spontaneous or following renal trauma) is rare. Rupture into the pelvicalyceal system can produce hematuria.

Infected cysts (rare) present with flank pain and fever. Very occasionally, large cysts can cause obstruction and hydronephrosis.

Differential diagnosis

- Renal cell carcinoma
- Early autosomal dominant polycystic kidney disease (ADPKD)—diffuse, multiple, or bilateral cysts; presence of hepatic cysts
- Complex renal cysts (i.e., those which contain blood, pus, or calcification)

Investigation

Renal ultrasound

Simple cysts are round or spherical, have a smooth and distinct outline, and are anechoic (no echoes within the cyst—i.e., sound waves are transmitted through the cyst). Evidence of calcification, septation, irregular margins, or clusters of cysts requires further investigation (CT ± aspiration, MRI). In the absence of these features no further investigation is required.

CT (see Table 7.1)

Simple cysts are seen as round, smooth-walled lesions with homogenous fluid in the cavity (with a typical density of −10 to +20 Hounsfield units), and with no enhancement after contrast (enhancement implies that the mass contains vascular tissue or communicates with the collecting system, i.e., that it is not a simple cyst).

Hyperdense cysts have a density of 20–90 Hounsfield units, do not enhance with contrast media, and are <3 cm in diameter.

Treatment

A simple cyst (round or spherical, smooth wall, distinct outline, and no internal echoes) requires no further investigation, no treatment, and no follow-up. In the rare situation where the cyst is thought to be the cause of symptoms (e.g., back or flank pain), treatment options include percutaneous aspiration ± injection of sclerosing agent or surgical excision of the cyst wall. In the rare event of cyst infection, percutaneous drainage and antibiotics are indicated.

Cysts with features on ultrasound suggesting possible malignancy (calcification, septation, irregular margins) should be investigated by CT with contrast.

Table 7.1 Bosniak classification of CT appearance of simple and complex cysts

Type	Description	Approx. % of such cysts that are malignant*	Treatment
I	Simple benign cyst with no smooth margins, no contrast enhancement, no septation, no calcification	None	None; no follow-up required
II	Smooth margins; thin septae; minimal calcification; no contrast enhancement Includes high-density (hyperdense) cysts	10%	Observation—repeat ultrasound looking for increase in size or development of malignant features
III	Irregular margins; moderate calcification; thick septation (septae >1mm thick)	40–50%	Surgical exploration ± partial nephrectomy
IV	Cystic malignant lesion; irregular margins and/ or solid enhancing elements	90%	Radical nephrectomy

* From Siegel et al. (1997). Study relating CTs of cysts where pathological identification had been performed. *AJR Am J Roentgenol* 169:813–818.

Cystic renal disease: calyceal diverticulum

A *calyceal diverticulum* is an outpocketing from the pelvicalyceal system, with which it communicates by way of a narrow neck. It is lined by a smooth layer of transitional epithelium and is covered by a thin layer of renal cortex.

The etiology of calyceal diverticula is unknown. They are usually asymptomatic and are discovered incidentally on an IVP. Symptoms may result from the development of a stone or infection within the diverticulum, presumably caused by urinary stasis.

Stones that form within the calyceal diverticulum may be treated by flexible ureteroscopy and laser lithotripsy or, if large, by percutaneous nephrolithotomy (PCNL) (if percutaneous access is possible). Extracorporeal shock wave lithotripsy (ESWL) may result in stone fragmentation, but it may be difficult for the stone fragments to get out of the diverticulum and they may simply reform into a larger stone.

Endoscopic dilatation or incision of the neck of the diverticulum may be attempted at the time of stone surgery to prevent recurrence, and this technique can also be employed if the diverticulum is thought to be the cause of recurrent urinary infection.

Open surgery has been used to remove stones and to de-roof calyceal diverticula.

Cystic renal disease: medullary sponge kidney (MSK)

Definition

MSK is a cystic condition of the kidneys characterized by dilatation of the distal collecting ducts associated with the formation of multiple cysts and diverticula within the medulla of the kidney.

Prevalence

Prevalence is difficult to know, as MSK may be asymptomatic (diagnosed on an IVP done for other reasons or at postmortem). It is estimated to affect between 1 in 5000 and 1 in 20,000 people in the general population, and 1 in 200 in those undergoing IVP (a select population). In 75% of cases both kidneys are affected.

Pathology

The renal medulla resembles a sponge in cross-section because of dilated collecting ducts in the renal papillae and the development of numerous small cysts. This is associated with urinary stasis and the formation of small calculi within the cysts.

It has a reported familial inheritance and is associated with other malformations (hemihypertrophy).

Presentation

The majority of patients are asymptomatic. When symptoms do occur, they include ureteric colic, renal stone disease (calcium oxalate ± calcium phosphate), UTI, and hematuria (microscopic or macroscopic). Up to 50% have hypercalciuria due to renal calcium leak or increased gastrointestinal calcium absorption.

Renal function is normal, unless obstruction occurs (secondary to renal pelvis or ureteric stones).

Differential diagnosis

This includes other causes of nephrocalcinosis (deposition of calcium in the renal medulla) (e.g., TB, healed papillary necrosis).

Investigation

Intravenous pyelogram (IVP)

The characteristic radiological features of MSK, as seen on IVP, are dilatation of the distal portion of the collecting ducts with numerous associated cysts and diverticula (the dilated ducts are said to give the appearance of bristles on a brush). The collecting ducts may become filled with calcifications, giving an appearance described as a bouquet of flowers or bunches of grapes.

Biochemistry

Levels of 24-hour urinary calcium may be elevated (hypercalciuria). Detection of hypercalciuria requires further investigation to exclude other causes (i.e., raised serum parathyroid hormone levels [PTH] indicate hyperparathyroidism).

Treatment

Asymptomatic MSK disease requires no treatment. General measures to reduce urine calcium levels help reduce the chance of calcium stone formation (high fluid intake, vegetarian diet, low salt intake, consumption of fruit and citrus fruit juices). Thiazide diuretics may be required for hypercalciuria resistant to dietary measures designed to lower urine calcium concentration.

Intrarenal calculi are often small and, as such, may not require treatment, but if indicated this can take the form of ESWL or flexible ureteroscopy and laser treatment.

Ureteric stones are again usually small and will therefore pass spontaneously in many cases, with a period of observation. Renal function tends to remain stable in the long term.

Acquired renal cystic disease (ARCD)

Definition and epidemiology

ARCD is cystic degenerative disease of the kidney with greater than 5 cysts visualized on CT scan. By definition, this is an acquired condition, in contrast to adult polycystic kidney disease (ADPKD), which is inherited (in an autosomal dominant fashion). It is predominantly associated with chronic and end-stage renal failure (originally, it was thought to specifically affect patients on hemodialysis).

It is clinically important because it may cause pain or hematuria and is associated with the development of benign and malignant renal tumors.

Approximately one-third of patients develop ARCD after 3 years of dialysis. The male-to-female ratio is 2:1.

Pathology

Usually multiple, bilateral cysts are found mainly within the cortex of small, contracted kidneys. Cysts vary in size (average 0.5–1 cm) and are filled with a clear fluid, which may contain oxalate crystals. They usually have cuboidal and columnar epithelial linings and are in continuity with renal tubules (and thus cannot be defined as simple cysts).

Atypical cysts have a hyperplastic lining of epithelial cells, which may represent a precursor for tumor formation. Renal transplantation can cause regression of cysts in the native kidneys.

Etiology

The exact pathogenesis is unknown, but several theories have been proposed. Obstruction or ischemia of renal tubules may induce cyst formation. Renal failure may predispose to the accumulation of toxic endogenous substances or metabolites that alter the release of growth factors and result in changes in sex steroid production or cause cell proliferation (secondary to immunosuppressive effects) that results in cyst formation.

Associated disorders

There is an increased risk of benign and malignant renal tumors. The chance of developing renal cell carcinoma is 3–6 times greater than that in the general population (males > females).

ARCD may also be associated with tubulointerstitial nephritis and membranoproliferative glomerulonephritis.

Presentation

Flank pain, UTI, macroscopic hematuria, renal colic (stone disease), and hypertension can occur.

Investigation

This depends on the presenting symptoms.

- For suspected UTI—culture urine
- For hematuria—urine cytology, flexible cystoscopy, and renal ultrasound. On ultrasound the kidneys are small and hyperechoic, with multiple cysts of varying size, many of which show calcification. If the nature of the cysts cannot be determined with certainty on ultrasound, arrange for a renal CT.

Treatment

Persistent macroscopic hematuria can become problematic, exacerbated by heparinization (required for hemodialysis). Options include transfer to peritoneal dialysis, renal embolization, or nephrectomy.

Infected cysts that develop into abscesses require percutaneous or surgical drainage. Radical nephrectomy is indicated for renal masses with features suspicious of malignancy.

Smaller asymptomatic masses require surveillance.

Autosomal dominant (adult) polycystic kidney disease (ADPKD)

Definition
ADPKD is an autosomal dominant inherited disorder leading to the development of multiple expanding renal parenchymal cysts.

Epidemiology
Incidence is 0.1%; 95% of cases are bilateral. Symptoms manifest in the fourth decade. ADPKD accounts for 10% of all cases of renal failure.

Pathology
The kidneys reach an enormous size due to multiple fluid-filled cysts and can easily be palpated on abdominal examination. Expansion of the cysts results in ischemic atrophy of the surrounding renal parenchyma and obstruction of normal renal tubules.

End-stage renal failure is inevitable and occurs around the age of 50 years.

Associated disorders
These include a 10–30% incidence of Circle of Willis berry aneurysms (associated with subarachnoid hemorrhage); cysts of the liver (33%), pancreas (10%), and spleen (<5%); renal adenoma; cardiac valve abnormalities; aortic aneurysms; and diverticular disease.

Etiology
PKD-1 gene defects (chromosome 16) account for 90% of cases; PKD-2 gene defects (chromosome 4) cause 10%, and now a third gene, PKD-3 is also implicated.

Pathogenesis theories include intrinsic basement membrane abnormalities; tubular epithelial hyperplasia (causing tubular obstruction and basement membrane weakness); and alterations in the supportive extracellular matrix due to defective proteins, all of which may cause cyst formation.

Presentation
Patients have a positive family history (50% inheritance); palpable abdominal masses; flank pain (due to mass effect, infection, stones, or following acute cystic distension due to hemorrhage or obstruction); macroscopic (and microscopic) hematuria; UTI; and hypertension (75%).

Renal failure may present with lethargy, nausea, vomiting, anemia, confusion, and seizures.

Differential diagnosis
This includes renal tumors; simple cysts; von Hippel–Landau syndrome (cerebellar and retinal hemangioblastomas; renal, adrenal, and pancreatic cysts); and tuberous sclerosis (adenoma sebaceum, epilepsy, learning difficulties, with polycystic kidneys and renal tumors).

Investigation

This depends on the presenting symptoms.
- For suspected UTI—culture urine
- For hematuria—urine cytology, flexible cystoscopy, and renal ultrasound. On ultrasound the kidneys are small and hyperechoic, with multiple cysts of varying size, many of which show calcification. If the nature of the cysts cannot be determined with certainty on ultrasound, arrange for a renal CT.
- Renal failure will be managed by a nephrologist. Anemia may occur, though ADPKD may cause increased erythropoietin production and polycythemia.
- Renal imaging (ultrasound and CT are useful for investigation of complications)

Treatment

The aim is to preserve renal function as long as possible (control hypertension and UTI). Infected cysts (abscesses) should be drained.

Persistent, heavy hematuria can be controlled by embolization or nephrectomy.

Progressive renal failure requires dialysis and, ultimately, renal transplantation.

Vesicoureteric reflux (VUR) in adults

VUR is the retrograde flow of urine from the bladder into the upper urinary tract with or without dilatation of the ureter, renal pelvis, and calyces. It can cause symptoms and may lead to renal failure (reflux nephropathy). In adults 10–15% of patients requiring hemodialysis or transplantation do so because of reflux nephropathy.

Pathophysiology

Reflux is normally prevented by low bladder pressures, efficient ureteric peristalsis, and the ability of the vesicoureteric junction (VUJ) to occlude the distal ureter during bladder contraction. This is assisted by the ureter passing obliquely through the bladder wall (the "intramural" ureter), which is 1–2 cm long. Normal intramural ureteric length to ureteric diameter ratio is 5:1.

VUR of childhood tends to resolve spontaneously with increasing age because as the bladder grows, the intramural ureter lengthens.

Classification

Primary

A primary anatomical (and therefore functional) defect is where the intramural length of the ureter is too short (ratio <5:1).

Secondary

A secondary defect is secondary to some other anatomical or functional problem:

- Bladder outlet obstruction (BPO, DSD due to neuropathic disorders,[1] posterior urethral valves, urethral stricture) that leads to elevated bladder pressures
- Poor bladder compliance or the intermittently elevated pressures of detrusor hyperreflexia (due to neuropathic disorders[1]—e.g., spinal cord injury, spina bifida)
- Iatrogenic reflux following TURP or TURBT (a tumor overlying the ureteric orifice)—this is rare; ureteric meatotomy (incision of the ureteric orifice) for removal of ureteric stones at the VUJ; following incision of a ureterocele; ureteroneocystostomy; after pelvic radiotherapy
- Inflammatory conditions affecting function of the VUJ: TB, schistosomiasis, UTI

Associated disorders

VUR is commonly seen in duplex ureters (the Meyer–Weigert law).[2] Cystitis can cause VUR through bladder inflammation, reduced bladder compliance, increased pressures, and distortion of the VUJ. Coexistence of UTI with VUR is a potent cause of pyelonephritis—reflux of infected urine under high pressure causes reflux nephropathy, resulting in renal scarring, hypertension, and renal impairment.

1 Neuropathic disorders therefore cause VUR because they lead to intermittently or chronically raised bladder pressure (due to BOO, poor compliance, and/or detrusor hyperreflexia).
2 The lower pole ureter inserts into the bladder in a proximal location to the upper pole ureter, which inserts distally—i.e., nearer the bladder neck. The lower pole ureter has a shorter intramural length and therefore refluxes. The upper pole ureter has a longer intramural length and tends to be obstructed.

Presentation

- VUR may be symptomless, being identified during VCUG, IVP, or renal ultrasound (which shows ureteric and renal pelvis dilatation) done for some other cause.
- UTI symptoms
- Flank pain associated with a full bladder or immediately after micturition

Symptoms of recurrent UTI or of flank pain may have been present for many years before the patient seeks medical advice. Even then it may take some time for a diagnosis of VUR to be made because a high index of suspicion is required and the definitive test for making a diagnosis of VUR (VCUG—see below) is invasive (although VUR may be diagnosed by the less invasive use of IVP).

Investigation

The definitive test for the diagnosis of VUR is cystography. VUR may be apparent during bladder filling or during voiding (voiding cystourethrography [VCUG]—also known as micturating cystourethrography [MCUG]).

Urodynamics establishes the presence of voiding dysfunction (e.g., DSD) if this is suspected from the clinical picture. If there is radiographic evidence of reflux nephropathy, check blood pressure, check the urine for proteinuria, measure serum creatinine, and arrange for a ^{99m}Tc-DMSA isotope study to assess renal cortical scarring and determine split renal function.

Management

VUR is harmful to the kidney:
- In the presence of infected urine
- Where bladder pressures are markedly elevated (due to severe BOO, poor compliance, or high-pressure hyperreflexic bladder contractions)

In the absence of urinary infection or severe outflow obstruction/raised bladder pressures, VUR is not harmful, at least in the short term (months).

Subsequent management depends on the following:
- The presence and severity of symptoms
- The presence of recurrent, bacteriologically proven urinary infection
- The presence of already established renal damage (radiological evidence of reflux nephropathy, hypertension, proteinuria—proteinuria is a poor prognostic factor in patients with VUR, indicating the likelihood of impending end-stage renal failure)

For the patient with primary VUR, recurrent UTIs with no symptoms between infections, no hypertension, and good renal function, treat the UTIs when they occur and consider low-dose antibiotic prophylaxis if UTIs occur frequently (say >3 per year). If the UTIs are regularly associated with constitutional disturbance (acute pyelonephritis rather than simple cystitis), then ureteric reimplantation is indicated.

For the patient with primary VUR and objective evidence of deterioration in the affected kidney (i.e., progressive radiological signs of reflux nephropathy or reduction in renal function), use ureteric reimplantation.

Reflux into a nonfunctioning kidney (<10% function on DMSA scan) with recurrent UTIs and/or hypertension requires nephroureterectomy.

Primary reflux with severe recurrent flank pain requires ureteric reimplantation.

Secondary reflux

For secondary reflux into a transplanted kidney, no treatment is needed.

For VUR in association with the neuropathic bladder, treat the underlying cause—relieve BOO and improve bladder compliance (options: intravesical Botox injections, augmentation cystoplasty, sacral deafferentation).

For VUR with no symptoms, no UTI, no high bladder pressures and no BOO, the management of these patients is controversial because it is not known whether low-pressure, sterile reflux causes deterioration in renal function over many years without treatment.

Grade I and II reflux (reflux of contrast into nondilated ureter) probably does not require surgery, and many urologists would not recommend surgery but would monitor the patient for infection, hypertension, and evidence of deterioration in the appearance and function of the kidneys.

Grade III or more may require surgical intervention, and many urologists would recommend ureteric reimplantation or a STING procedure (see Fig. 7.1 for grading system for reflux).

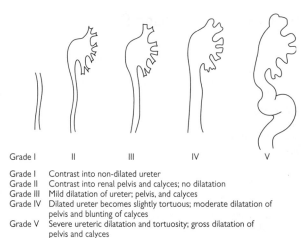

Grade I   II   III   IV   V

Grade I   Contrast into non-dilated ureter
Grade II   Contrast into renal pelvis and calyces; no dilatation
Grade III   Mild dilatation of ureter; pelvis, and calyces
Grade IV   Dilated ureter becomes slightly tortuous; moderate dilatation of
                pelvis and blunting of calyces
Grade V   Severe ureteric dilatation and tortuosity; gross dilatation of
                pelvis and calyces

Figure 7.1 International reflux classification

Ureteropelvic junction (UPJ) obstruction in adults

Ureteropelvic junction (UPJ) obstruction is an obstruction of the proximal ureter at the junction with the renal pelvis resulting in a restriction of urine flow. It is known as *pelviureteric junction obstruction* (PUJO) outside of the United States.

Epidemiology

This affects more males than females (5:2 ratio). In unilateral cases, the left side is affected more often than the right; 10–15% of cases are bilateral.

Etiology

Congenital

- *Intrinsic:* Smooth muscle defect results in an aperistaltic segment of ureter at the UPJ.
- *Extrinsic:* compression from lower renal pole vessel over which the UPJ runs. It is unlikely that these vessels are the primary cause of the obstruction. It is more probable that UPJ obstruction leads to a dilated UPJ and ballooning of the renal pelvis over the lower pole vessels, which may contribute to, but is not the primary cause of, the obstruction.
- *Acquired:* UPJ stricture secondary to ureteral manipulation (e.g., ureteroscopy); trauma from passage of calculi; fibroepithelial polyps; TCC of urothelium at UPJ; external compression of ureter by retroperitoneal fibrosis or malignancy

Presentation

Patients present with flank pain precipitated by a diuresis (high fluid intake; especially precipitated by consumption of alcohol), flank mass, UTI, and hematuria (after minor trauma). It may also be associated with vesicoureteric reflux (VUR).

Investigation

Renal ultrasound shows renal pelvis dilatation in the absence of a dilated ureter. IVP demonstrates delay of excretion of contrast and a dilated pelvicalyceal system. Arrange for a CT, to exclude a small, radiolucent stone, urothelial TCC, or retroperitoneal pathology that may be the cause of the obstruction at the UPJ.

MAG3 renography with administration of Lasix to establish a maximum diuresis is the definitive diagnostic test for UPJ obstruction. Radioisotope accumulates in the renal pelvis, and following IV Lasix it continues to accumulate (a rising curve).

Many urologists perform retrograde pyelography to establish the exact site of the obstruction, but they do this at the time of UPJ repair to avoid introducing infection into an obstructed renal pelvis.

Treatment

Surgery

Surgery is indicated for recurrent episodes of bothersome pain, renal impairment, when a stone has developed in the obstructed kidney, and when infection (pyonephrosis) has supervened.

In the absence of symptoms, consider watchful waiting with serial MAG3 renograms. If renal function remains stable and the patient remains free of symptoms, there is no need to operate.

Endoscopic treatment of a UPJ obstruction is called an *endopyelotomy* (or pyelolysis). Various techniques have been described, but the essential principle is the same—full-thickness incision through the obstructing proximal ureter, from within the lumen of the ureter down into the peripelvic and periureteral fat, using a sharp knife or holmium:YAG laser. The incision is stented for 4 weeks to allow re-epithelialization of the UPJ. The procedure is relatively minimally invasive and is generally not used for UPJ obstruction >2 cm in length.

The incision may be made percutaneously or by a retrograde approach via a rigid or flexible ureteroscope, or by using a specially designed endopyelotomy balloon (the Acucise® technique). An angioplasty-type balloon over which a cautery wire runs is inflated across the UPJ. Passage of an electrical current heats the wire and this cuts through the obstructing ring of tissue at the UPJ.

The presence of a combination of UPJ obstruction and a renal stone that is suitable for PCNL is an indication for combined PCNL and percutaneous endopyelotomy.

Success rates in terms of relieving obstruction are as follows: percutaneous endopyelotomy, 60–100% (mean 70%); cautery wire balloon endopyelotomy, 70%; ureteroscopic endopyelotomy, 80%.

Pyeloplasty

- *Open* pyeloplasty has success rates of 95% and may also be used after endopyelotomy failure or as a first-line technique.
- *Laparoscopic or robotic-assisted* pyeloplasty has the advantage of accelerated patient recovery, with success rates of 95%.
- *Common techniques* include dismembered pyeloplasty (also known as the Anderson–Hynes pyeloplasty: the narrowed area of UPJ is excised, the proximal ureter is spatulated and anastomosed to the renal pelvis), flap pyeloplasty (Culp), and Y-V-plasty (Foley).

Anomalies of renal ascent and fusion: horseshoe kidney, pelvic kidney, malrotation

Abnormalities of renal ascent and fusion occur in weeks 6–9 of gestation, when the embryonic kidney is ascending to its definitive lumbar position (ascending as a result of rapid caudal growth of the embryo).

Horseshoe kidney

This is the most common example of renal fusion. Prevalence is 1 in 400, with a male-to-female ratio 2:1.

The kidneys lie vertically (instead of obliquely) and are joined at their lower poles (in 95%) by midline parenchymal tissue (the isthmus). The inferior mesenteric artery obstructs ascent of the isthmus. Consequently, the horseshoe kidney lies lower in the abdomen (at L3 or L4 vertebral level).

Normal rotation of the kidney is also prevented, thus the renal pelvis lies anteriorly, with the ureters also passing anteriorly over the kidneys and isthmus (but entering the bladder normally). Blood supply is variable, usually from one or more renal arteries or their branches, or from branches off the aorta or inferior mesenteric artery (see Fig. 7.2).

A proportion of individuals with horseshoe kidneys have associated congenital abnormalities (Turner syndrome, trisomy 18, genitourinary anomalies, ureteric duplication), vesicoureteric reflux, UPJ obstruction, and renal tumors (including Wilm tumors).

Most patients with horseshoe kidneys remain asymptomatic; however, infection and calculi may develop and cause symptoms. The diagnosis is usually suggested on renal ultrasound and confirmed by IVP (calyces of the lower renal pole are seen to point medially, and lie medially in relation to the ureters) or CT. Renal function is usually normal.

Pelvic kidney

This represents a form of renal ectopia. Prevalence is 1 in 2000–3000, with both sexes affected equally.

The left kidney is affected more often than the right, and bilateral cases are seen in <10%. The affected kidney is smaller, with the renal pelvis positioned anteriorly (instead of medially), and the ureter is short but enters the bladder normally.

Pelvic kidneys lie opposite the sacrum and below the aortic bifurcation and are supplied by adjacent (aberrant) vessels (see Fig. 7.3). There is an increased risk of congenital anomalies, including contralateral renal agenesis and genital malformations.

Most cases are asymptomatic. Diagnosis is made on renal ultrasound scan, IVP, or renography. Complications include obstruction, hydronephrosis, and infection.

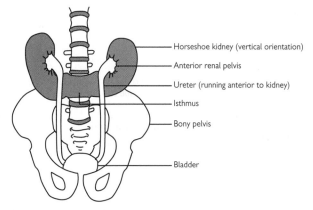

Figure 7.2 Horseshoe kidney.

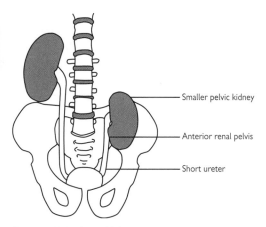

Figure 7.3 Pelvic (ectopic) kidney.

Malrotation

The kidney is located in a normal position, but the renal pelvis fails to rotate from an anterior to a medial orientation. Prevalence is ~1 in 1000, with a male-to-female ratio of 2:1. The renal shape may be altered (flattened, oval, triangular, or elongated) and the kidney retains its fetal lobulated outline (see Fig. 7.4).

It is associated with increased deposition of fibrous tissue around the renal hilum, which can produce symptoms due to ureteric or UPJ obstruction (causing hydronephrosis, infection, or stone formation). Most patients, however, remain asymptomatic.

The diagnosis is made on renal ultrasound scan, IVP, or retrograde pyelography.

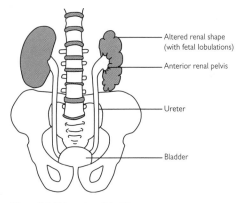

Altered renal shape
(with fetal lobulations)

Anterior renal pelvis

Ureter

Bladder

Figure 7.4 Malrotation of the kidney.

Renal duplications

Definitions

A duplex kidney has an upper pole and a lower pole, each with its own separate pelvicalyceal system and ureter. The two ureters may join to form a single ureter at the pelviureteric junction (bifid system) or more distally (bifid ureter) before entering the bladder through one ureteric orifice.

Alternatively, the two ureters may pass down individually to the bladder (complete duplication). In this case, the Weigert–Meyer rule states that the upper-pole ureter always opens onto the bladder medially and inferiorly to the ureter of the lower pole, thereby predisposing to ectopic placement of the ureteric orifice and obstruction (due to the longer intramural course of the ureter through the bladder wall).

The lower-pole ureter opens onto the bladder laterally and superiorly, reducing the intramural ureteric length, which predisposes to vesicoureteric reflux (in up to 85%).

Epidemiology

Ureteric duplication occurs in 1 in 125 individuals, with a female-to-male ratio of 2:1. Unilateral cases are more common than bilateral cases, with right and left sides affected equally.

Risk of other congenital malformations is increased.

Embryology

In duplication, two ureteric buds arise from the mesonephric duct (week 4 gestation). The ureteric bud situated more distally (lower-pole ureter) enters the bladder first and therefore migrates a longer distance, resulting in the superior and lateral position of the ureteric orifice.

The proximal bud (upper-pole ureter) has less time to migrate, and consequently the ureteric orifice is inferior and medial (ectopic). Interaction of each ureteric bud with the same metanephric tissue creates separate collecting systems within the same renal unit.

With bifid ureters, a single ureteric bud splits after it has emerged from the mesonephric duct.

Complications

Ectopic ureters are associated with both upper renal-pole hydronephrosis (secondary to obstruction) and hypoplasia or dysplasia (renal maldevelopment related to ectopic displacement of ureteric orifice).

Lower-pole ureters are prone to reflux, resulting in hydroureter and hydronephrosis.

Bifid ureters can get urine continuously passing from one collecting system to the other, causing urinary stasis (predisposing to infection).

Presentation

Patients have symptoms of UTI or flank pain, or an asymptomatic incidental finding.

Investigation

- Renal ultrasound scan demonstrates ureteric duplication ± dilatation and hydronephrosis.
- IVP decreased contrast excretion from renal upper pole ± hydron-epFlankhrosis (which may displace the lower pole downward and outward, producing a "drooping lily" appearance).
- Micturating cystourethrography (MCUG) will determine whether reflux is present.
- CT and MRI reveal detailed anatomical information.
- Isotope renogram (^{99m}Tc-DMSA) assesses renal function.

Treatment

In symptomatic patients, the aim is to reduce obstruction and reflux and to improve function. Common sheath ureteric reimplantation (where a cuff of bladder tissue is taken that encompasses both duplicated ureters) can treat both conditions.

Where an ectopic ureter is associated with a poorly functioning renal upper pole, open or laparoscopic heminephrectomy with excision of the associated ureter may be considered.

Stone disease

Kidney stones: epidemiology 356
Kidney stones: types and predisposing factors 358
Kidney stones: mechanisms of formation 360
Factors predisposing to specific stone types 362
Evaluation of the stone former 366
Kidney stones: presentation and diagnosis 368
Kidney stone treatment options: watchful waiting 370
Stone fragmentation techniques: extracorporeal lithotripsy
    (ESWL) 372
Intracorporeal techniques of stone fragmentation
    (fragmentation within the body) 374
Kidney stone treatment: flexible ureteroscopy and laser
    treatment 378
Kidney stone treatment: percutaneous nephrolithotomy
    (PCNL) 380
Kidney stones: open stone surgery 383
Kidney stones: medical therapy (dissolution therapy) 384
Ureteric stones: presentation 386
Ureteric stones: diagnostic radiological imaging 388
Ureteric stones: acute management 390
Ureteric stones: indications for intervention to relieve
    obstruction and/or remove the stone 392
Ureteric stone treatment 394
Treatment options for ureteric stones 396
Prevention of calcium oxalate stone formation 398
Bladder stones 400
Management of ureteric stones in pregnancy 402

Kidney stones: epidemiology

Approximately 10% of Caucasian men will develop a kidney stone by the age of 70. Within 1 year of a calcium oxalate stone, 10% of men will form another calcium oxalate stone, and 50% will have formed another stone within 10 years.

The prevalence of renal tract stone disease is determined by factors *intrinsic* to the individual and by *extrinsic* (environmental) factors. A combination of factors often contributes to the risk of stone formation.

Intrinsic factors

Age

Peak incidence of stones occurs between the ages of 20 and 50 years.

Sex

Males are affected 3 times as frequently as females. Testosterone may cause increased oxalate production in the liver (predisposing to calcium oxalate stones) and women have higher urinary citrate concentrations (citrate inhibits calcium oxalate stone formation).

Genetic

Kidney stones are relatively uncommon in Native Americans, Black Africans, and U.S. Blacks, and more common in Caucasians and Asians. About 25% of patients with kidney stones report a family history of stone disease (the relative risk of stone formation remaining high after adjusting for dietary calcium intake).

Familial renal tubular acidosis (predisposing to calcium phosphate stones) and cystinuria (predisposing to cystine stones) are inherited.[1]

Extrinsic (environmental) factors

Geographical location, climate, and season

The relationship between these factors and stone risk is complex. While renal stone disease is more common in hot climates, some endogenous populations of hot climates have a low incidence of stones (e.g., Black Africans, Aborigines), and many temperate areas have a high incidence of stones (e.g., Northern Europe and Scandinavia). This may relate to Western lifestyle—excess food, inadequate fluid intake, limited exercise—combined with a genetic predisposition to stone formation.

Ureteric stones become more prevalent during the summer

The highest incidence occurs a month or so after peak summertime temperatures, presumably because of higher urinary concentration in the summer (encourages crystallization). Concentrated urine has a lower pH, encouraging cystine and uric acid stone formation.

Exposure to sunlight may also increase endogenous vitamin D production, leading to hypercalciuria.

---

1 Curhan GC, Willett WC, Rimm EB, Stampfer MJ (1997). Family history and risk of kidney stones. *J Am Soc Nephrol*, 8:1568–1573.

Water intake

Low fluid intake (<1200 mL/day) predisposes to stone formation.[2] Increasing water hardness (high calcium content) may reduce risk of stone formation, by decreasing urinary oxalate.

Diet

High animal protein intake increases risk of stone disease (high urinary oxalate, low pH, low urinary citrate).[3,4] High salt intake causes hypercalciuria. Contrary to conventional teaching, low-calcium diets predispose to calcium stone disease, and high-calcium intake is protective.[5]

Occupation

Sedentary occupations predispose to stones more than manual work.

2 Borghi L, et al. (1996) Urinary volume, water and recurrences in idiopathic calcium nephrolithiasis: a 5-year randomized prospective study. *J Urol* 155:839–843.
3 Curhan GC, et al. (1997) Comparison of dietary calcium with supplemental calcium and other nutrients as factors affecting the risk for kidney stones in women. *Ann Intern Med* 126:497–504.
4 Borghi L, et al. (2002) Comparison of 2 diets for the prevention of recurrent stones in idiopathic hypercalciuria. *N Engl J Med* 346:77–84.
5 Curhan GC, et al. (1993) A prospective study of dietary calcium and other nutrients and the risk of symptomatic kidney stones. *N Engl J Med* 328:833–838.

Kidney stones: types and predisposing factors

Stones may be classified according to composition (Table 8.1), X-ray appearance, or size and shape.

Other rare stone types (all radiolucent) include indinavir (a protease inhibitor for treatment of HIV), triamterene (a relatively insoluble potassium-sparing diuretic, most of which is excreted in urine), and xanthine.

Radiodensity on X-ray

Three broad categories of stones are described, based on their X-ray appearance. This gives some indication of the likely stone composition and helps to some extent to determine treatment options.

However, in only 40% of cases is stone composition correctly identified from visual estimation of radiodensity on plain X-ray.[1]

Radio-opaque

Opacity implies presence of substantial amounts of calcium within the stone. Calcium phosphate stones are the most radiodense stones, almost as dense as bone. Calcium oxalate stones are slightly less radiodense.

Relatively radiolucent

Cystine stones are relatively radiodense because they contain sulfur (Fig. 8.1). Magnesium ammonium phosphate (struvite) stones are less radiodense than calcium-containing stones.

Completely radiolucent

Uric acid, triamterene, xanthine, indinavir stones are in this category (cannot be seen even on CTU).

Table 8.1 Composition of kidney stones

Stone composition	% of all renal calculi*
Calcium oxalate	85%
Uric acid[†]	5–10%
Calcium phosphate + calcium oxalate	10%
Pure calcium phosphate	Rare
Struvite (infection stones)	2–20%
Cystine	1%

* The precise distribution of stone types will vary depending on the characteristics of the study population (geographical location, racial distribution, etc.). Hence, the quoted figures do not equate to 100.

†~80% of uric acid stones are pure uric acid; 20% contain some calcium oxalate.

1 Ramakumar S, Patterson DE, LeRoy AJ, et al. (1999) Prediction of stone composition from plain radiographs: a prospective study. *J Endosc Urol* 13:397–401.

Size and shape

Stones can be characterized by their size, in centimeters. Stones that grow to occupy the renal collecting system (the pelvis and one or more renal calyx) are known as staghorn calculi, since they resemble the horns of a stag (Fig. 8.2). They are most commonly composed of struvite—magnesium ammonium phosphate (being caused by infection and forming under the alkaline conditions induced by urea-splitting bacteria), but may consist of uric acid, cystine, or calcium oxalate monohydrate.

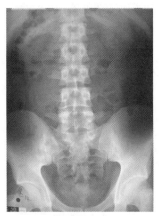

Figure 8.1 A left cystine stone, barely visible just below the midpoint of the 12th rib.

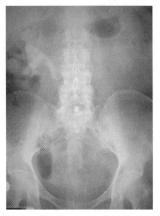

Figure 8.2 A large, right staghorn calculus.

Kidney stones: mechanisms of formation

Urine is said to be saturated with, for example, calcium and oxalate, when the product of the concentrations of calcium and oxalate exceeds the solubility product (K_{sp}). Below the solubility product, crystals of calcium and oxalate will not form and the urine is undersaturated. Above the solubility product, crystals of calcium and oxalate should form, but they do not because of the presence of *inhibitors* of crystal formation.

However, above a certain concentration of calcium and oxalate, inhibitors of crystallization become ineffective, and crystals of calcium oxalate start to form. The concentration of calcium and oxalate at which this is reached (i.e., at which crystallization starts) is known as the *formation product* (K_f), and the urine is said to be *supersaturated* with the substance or substances in question at concentrations above this level.

Urine is described as being *metastable* for calcium and oxalate at concentrations between the solubility product of calcium and oxalate and the formation product (see Box 8.1).

The ability of urine to hold more solute in solution than can pure water is due partly to the presence of various inhibitors of crystallization (e.g., citrate forms a soluble complex with calcium, preventing it from combining with oxalate or phosphate to form calcium oxalate or calcium phosphate stones). Other inhibitors of crystallization include magnesium, glycosaminoglycans, and Tamm–Horsfall protein.

Periods of intermittent supersaturation of urine with various substances can occur as a consequence of dehydration and following meals.

The earliest phase of crystal formation is known as *nucleation*. Crystal nuclei usually form on the surfaces of epithelial cells or on other crystals. Crystal nuclei form into clumps—a process known as *aggregation*. Citrate and magnesium inhibit not only crystallization but also aggregation.

Box 8.1 Steps leading to stone formation

- Calcium and oxalate concentration < solubility product → NO STONE FORMATION
- Metastable calcium and oxalate concentrations → NO STONE FORMATION
- Calcium and oxalate concentrations > formation product → STONE FORMATION

In the urine of subjects who do not form stones, the concentrations of most stone components are between K_{sp} and K_f.

Factors predisposing to specific stone types

Calcium oxalate (~85% of stones)

Hypercalciuria

Excretion of >7 mmol of calcium per day in men and >6 mmol/day in women. A major risk factor for calcium oxalate stone formation is when it increases the relative supersaturation of urine. About 50% of patients with calcium stone disease have hypercalciuria. There are three types:

• Absorptive—increased intestinal absorption of calcium
• Renal—renal leak of calcium
• Resorptive—increased demineralization of bone (due to hyperparathyroidism)

Hypercalcemia

Almost all patients with hypercalcemia who form stones have primary hyperparathyroidism. Of hyperparathyroid patients, about 1% form stones (the other 99% do not because of early detection of hyperparathyroidism by screening serum calcium).

Hyperoxaluria

This is due to the following:

• Altered membrane transport of oxalate leading to increased renal leak of oxalate
• Primary hyperoxaluria—increased hepatic oxalate production; rare
• Increased oxalate absorption in short bowel syndrome or malabsorption (enteric hyperoxaluria)—the colon is exposed to more bile salts and this increases its permeability to oxalate.

Hypocitraturia

This is low urinary citrate excretion. Citrate forms a soluble complex with calcium and prevents complexing of calcium with oxalate to form calcium oxalate stones.

Hyperuricosuria

High urinary uric acid levels lead to formation of uric acid crystals, on the surface of which calcium oxalate crystals form.

Uric acid (~5–10% of stones)

Humans are unable to convert uric acid (which is relatively insoluble) into allantoin (which is very soluble). Human urine is supersaturated with insoluble uric acid. Uric acid exists in two forms in urine—uric acid and sodium urate. Sodium urate is 20 times more soluble than uric acid.

At a urine pH of 5, <20% of uric acid is present as soluble sodium urate. At urine pH 5.5, half the uric acid is ionized as sodium urate (soluble) and half is nonionized as free uric acid (insoluble). At a urine pH of 6.5, >90% of uric acid is present as soluble sodium urate.

Thus, uric acid is essentially insoluble in acid urine and soluble in alkaline urine. Human urine is acidic (because the end products of metabolism are acid) and this low pH, combined with supersaturation of urine with uric acid, predisposes to uric acid stone formation.

Approximately 20% of patients with gout have uric acid stones. Patients with uric acid stones may have the following:

- **Gout.** 50% of patients with uric acid stones have gout. The chance of forming a uric acid stone if you have gout is on the order of 1% per year from the time of the first attack of gout.
- **Myeloproliferative disorders.** Particularly following treatment with cytotoxic drugs, cell necrosis results in release of large quantities of nucleic acids that are converted to uric acid. A large plug of uric acid crystals may form in the collecting system of the kidney, in the absence of ureteric colic, causing oliguria or anuria.
- **Idiopathic uric acid stones** (no associated condition)

Calcium phosphate (calcium phosphate + calcium oxalate = 10% of stones)

These stones occur in patients with renal tubular acidosis (RTA), a defect of renal tubular H^+ secretion resulting in impaired ability of the kidney to acidify urine. The urine is thus of high pH, and the patient has a metabolic acidosis. The high urine pH increases supersaturation of the urine with calcium and phosphate, leading to their precipitation as stones.

Types of renal tubular acidosis

- **Type 1 or distal RTA:** The distal tubule is unable to maintain a proton gradient between the blood and the tubular fluid. Of such patients, 70% have stones. Urine pH is >5.5, the patient has a metabolic acidosis and hypokalemia, urinary citrate is low, and hypercalciuria is present.
- **Type 2 or proximal RTA** is due to failure of bicarbonate resorption in the proximal tubule. There is associated increased urinary citrate excretion, which protects against stone formation.
- **Type 3:** A variant of type 1 RTA
- **Type 4** is seen in diabetic nephropathy and interstitial renal disease. These patients do not make stones.

If urine pH is >5.5, use the ammonium chloride loading test. Urine pH that remains above 5.5 after an oral dose of ammonium chloride = incomplete distal RTA.

Struvite (infection or triple phosphate stones) (2–20% of stones)

These stones are composed of magnesium, ammonium, and phosphate. They form as a consequence of urease-producing bacteria that produce ammonia from breakdown of urea (urease hydrolyses urea to carbon dioxide and ammonium) and, in so doing, alkalinize urine as in the following equation:

$$NH_2-O-NH_2 + H_2O \rightarrow 2NH_3 + CO_2$$

Under alkaline conditions, crystals of magnesium, ammonium, and phosphate precipitate.

Cystine (1% of all stones)

These stones occur only in patients with cystinuria—an inherited (autosomal recessive) disorder of transmembrane cystine transport, resulting in decreased absorption of cystine from the intestine and in the proximal tubule of the kidney.

Cystine is very insoluble, so reduced absorption of cystine from the proximal tubule results in supersaturation with cystine and cystine crystal formation. Cystine is poorly soluble in acid urine (300 mg/L at pH 5, 400 mg/L at pH 7).

Evaluation of the stone former

Determination of stone type and a metabolic evaluation allows identification of the factors that led to stone formation, so advice can be given to prevent future stone formation.

Metabolic evaluation depends, to an extent, on the stone type (see Table 8.2). In many cases a stone is retrieved. Stone type is analyzed by polarizing microscopy, X-ray diffraction, and infrared spectroscopy, rather than by chemical analysis. Where no stone is retrieved, its nature must be inferred from its radiological appearance (e.g., a completely radiolucent stone is likely to be composed of uric acid) or from more detailed metabolic evaluation.

In most patients, multiple factors are involved in the genesis of kidney stones and, as a general guide, the following evaluation is appropriate in most patients.

Risk factors for stone disease
- *Diet:* Enquire about volume of fluid intake, meat consumption (causes hypercalciuria, high uric acid levels, low urine pH, low urinary citrate), multivitamins (vitamin D increases intestinal calcium absorption), high doses of vitamin C (ascorbic acid causes hyperoxaluria).
- *Drugs:* Corticosteroids (increase enteric absorption of calcium, leading to hypercalciuria); chemotherapeutic agents (breakdown products of malignant cells leads to hyperuricemia).
- *Urinary tract infection:* Urease-producing bacteria *(Proteus, Klebsiella, Serratia, Enterobacter)* predispose to struvite stones.
- *Mobility:* Low activity levels predispose to bone demineralization and hypercalciuria.
- *Systemic disease:* gout, primary hyperparathyroidism, sarcoidosis
- *Family history:* cystinuria, RTA
- *Renal anatomy:* UPJ, horseshoe kidney, medullary sponge kidney (up to 2% of patients with calcium-containing stones have MSK)
- *Previous bowel resection or inflammatory bowel disease* causes intestinal hyperoxaluria.

Metabolic evaluation of the stone former
Patients can be categorized as low risk or high risk for subsequent stone formation. High risk includes previous history of a stone, family history of stones, gastrointestinal (GI) disease, gout, chronic UTI, nephrocalcinosis.

Low-risk patient evaluation
Assess urea and electrolytes, CBC (to detect undiagnosed hematological malignancy), serum calcium (corrected for serum albumin), and uric acid, as well as urine culture, and urine dipstick for pH (see below).

High-risk patient evaluation
Evaluation is the same as for low-risk patients plus 24-hour urine for calcium, oxalate, uric acid, and cystine, and evaluation for RTA.

Table 8.2 Characteristics of stone types

Stone type	Urine acidity	Mean urine pH (SEM)
Calcium oxalate	Variable	6 (± 0.4)
Calcium phosphate	Tendency toward alkaline urine	>5.5
Uric acid	Acid	5.5 (± 0.4)
Struvite	Alkaline*	—
Cystine	Normal (5–7)	—

* Urine pH must be above 7.2 for deposition of struvite crystals.

Urine pH

Urine pH in normal individuals shows variation, pH 5–7. After a meal, pH is initially acid because of acid production from metabolism of purines (nucleic acids in, for example, meat). This is followed by an alkaline tide, with pH rising to >6.5.

Urine pH can help establish what type of stone the patient may have (if a stone is not available for analysis) and can help the urologist and patient in determining whether preventative measures are likely to be effective or not.

- pH <6 in a patient with radiolucent stones suggests the presence of uric acid stones.
- pH consistently >5.5 suggests type 1 (distal) RTA (~70% of such patients will form calcium phosphate stones).

Evaluation for RTA

Evaluate for RTA if there are calcium phosphate stones, bilateral stones, nephrocalcinosis, MSK, or hypocitraturia.

- If fasting morning urine pH (i.e., first urine of the day) is >5.5, the patient has complete distal RTA.
- First and second morning urine pH is a useful screening test for detection of incomplete distal RTA; over 90% of cases of RTA have a pH >6 on both specimens. The ammonium chloride loading test involves an oral dose of ammonium chloride (0.1 g/kg; an acid load). If serum pH falls <7.3 or serum bicarbonate falls <16 mmol/L, but urine pH remains >5.5, the patient has incomplete distal RTA.

Diagnostic tests for suspected cystinuria

These include the cyanide-nitroprusside colorimetric test (cystine spot test). If positive, a 24-hour urine collection is done. A 24-hour cystine >250 mg is diagnostic of cystinuria.[1]

1 Millman S, Strauss AL, Parks JH, Coe FL (1982). Pathogenesis and clinical course of mixed calcium oxalate and uric acid nephrolithiasis. Kidney Int 22:366–370.

Kidney stones: presentation and diagnosis

Kidney stones may present with symptoms or be found incidentally during investigation of other problems. Presenting symptoms include pain or hematuria (microscopic or occasionally macroscopic). Struvite staghorn calculi classically present with recurrent UTIs. Malaise, weakness, and loss of appetite can also occur.

Less commonly, struvite stones present with infective complications (pyonephrosis, perinephric abscess, septicemia, xanthogranulomatous pyelonephritis).

Diagnostic tests

- **Plain abdominal radiography:** Calculi that contain calcium are radiodense. Sulfur-containing stones (cystine) are relatively radiolucent on plain radiography.
- Radiodensity of stones in decreasing order is calcium phosphate > calcium oxalate > struvite (magnesium ammonium phosphate) >> cystine.
- Completely radiolucent stones (e.g., uric acid, triamterene, indinavir) are usually suspected on the basis of the patient's history and/or urine pH (pH <6: gout; drug history: triamterene, indinavir), and the diagnosis may be confirmed by ultrasound, computed tomographic urography (CTU), or magnetic resonance urography (MRU).
- **Renal ultrasound:** Its sensitivity for detecting renal calculi is ~95%.[1] A combination of plain abdominal radiography and renal ultrasonography is a useful screening test for renal calculi.
- **IVP** is increasingly being replaced by CTU. IVP is useful for patients with suspected indinavir stones (which are not visible on CT).
- **CTU** is a very accurate method of diagnosing all but indinavir stones. It allows accurate determination of stone size and location and good definition of pelvicalyceal anatomy.
- **MRU** cannot visualize stones but is able to demonstrate the presence of hydronephrosis.

---

1 Haddad MC, Sharif HS, Abomelha ME, et al. (1992) Management of renal colic: redefining the role of the urogram. *Radiology* 184:35–36.

Kidney stone treatment options: watchful waiting

The traditional indications for intervention are pain, infection, and obstruction. Hematuria caused by a stone is only very rarely severe or frequent enough to be the only reason to warrant treatment.

Before embarking on treatment of a stone that you think is the cause of the patient's pain or infections, warn the patient that though you may be able to remove the stone successfully, their pain or infections may persist (i.e., the stone may be coincidental to their pain or infections, which may be due to something else).

Remember, UTIs are common in women, as are stones, and it is not therefore surprising that the two may coexist in the same patient but be otherwise unrelated.

Options for stone treatment are watchful waiting, extracorporeal shock wave (ESWL), flexible ureteroscopy, percutaneous nephrolithotomy (PCNL), open surgery, and medical dissolution therapy.

When to watch and wait—and when not to

It is not necessary to treat every kidney stone. As a rule of thumb, the younger the patient, the larger the stone, and the more symptoms it is causing, the more inclined we are to recommend treatment.

Thus, one would probably do nothing about a 1 cm asymptomatic stone in the kidney of a 95-year-old patient. On the other hand, a 1 cm stone in an asymptomatic 20-year-old runs the risk over the remaining (many) years of the patient's life of causing problems. It could drop into the ureter, causing ureteric colic, or it could increase in size and affect kidney function or cause pain.

Asymptomatic stones followed over a 3-year period are more likely to require intervention (surgery or ESWL) or to increase in size or cause pain if they are >4 mm in diameter and if they are located in a middle or lower pole calyx.[1] The approximate risks, over 3 years of follow-up, of requiring intervention, of developing pain, or of increase in stone size, relative to stone size, is shown in Table 8.3.

Another factor determining the need for treatment is the patient's job. Airline pilots are not allowed to fly if they have kidney stones, for fear that the stones could drop into the ureter at 30,000 ft, with disastrous consequences.

Some stones are definitely not suitable for watchful waiting. Untreated struvite (i.e., infection related) staghorn calculi will eventually destroy the kidney if untreated and are a significant risk to the patient's life. Watchful waiting is therefore NOT recommended for staghorn calculi unless patient comorbidity is such that surgery would be a higher risk than watchful waiting.

1 Burgher A, et al. (2004). Progression of nephrolithiasis: long-term outcomes with observation of asymptomatic calculi. *J Endourol* 18:534–539.

Table 8.3 Approximate 3-year risk of intervention, pain, or increase in stone size

	Stone size			
	<5 mm	**5–10 mm**	**11–15 mm**	**>15 mm**
% Requiring intervention	20%	25%	40%	30%
% Causing pain	40%	40%	40%	60%
% Increasing in size	50%	55%	60%	70%

Historical series suggest that ~30% of patients with staghorn calculi who did not undergo surgical removal died of renal-related causes—renal failure and urosepsis (septicemia, pyonephrosis, perinephric abscess).[2,3] A combination of a neurogenic bladder and staghorn calculus seems to be particularly associated with a poor outcome.[4]

2 Blandy JP, Singh M (1976). The case for a more aggressive approach to staghorn stones. *J Urol* 115:505–506.
3 Rous SN, Turner WR (1977). Retrospective study of 95 patients with staghorn calculus disease. *J Urol* 118:902.
4 Teichmann J (1995). Long-term renal fate and prognosis after staghorn calculus management. *J Urol* 153:1403–1407.

Stone fragmentation techniques: extracorporeal lithotripsy (ESWL)

The technique of focusing externally generated shock waves at a target (the stone) was first used in humans in 1980. The first commercial lithotriptor, the Dornier HM3, became available in 1983.[1] ESWL revolutionized kidney and ureteric stone treatment.

Three methods of shock wave generation are commercially available—electrohydraulic, electromagnetic, and piezoelectric.

Electrohydraulic

Application of a high-voltage electrical current between 2 electrodes about 1 mm apart under water causes discharge of a spark. Water around the tip of the electrode is vaporized by the high temperature, resulting in a rapidly expanding gas bubble. The rapid expansion and then rapid collapse of this bubble generates a shock wave that is focused by a metal reflector shaped as a hemi-ellipsoid.

This method was used in the original Dornier HM3 lithotriptor.

Electromagnetic

Two electrically conducting cylindrical plates are separated by a thin membrane of insulating material. Passage of an electrical current through the plates generates a strong magnetic field between them, the subsequent movement of which generates a shock wave. An acoustic lens is used to focus the shock wave.

Piezoelectric

A spherical dish is covered with about 3000 small ceramic elements, each of which expands rapidly when a high voltage is applied across them. This rapid expansion generates a shock wave. X-ray, ultrasound, or combinations of both are used to locate the stone on which the shock waves are focused.

Older machines required general or regional anesthesia because the shock waves were powerful and caused severe pain.

Newer lithotriptors generate less powerful shock waves, allowing ESWL with oral or parenteral analgesia in many cases, but they are less efficient at stone fragmentation.

Efficacy of ESWL

The likelihood of fragmentation with ESWL depends on stone size and location, anatomy of renal collecting system, degree of obesity, and stone composition. ESWL is most effective for stones <2 cm in diameter, in favorable anatomical locations. It is less effective for stones >2 cm diameter, in lower-pole stones in a calyceal diverticulum (poor drainage), and those composed of cystine or calcium oxalate monohydrate (very hard).

Stone-free rates for solitary kidney stones are 80% for stones <1 cm in diameter, 60% for those between 1 and 2 cm, and 50% for those >2 cm in diameter. Lower stone-free rates as compared with open surgery or PCNL are accepted because of the minimal morbidity of ESWL.

1 Chaussy CG, Brendel W, Schmidt E (1980). Extracorporeal induced destruction of kidney stones by shock waves. *Lancet* 2:1265–1268.

There have been no randomized studies comparing stone-free rates between different lithotriptors. In nonrandomized studies, rather surprisingly, when it comes to efficacy of stone fragmentation, older (the original Dornier HM3 machine) is better (but with higher requirement for analgesia and sedation or general anesthesia). Less powerful (modern) lithotriptors have lower stone-free rates and higher retreatment rates.

Side effects of ESWL

ESWL causes a certain amount of structural and functional renal damage (found more frequently the harder you look). Hematuria (microscopic, macroscopic) and edema are common, perirenal hematomas less so (0.5% detected on ultrasound with modern machines, although reported in as many as 30% with the Dornier HM3).

Effective renal plasma flow (measured by renography) has been reported to fall in ~30% of treated kidneys. There are data suggesting that ESWL may increase the likelihood of development of hypertension.

Acute renal injury may be more likely to occur in patients with pre-existing hypertension, prolonged coagulation time, coexisting coronary heart disease, or diabetes and in those with solitary kidneys.

Contraindications to ESWL

Absolute contraindications are pregnancy and uncorrected blood clotting disorders (including anticoagulation).

Procedure-specific consent form: potential complications after ESWL

Common
- Bleeding on passing urine for short period after procedure
- Pain in the kidney as small fragments of stone pass after fragmentation
- UTI from bacteria released from the stone, needing antibiotic treatment.

Occasional
- Stone will not break as too hard, requiring an alternative treatment
- Repeated ESWL treatments may be required
- Recurrence of stones

Rare
- Kidney damage (bruising) or infection, needing further treatment
- Stone fragments occasionally get stuck in the tube (ureter) between the kidney and the bladder, requiring hospital admission and sometimes surgery to remove the stone fragment
- Severe infection requiring intravenous antibiotics and sometimes drainage of the kidney by a small drain placed through the back into the kidney.

Alternative therapy

Endoscopic surgery, open surgery, or observation can be used to allow spontaneous passage.

Intracorporeal techniques of stone fragmentation (fragmentation within the body)

Electrohydraulic lithotripsy (EHL)

EHL was the first technique developed for intracorporeal lithotripsy. A high voltage applied across a concentric electrode under water generates a spark. This vaporizes water, and the subsequent expansion and collapse of the gas bubble generates a shock wave.

EHL is an effective form of stone fragmentation. The shock wave is not focused, so the EHL probe must be applied within 1 mm of the stone to optimize stone fragmentation.

EHL has a narrower safety margin than that of pneumatic, ultrasonic, or laser lithotripsy and should be kept as far away as possible from the wall of the ureter, renal pelvis, or bladder to limit damage to these structures, and at least 2 mm away from the cystoscope, ureteroscope, or nephroscope to prevent lens fracture.

Principal uses are for bladder stones (wider safety margin than in the narrower ureter).

Pneumatic (ballistic) lithotripsy

A metal projectile contained within the handpiece is propelled backward and forward at great speed by bursts of compressed air (see Fig. 8.3). It strikes a long, thin, metal probe at one end of the handpiece at 12Hz (12 strikes/second) transmitting shock waves to the probe, which, when in contact with a rigid structure such as a stone, fragments the stone.

This technique is used for stone fragmentation in the ureter (using a thin probe to allow insertion down a ureteroscope) or kidney (a thicker probe may be used, with an inbuilt suction device—Lithovac—to remove stone fragments).

Pneumatic lithotripsy is very safe, since the excursion of the end of probe is about a millimeter, and it bounces off the pliable wall of the ureter. Ureteric perforation is therefore rare.

The device is low cost and requires low maintenance. However, its ballistic effect has a tendency to cause stone migration into the proximal ureter or renal pelvis, where the stone may be inaccessible to further treatment. The metal probe cannot bend around corners, so it cannot be used for ureteroscopic treatment of stones within the kidney or with a flexible ureteroscope.

Its principal use is for ureteric stones.

Ultrasonic lithotripsy

An electrical current applied across a piezoceramic plate located in the ultrasound transducer generates ultrasound waves of a specific frequency (23,000–25,000 Hz). The ultrasound energy is transmitted to a hollow metal probe, which in turn is applied to the stone (see Fig. 8.4).

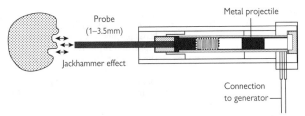

Figure 8.3 The Lithoclast: a pneumatic lithotripsy device. This figure was published in Walsh PC, et al. *Campbell's Urology*, 8th edition, pp. 3395–979. Copyright Elsevier 2002.

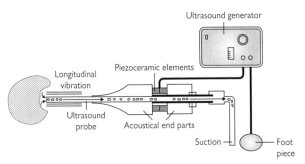

Figure 8.4 The Calcuson: an ultrasonic lithotripsy device. This figure was published in Walsh PC, et al. *Campbell's Urology*, 8th edition, pp. 3395–979. Copyright Elsevier 2002.

The stone resonates at high frequency and this causes it to break into small fragments (the opera singer breaking a glass) that are then sucked out through the center of the hollow probe. Soft tissues do not resonate when the probe is applied to them and thus are not damaged.

This technique can only be used down straight, rigid instruments.

Principal uses include fragmentation of renal calculi during PCNL.

Laser lithotripsy

The holmium:YAG laser is principally a photothermal mechanism of action, causing stone vaporization. It has minimal shock-wave generation and therefore less risk of causing stone migration. The laser energy is delivered down fibers that vary in diameter from 200 to 360 microns. The 200-micron fiber is very flexible and can be used to gain access to stones even within the lower pole of the kidney (see Figs. 8.5 and 8.6).

The zone of thermal injury is limited to 0.5–1 mm from the laser tip. No stone can withstand the heat generated by the Ho:YAG laser. Laser lithotripsy takes time; however, since the thin laser fiber must be "painted" over the surface of the stone to vaporize it.

Principal uses are for ureteric stones and small intrarenal stones.

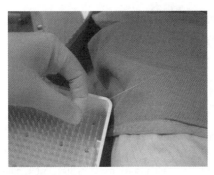

Figure 8.5 A laser fiber.

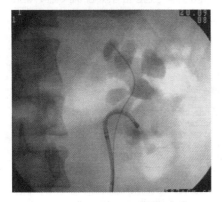

Figure 8.6 Access to the lower pole of the kidney with a flexible ureteroscope.

Kidney stone treatment: flexible ureteroscopy and laser treatment

The development of small-caliber ureteroscopes with active deflecting mechanisms and instrument channels, in combination with the development of laser technology, small-diameter laser fibers, and stone baskets and graspers, has opened the way for intracorporeal, endoscopic treatment of kidney stones.

Access to virtually the entire collecting system is possible with modern instruments. The holmium:YAG laser has a minimal effect on tissues at distances of 2–3 mm from the laser tip and so collateral tissue damage is minimal with this laser type.

Flexible ureteroscopy and laser fragmentation offers a more effective treatment option than ESWL, with a lower morbidity than PCNL, but usually requires a general anesthetic (some patients will tolerate it with sedation alone). It can also allow access to areas of the kidney where ESWL is less efficient or where PCNL cannot reach. It is most suited to stones <2 cm in diameter.

Indications for flexible ureteroscopic kidney stone treatment

- ESWL failure
- Lower pole stone (reduces likelihood of stone passage post- ESWL—fragments have to pass uphill)
- Cystine stones
- Obesity such that PCNL access is technically difficult or impossible (nephroscopes may not be long enough to reach stone)
- Obesity such that ESWL is technically difficult or impossible. BMI >28 is associated with lower ESWL success rates. Treatment distance may exceed focal length of lithotriptor.
- Musculoskeletal deformities such that stone access by PCNL or ESWL is difficult or impossible (e.g., kyphoscoliosis)
- Stone in a calyceal diverticulum (accessing stones in small diverticulae in upper and anterior calyces is difficult and carries significant risks)
- Stenosis of a calyceal infundibulum or tight angle between renal pelvis and infundibulum. The flexible ureteroscope can negotiate acute angles and the laser can be used to divide obstructions.
- Bleeding diathesis where reversal of this diathesis is potentially dangerous or difficult
- Horseshoe or pelvic kidney. ESWL fragmentation rates are only 50% in such cases[1] due to difficulties of shock-wave transmission through overlying organs (bowel). PCNL for such kidneys is difficult because of bowel proximity and variable blood supply (blood supply derived from multiple sources).
- Patient preference

---

1 Kupeli B, Isen K, Biri H, et al. (1999). Extracorporeal shockwave lithotripsy in anomalous kidneys. *J Endourol* 13:39–52.

Disadvantages

Efficacy diminishes as stone burden increases—it simply takes a long time to paint the surface of the stone with laser energy, causing fragmentation.

A dust cloud is produced as the stone fragments, and this temporarily obscures the view until it has been washed away by irrigation. Stone fragmentation rates for those expert in flexible ureteroscopy are ~70–80% for stones <2 cm in diameter and 50% for those >2 cm in diameter,[2] and ~10% of patients will require two or more treatment sessions.

2 Dasgupta P, et al. (2004). Flexible ureterorenoscopy: prospective analysis of the Guy's experience. *Ann R Coll Surg* 86:367–370.

Kidney stone treatment: percutaneous nephrolithotomy (PCNL)

Technique

PCNL is the removal of a kidney stone via a track developed between the surface of the skin and the collecting system of the kidney. The first step requires inflation of the renal collecting system (pelvis and calyces) with fluid or air instilled via a ureteric catheter inserted cystoscopically (Fig. 8.7). This makes subsequent percutaneous puncture of a renal calyx with a nephrostomy needle easier (Fig. 8.8).

Once the nephrostomy needle is in the calyx, a guide wire is inserted into the renal pelvis to act as a guide over which the track is dilated (Fig. 8.9). An access sheath is passed down the track and into the calyx, and through this a nephroscope can be advanced into the kidney (Fig. 8.10). An ultrasonic lithotripsy probe is used to fragment the stone and remove the debris.

A posterior approach is most commonly used, below the 12th rib (to avoid the pleura and far enough away from the rib to avoid the intercostals, vessels, and nerve). The preferred approach is through a posterior calyx, rather than into the renal pelvis, because this avoids damage to posterior branches of the renal artery that are closely associated with the renal pelvis. General anesthesia is usual, though regional or even local anesthesia (with sedation) can be used.

Indications for PCNL

PCNL is generally recommended for stones >3 cm in diameter and those that have failed ESWL and/or an attempt at flexible ureteroscopy and laser treatment. It is the first-line option for staghorn calculi,[1] with ESWL and/or repeat PCNL being used for residual stone fragments.

For stones 2–3 cm in diameter, options include ESWL (with a JJ stent in situ), flexible ureteroscopy and laser treatment, and PCNL. PCNL gives the best chance of complete stone clearance with a single procedure, but this is achieved at a higher risk of morbidity.

Some patients will opt for several sessions of ESWL or flexible ureteroscopy/laser treatment and the possible risk of ultimately requiring PCNL because of failure of ESWL or laser treatment, rather than proceeding with PCNL up front.

About half of stones >2 cm in diameter will be fragmented by flexible ureteroscopy and laser treatment.

Outcomes of PCNL

For small stones, the stone-free rate after PCNL is on the order of 90–95%. For staghorn stones, the stone-free rate of PCNL, combined with postoperative ESWL for residual stone fragments, is on the order of 80–85%.

---

1 Segura JW, Preminger GM, Assimos DG, et al. (1994). Nephrolithiasis clinical guidelines panel summary report on the management of staghorn calculi. *J Urol* 151:1648–1651.

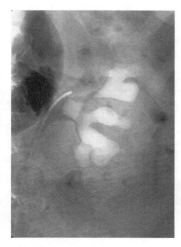

Figure 8.7 A ureteric catheter is inserted into the renal pelvis to dilate it with air or fluid.

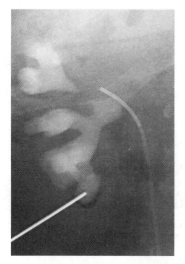

Figure 8.8 A nephrostomy needle has been inserted into a calyx.

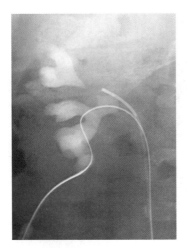

Figure 8.9 A guide wire is inserted into the renal pelvis and down the ureter; over this guide wire the track is dilated.

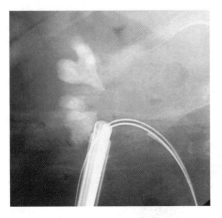

Figure 8.10 An access sheath is passed down the track and into the calyx, and through this a nephroscope can be advanced into the kidney.

Kidney stones: open stone surgery

Indications
- Complex stone burden (projection of stone into multiple calyces, such that multiple PCNL tracks would be required to gain access to all the stone)
- Failure of endoscopic treatment (technical difficulty gaining access to the collecting system of the kidney)
- Anatomic abnormality that precludes endoscopic surgery (e.g., retrorenal colon)
- Body habitus that precludes endoscopic surgery (e.g., gross obesity, kyphoscoliosis—open stone surgery can be difficult)
- Patient request for a single procedure where multiple PCNLs might be required for stone clearance
- Nonfunctioning kidney

Nonfunctioning kidney
When the kidney is not working, the stone may be left in situ if it is not causing symptoms (e.g., pain, recurrent urinary infection, hematuria). However, staghorn calculi should be removed, unless the patient has comorbidity that would preclude safe surgery, because of the substantial risk of developing serious infective complications.

If the kidney is nonfunctioning, the simplest way of removing the stone is to remove the kidney.

Functioning kidneys with either an open or laparoscopic technique—options for stone removal
Small to medium-sized stones
- Pyelolithotomy
- Radial nephrolithotomy

Staghorn calculi
- Anatrophic (avascular) nephrolithotomy
- Extended pyelolithotomy with radial nephrotomies (small incisions over individual stones)
- Excision of the kidney, bench surgery to remove the stones, and autotransplantation

Specific complications of open stone surgery
Complications include wound infection (the stones operated on are often infection stones), flank hernia, and wound pain. (With PCNL these problems do not occur; blood transfusion rate is lower, analgesic requirement is less, mobilization is more rapid, and discharge is earlier—all of which account for PCNL having replaced open surgery as the mainstay of treatment of large stones.)

There is a significant chance of stone recurrence after open stone surgery (as for any other treatment modality) and the scar tissue that develops around the kidney will make subsequent open stone surgery technically more difficult.

Kidney stones: medical therapy (dissolution therapy)

Uric acid and cystine stones are potentially suitable for dissolution therapy. Calcium within either stone type reduces the chances of successful dissolution.

Uric acid stones

Urine is frequently supersaturated with uric acid (derived from a purine-rich diet—i.e., animal protein). Half of patients who form uric acid stones have gout. The other 50% do so because of a high protein and low fluid intake (Western lifestyle). In patients with gout, the risk of developing stones is ~1% per year after the first attack of gout.

Uric acid stones form in concentrated, acid urine. Dissolution therapy is based on hydration, urine alkalinization, allopurinol, and dietary manipulation—the aim being to reduce urinary uric acid saturation.

The patient should maintain a high fluid intake (urine output 2–3 L/day) and alkalinize the urine to pH 6.5–7 (sodium bicarbonate 650 mg 3 or 4 times daily or potassium citrate 30–60 mEq/day, equivalent to 15–30 mL of a potassium citrate solution 3 or 4 times daily).

In those with hyperuricemia or urinary uric acid excretion >1200 mg/day, add allopurinol 300–600 mg/day (inhibits conversion of hypoxanthine and xanthine to uric acid). Dissolution of large stones (even staghorn calculi) is possible with this regimen.

Cystine stones

Cystinuria is an inherited kidney and intestinal transepithelial transport defect for the amino acids cystine, ornithine, lysine, and arginine, ("COLA") leading to excessive urinary excretion of cystine. It has autosomal recessive inheritance, with prevalence of 1 in 700 being homozygous (i.e., both genes defective). It occurs equally in both sexes. About 3% of adult stone formers are cystinuric and 6% of stone-forming children.

Most cystinuric patients excrete about 1 g of cystine per day, which is well above the solubility of cystine. Cystine solubility in acid solutions is low (300 mg/L at pH 5, 400 mg/L at pH 7). Patients with cystinuria present with renal calculi, often in their teens or 20's. Cystine stones are relatively radiodense because they contain sulfur atoms.

The cyanide nitroprusside test will detect most homozygote stone formers and some heterozygotes (false positives occur in the presence of ketones).

Treatment of existing stones and prevention of further stones
The aim is to do the following:
- Reduce cystine excretion (dietary restriction of the cystine precursor amino acid methionine and also of sodium intake to <100 mg/day)
- Increase solubility of cystine by alkalinization of the urine to >pH 7.5, maintenance of a high fluid intake, and use of drugs that convert cystine to more soluble compounds.

D-penicillamine, N-acetyl-D-penicillamine, and mercaptopropionylglycine bind to cystine—the compounds so formed are more soluble in urine than cystine alone. D-penicillamine has potentially unpleasant and serious side effects (allergic reactions, nephrotic syndrome, pancytopenia, proteinuria, epidermolysis, thrombocytosis, hypogeusia).

Therefore, it is reserved for cases where alkalinization therapy and high fluid intake fail to dissolve the stones.

Treatment for failed dissolution therapy

Cystine stones are very hard and are therefore relatively resistant to ESWL. Nonetheless, for small cystine stones, a substantial proportion will still respond to ESWL. Flexible ureteroscopy (for small) and PCNL (for larger) cystine stones are used where ESWL fragmentation has failed.

Ureteric stones: presentation

Ureteric stones usually present with sudden onset of severe flank pain that is colicky (waves of increasing severity are followed by a reduction in severity, but it seldom goes away completely). It may radiate to the groin as the stone passes into the lower ureter.

Approximately 50% of patients with classic symptoms for a ureteric stone do not have a stone confirmed on subsequent imaging studies, nor do they physically ever pass a stone.

Examination

Spend a few seconds looking at the patient. Ureteric stone pain is colicky—the patient moves around, trying to find a comfortable position. The patient may be doubled-up with pain.

Patients with conditions causing peritonitis (e.g., appendicitis, a ruptured ectopic pregnancy) lie very still: movement and abdominal palpation are very painful.

Pregnancy test

Arrange for a pregnancy test in premenopausal women (this is mandatory in any premenopausal woman who is going to undergo imaging using ionizing radiation). If positive, refer to a gynecologist; if negative, obtain imaging to determine whether the patient has a ureteric stone.

Dipstick or microscopic hematuria

Many patients with ureteric stones have dipstick or microscopic hematuria (and, more rarely, macroscopic hematuria), but 10–30% have no blood in their urine.[1,2] The sensitivity of dipstick hematuria for detecting ureteric stones presenting acutely is ~95% on the first day of pain, 85% on the second day, and 65% on the third and fourth days.[2] Therefore, patients with a ureteric stone whose pain started 3–4 days ago may not have blood detectable in their urine.

Dipstick testing is slightly more sensitive than urine microscopy for detecting stones (80% vs. 70%) because blood cells lyse, and therefore disappear, if the urine specimen is not examined under the microscope within a few hours. Both ways of detecting hematuria have roughly the same specificity for diagnosing ureteric stones (~60%).

Remember, blood in the urine on dipstick testing or microscopy may be a coincidental finding because of non-stone urological disease (e.g., neoplasm, infection) or a false-positive test (no abnormality is found in ~70% of patients with microscopic hematuria, despite full urological investigation).

1 Luchs JS, Katz DS, Lane DS, et al. (2002). Utility of hematuria testing in patients with suspected renal colic: correlation with unenhanced helical CT results. *Urology* 59:839.

2 Kobayashi T, Nishizawa K, Mitsumori K, Ogura K (2003). Impact of date of onset on the absence of hematuria in patients with acute renal colic. *J Urol* 170:1093–1096.

Temperature

The most important aspect of examination in a patient with a ureteric stone confirmed on imaging is to measure their temperature. If the patient has a stone and a fever, they may have infection proximal to the stone. This is considered a urological emergency.

A fever in the presence of an obstructing stone is an indication for urine and blood culture, intravenous fluids and antibiotics, and nephrostomy drainage if the fever does not resolve within a matter of hours.

Ureteric stones: diagnostic radiological imaging

The intravenous pyelogram (IVP), for many years the mainstay of imaging in patients with flank pain, has been replaced by CT urography (CTU) (Fig. 8.11). Compared with IVP, CTU

- Has greater specificity (95%) and sensitivity (97%) for diagnosing ureteric stones[1]—it can identify other, non-stone causes of flank pain (Fig. 8.12).
- Requires no contrast administration, avoiding the chance of a contrast reaction (risk of fatal anaphylaxis following the administration of low-osmolality contrast media for IVP is on the order of 1 in 100,000).[2]
- Is faster, taking just a few minutes to image the kidneys and ureters. An IVP, particularly when delayed films are required to identify a stone causing high-grade obstruction, may take hours to identify the precise location of the obstructing stone.
- Is equivalent in cost to that of IVP, in hospitals where high volumes of CT scans are done.[3]

If you only have access to IVP, remember that it is contraindicated in patients with a history of previous contrast reactions and should be avoided in those with hay fever, a strong history of allergies, or asthma who have not been pretreated with high-dose steroids 24 hours before the IVP. Patients taking metformin for diabetes should stop this for 48 hours prior to an IVP. Clearly, being able to perform an alternative test, such as CTU in such patients, is very useful.

Where 24-hour CTU access is not available, admit patients with suspected ureteric colic for pain relief and arrange for a CTU the following morning. When CT urography is not immediately available (between the hours of midnight and 8 a.m.), we obtain urgent abdominal ultrasonography in all patients aged >50 years who present with flank pain suggestive of a possible stone, to exclude serious pathology such as a leaking abdominal aortic aneurysm and to demonstrate any other gross abnormalities due to non-stone associated flank pain.

Plain abdominal X-ray and renal ultrasound are not sufficiently sensitive or specific for their routine use for diagnosing ureteric stones.

MR urography

MRU is a very accurate way of determining whether a stone is present in the ureter or not.[4] However, cost and restricted availability limit its usefulness as a routine diagnostic method of imaging in cases of acute flank pain. This situation may change as MR scanners become more widely available.

1 Smith RC, Verga M, McCarthy S, Rosenfield AT (1996). Diagnosis of acute flank pain: value of unenhanced helical CT. *Am J Roentgen* 166:97–101.
2 Caro JJ, Trindale E, McGregor M (1991). The risks of death and severe non-fatal reactions with high vs low osmolality contrast media. *Am J Roentgen* 156:825–832.
3 Thomson JM, Glocer J, Abbott C, et al. (2001) Computed tomography versus intravenous urography in diagnosis of acute flank pain from urolithiasis: a randomized study comparing imaging costs and radiation dose. *Australas Radiol* 45:291–297.
4 Louca G, Liberopoulos K, Fidas A, et al. (1999) MR urography in the diagnosis of urinary tract obstruction. *Eur Urol* 35:102–108.

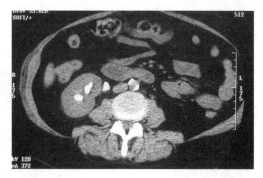

Figure 8.11 CT urogram.

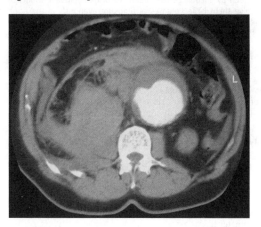

Figure 8.12 A leaking aortic aneurysm identified on a CTU in a patient with flank pain.

Ureteric stones: acute management

While appropriate imaging studies are being organized, pain relief should be given.

- A nonsteroidal anti-inflammatory (NSAID) (e.g., diclofenac—Voltaren or ketorolac tromethamine—Toradol) by intramuscular or intravenous injection, by mouth or per rectum, provides rapid and effective pain control. Its analgesic effect is partly anti-inflammatory, partly by reducing ureteric peristalsis.
- When NSAIDs are inadequate, opiate analgesics such as dilaudid or morphine are added.
- Calcium channel antagonists (e.g., nifedipine) may reduce the pain of ureteric colic by reducing the frequency of ureteric contractions.[1,2] This is used for upper ureteral stones, whereas α-blockers (e.g., Flomax and Uroxatral) may be used for distal ureteral stones.

There is no need to encourage the patient to drink copious amounts of fluids or to give them large volumes of fluids intravenously in the hope that this will flush out the stone. Renal blood flow and urine output from the affected kidney fall during an episode of acute, partial obstruction due to a stone.

Excess urine output will tend to cause a greater degree of hydronephrosis in the affected kidney, which will make ureteric peristalsis even less efficient than it already is. Peristalsis, the forward propulsion of a bolus of urine down the ureter, can only occur if the walls of the ureter above the bolus of urine can coapt, i.e., close firmly together. If they cannot, as occurs in a ureter distended with urine, the bolus of urine cannot move distally.

Watchful waiting

In many instances, small ureteric stones will pass spontaneously within days or a few weeks, with analgesic supplements for exacerbations of pain.

Chances of spontaneous stone passage depend principally on stone size. Between 90% and 98% of stones measuring <4 mm will pass spontaneously.[3,4] Average time for spontaneous stone passage for stones 4–6 mm in diameter is 3 weeks.

Stones that have not passed in 2 months are unlikely to do so. Therefore, accurate determination of stone size (on plain abdominal X-ray or by CTU) helps predict chances of spontaneous stone passage.

1 B Borghi L, et al. (1994). Nifedipine and methylprednisolone in facilitating ureteral stone passage: a randomised, double-blind, placebo controlled study. *J Urol* 152:1095–1098.

2 Porpiglia F, et al. (2000). Effectiveness of nifedipine and deflazacort in the management of distal ureteric stones. *Urology* 56:579–582.

3 Segura JW, et al. (1997). Ureteral stones guidelines panel summary report on the management of ureteral calculi. *J Urol* 158:1915–1921.

4 Miller OF, et al. (1999). Time to stone passage for observed ureteral calculi. *J Urol* 162:688–691.

Nifedipine[1,2] and tamsulosin or alfuzosin (an α-adrenergic adrenoceptor blocking drug) may assist spontaneous stone passage and reduce frequency of ureteric colic.[5] Nitroglycerine patches do not aid stone passage or reduce the frequency of pain episodes.[6]

5 Dellabella M, et al. (2003). Efficacy of tamsulosin in the medical management of juxtavesical ureteral stones. *J Urol* 170:2202–2205.
6 Hussain Z, et al. (2001). Use of glyceryl trinitrate patches in patients with ureteral stones: a randomized, double-blind, placebo-controlled study. *Urology* 58:521–225.

Ureteric stones: indications for intervention to relieve obstruction and/or remove the stone

- Pain that fails to respond to analgesics or recurs and cannot be controlled with additional pain relief.
- Fever. Have a low threshold for draining the kidney (usually done by percutaneous nephrostomy).
- Impaired renal function (solitary kidney obstructed by a stone, bilateral ureteric stones, or pre-existing renal impairment that gets worse as a consequence of a ureteric stone). The threshold for intervention is lower.
- Prolonged unrelieved obstruction. This can result in long-term loss of renal function.[1] How long it takes for this loss of renal function to occur is uncertain, but generally speaking, the period of watchful waiting for spontaneous stone passage tends to be limited to 4–6 weeks.
- Social reasons. Young, active patients may opt for surgical treatment because they need to get back to work or their childcare duties, whereas some patients will be happy to sit things out. Airline pilots and some other professions are unable to work until they are stone free.

Emergency temporizing and definitive treatment of the stone

When the pain of a ureteric stone fails to respond to analgesics or renal function is impaired because of the stone, then temporary relief of the obstruction can be obtained by insertion of a JJ stent or percutaneous nephrostomy tube. (Percutaneous nephrostomy tube can restore efficient peristalsis by restoring the ability of the ureteric wall to coapt.)

JJ stent insertion or percutaneous nephrostomy tube can be done quickly, but the stone is still present (Fig. 8.13). It may pass down and out of the ureter with a stent or nephrostomy in situ, but in many instances it simply sits where it is and subsequent definitive treatment is still required.

While JJ stents can relieve stone pain, they can cause bothersome irritative bladder symptoms (pain in the bladder, frequency, and urgency). JJ stents do make subsequent stone treatment in the form of ureteroscopy technically easier by causing passive dilatation of the ureter.

The patient may elect to proceed to definitive stone treatment by immediate ureteroscopy (for stones at any location in the ureter) or ESWL (if the stone is in the upper and lower ureter—ESWL cannot be used for stones in the mid-ureter because this region is surrounded by bone, which prevents penetration of the shock waves) (Fig. 8.14).

Local facilities and expertise will determine whether definitive treatment can be offered immediately. Not all hospitals have access to ESWL or endoscopic surgeons 365 days a year.

---

1 Holm–Nielsen A, Jorgensen T, Mogensen P, Fogh J (1981). The prognostic value of probe renography in ureteric stone obstruction. *Br J Urol* 53:504–507.

Emergency treatment of an obstructed, infected kidney

The rationale for performing percutaneous nephrostomy rather than JJ stent insertion for an infected, obstructed kidney is to reduce the likelihood of septicemia occurring as a consequence of showering bacteria into the circulation. It is thought that this is more likely to occur with JJ stent insertion than with percutaneous nephrostomy insertion.

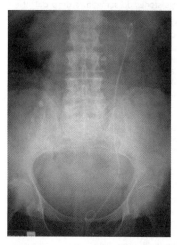

Figure 8.13 A JJ stent.

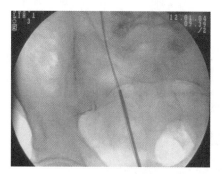

Figure 8.14 Ureteroscopic stone fragmentation for a lower ureteric stone.

Ureteric stone treatment

Many ureteric stones are 4 mm in diameter or smaller and most such stones (90%+) will pass spontaneously, given a few weeks of watchful waiting, with analgesics for exacerbations of pain.[1,2]

Average time for spontaneous stone passage for stones 4–6 mm in diameter is 3 weeks. Stones that have not passed in 2 months are much less likely to do so, though large stones do sometimes drop out of the ureter at the last moment.

Indications for stone removal

- Pain that fails to respond to analgesics or recurs and cannot be controlled with additional pain relief
- Impaired renal function (solitary kidney obstructed by a stone, bilateral ureteric stones, or pre-existing renal impairment that gets worse as a consequence of a ureteric stone)
- Prolonged unrelieved obstruction (generally speaking, ~4–6 weeks)
- Social reasons. Young, active patients may opt for surgical treatment because they need to get back to work or their childcare duties, whereas some patients will be happy to sit things out. Airline pilots and some other professions are unable to work until they are stone free.

These indications need to be related to the individual patient—their stone size, their renal function, presence of a normal contralateral kidney, their tolerance of exacerbations of pain, their job and social situation, and local facilities (the availability of surgeons with appropriate skill and equipment to perform endoscopic stone treatment).

Twenty years ago, when the only options were watchful waiting or open surgical removal of a stone (open ureterolithotomy), surgeons and patients were inclined to sit it out for a considerable time in the hope that the stone would pass spontaneously.

Currently, the advent of ESWL and of smaller ureteroscopes with efficient stone fragmentation devices (e.g., the holmium laser) has made stone treatment and removal a far less morbid procedure, with a far smoother and faster post-treatment recovery. It is easier for both the patient and the surgeon to opt for intervention, in the form of ESWL or surgery, as a quicker way of relieving them of their pain, and a way of avoiding unpredictable and unpleasant exacerbations of pain.

It is clearly important for the surgeon to inform the patient of the outcomes and potential complications of intervention, particularly given the fact that many of stones would pass spontaneously if left a little longer.

---

1 Segura JW, et al. (1997). Ureteral stones guidelines panel summary report on the management of ureteral calculi. *J Urol* 158:1915–1921.
2 Miller OF, et al. (1999). Time to stone passage for observed ureteral calculi. *J Urol* 162:688–691.

Treatment options for ureteric stones

- ESWL: in situ; after push-back into the kidney (i.e., into the renal pelvis or calyces); or after JJ stent insertion
- Ureteroscopy
- PCNL
- Open ureterolithotomy
- Laparoscopic ureterolithotomy

Basketing of stones (blind or under radiographic control) are historical treatments (the potential for serious ureteric injury is significant).

The ureter can be divided into two halves (proximal and distal to the iliac vessels) or in thirds (upper third from the UPJ to the upper edge of the sacrum; middle third from the upper to the lower edge of the sacrum; lower third from the lower edge of the sacrum to the VUJ).

AUA guidelines panel recommendations[1]

These guidelines should be interpreted in light of the following:

- Recent (within the last 5 years or so) improvements in ureteroscope design
- Local facilities and expertise

Smaller ureteroscopes with improved optics and larger instrument channels and the advent of holmium laser lithotripsy have improved the efficacy of ureteroscopic stone fragmentation (to ~95% stone clearance) and reduced its morbidity. As a consequence, many surgeons and patients will opt for ureteroscopy, with its potential for a one-off treatment, over ESWL, which requires more than one treatment and post-treatment imaging is needed to confirm stone clearance (with ureteroscopy you can directly see that the stone has gone).

Most urology departments do not have unlimited access to ESWL and patients may therefore opt for ureteroscopic stone extraction.

The stone clearance rates for ESWL are stone-size dependent. ESWL is more efficient for stones <1 cm in diameter than for those >1 cm in size. Conversely, the outcome of ureteroscopy is somewhat less dependent on stone size.

Recommendations

Proximal ureteric stones

- <1 cm diameter: ESWL (in situ, push-back)
- >1 cm diameter: ESWL, ureteroscopy, PCNL

JJ stent insertion does not increase stone-free rates and is therefore not required in routine cases. It is indicated for pain relief, relief of obstruction, and in those with solitary kidneys.

Distal ureteric stones

- Both ESWL and ureteroscopy are acceptable options.
- Stone-free rate <1 cm: 80–90% for both ESWL and ureteroscopy; >1 cm: 75% for both ESWL and ureteroscopy.

1 Segura JW, Preminger GM, Assimos DG, et al. (1997) Ureteral stones clinical guidelines panel summary report on the management of ureteral calculi. *J Urol* 158:1915–1921.

Failed initial ESWL is associated with a low success rate for subsequent ESWL. Therefore, if ESWL has no effect after one or two treatments, change tactics.[2]

Open ureterolithotomy and laparoscopic ureterolithotomy are used when ESWL or ureteroscopy have been tried and failed or were not feasible.

2 Pace KT. et al. (2000). Low success rate of repeat shock wave lithotripsy for uretal stones after failed initial treatment. *J Urol* 164:1905–1907.

Prevention of calcium oxalate stone formation

A series of landmark papers from Harvard Medical School[1] and other groups help us to give rational advice on reducing the risk of future stone formation in those who have formed one or more stones. The Harvard studies stratified risk of stone formation on the basis of intake of calcium and other nutrients (Nurses Health Study, $n = 81,000$ women; equivalent male study, $n = 45,000$).

Low fluid intake

Low fluid intake may be the single most important risk factor for recurrent stone formation. High fluid intake is protective,[1] by reducing urinary saturation of calcium, oxalate, and urate.

Time to recurrent stone formation is prolonged from 2 to 3 years in previous stone formers randomized to high fluid vs. low fluid intake (averaging about 2.5 vs. 1 L/day) and over 5 years, risk of recurrent stones was 27% in low-volume controls compared with 12% in high-volume patients.[2]

Dietary calcium

Conventional teaching was that high calcium intake increases the risk of calcium oxalate stone disease. The Harvard Medical School studies have shown that *low* calcium intake is, paradoxically, associated with an *increased* risk of forming kidney stones, in both men and women (relative risk of stone formation for the highest quintile of dietary calcium intake vs. the lowest quintile = 0.65; 95% confidence intervals 0.5 to 0.83—i.e., high calcium intake was associated with a *low* risk of stone formation).

Calcium supplements

In the Harvard studies,[3] the relative risk of stone formation in women on supplemental calcium compared with those not on calcium was 1.2 (95% confidence intervals 1.02–1.4). In 67% of women on supplements, the calcium was either not consumed with a meal or was consumed with a meal with low oxalate content. It is possible that consuming calcium supplements with a meal or with oxalate-containing foods could reduce this small risk of inducing kidney stones.

Other dietary risk factors related to stone formation

Increased risk of stone formation (relative risk of stone formation shown in brackets for highest to lowest quintiles of intake of particular dietary factor):
- Sucrose [1.5]
- Sodium [1.3]: high sodium intake (leading to natriuresis) causes hypercalciuria
- Potassium [0.65]

1 Curhan GC, et al. (1993). A prospective study of dietary calcium and other nutrients and the risk of symptomatic kidney stones. *N Engl J Med* 328:833–38.
2 Borghi L, et al. (1996). Urinary volume, water and recurrences in idiopathic calcium nephrolithiasis: A 5-year randomized prospective study. *J Urol* 155:839–843.
3 Curhan G, et al. (1997). Comparison of dietary calcium with supplemental calcium and other nutrients as factors affecting the risk for kidney stones in women. *Ann Intern Med* 126:497–504.

Animal proteins

High intake of animal proteins causes increased urinary excretion of calcium, reduced pH, high urinary uric acid, and reduced urinary citrate, all of which predispose to stone formation.[4]

Alcohol

Curhan's studies from Harvard[5] suggest small quantities of wine decrease risk of stones.

Vegetarian diet

Vegetable proteins contain less of the amino acids phenylalanine, tyrosine, and tryptophan that increase the endogenous production of oxalate. A vegetarian diet may protect against the risk of stone formation.[6,7]

Dietary oxalate

A small increase in urinary oxalate concentration increases calcium oxalate supersaturation much more than an increase in urinary calcium concentration. Mild hyperoxaluria is one of the main factors leading to calcium stone formation.[8]

4 Kok DJ (1990). The effects of dietary excesses in animal protein and in sodium on the composition and crystallization kinetics of calcium oxalate monohydrate in urines of healthy men. *J Clin Endocrinol Metab* 71:861–867.
5 Curhan G, et al. (1998). Beverage use and risk for kidney stones in women. *Ann Intern Med* 128:534–540.
6 Robertson WG, et al. (1982). Prevalence of urinary stone disease in vegetarians. *Eur Urol* 8:334–339.
7 Borghi, L (2002). Comparison of two diets for prevention of recurrent stones in idiopathic hypercalciuria. *N Engl J Med* 346:77–84.
8 Robertson WG, Peacock M, Ouimet D, et al. (1981). The main risk for calcium oxalate stone disease in man: hypercalciuria or mild hyperoxaluria? In Smith LH, Robertson WG, Finlayson B (Eds.), *Urolithiasis: Clinical and Basic Research.* New York: Plenum Press, pp. 3–12.

Bladder stones

Composition
Bladder stones consist of struvite (i.e., they are infection stones) or uric acid (in noninfected urine).

Adults
Bladder calculi are predominantly a disease of men aged >50 and with bladder outlet obstruction due to benign prostatic enlargement (BPE). They also occur in the chronically catheterized patient (e.g., spinal cord injury patients), in whom the chance of developing a bladder stone is 25% over 5 years (similar risk whether urethral or suprapubic location of the stone).[1]

Children
Bladder stones are still common in Thailand, Indonesia, North Africa, the Middle East, and Burma. In these endemic areas they are usually composed of a combination of ammonium urate and calcium oxalate. A low-phosphate diet in these areas (a diet of breast milk and polished rice or millet) results in high peaks of ammonia excretion in the urine.

Symptoms
Bladder stones may be symptomless (incidental finding on KUB X-ray or bladder ultrasound or on cystoscopy) and is the common presentation in spinal patients who have limited or no bladder sensation.

In the neurologically intact patient, suprapubic or perineal pain, hematuria, urgency and/or urge incontinence, recurrent UTI, and LUTS (hesitancy, poor flow) may occur.

Diagnosis
If you suspect a bladder stone, it will be visible on KUB X-ray or renal ultrasound (Fig. 8.15).

Treatment
Most stones are small enough to be removed cystoscopically (endoscopic cystolitholapaxy), using stone-fragmenting forceps for stones that can be engaged by the jaws of the forceps and EHL or pneumatic lithotripsy for those that cannot. Large stones (see Fig. 8.15) can be removed by open surgery (open cystolitholapaxy).

1 Ord J (2003). Bladder management and risk of bladder stone formation in spinal cord injured patients. *J Urol.* 170:1734–1737.

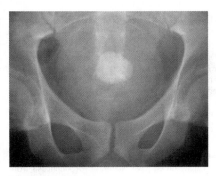

Figure 8.15 A bladder stone.

Management of ureteric stones in pregnancy

While hypercalciuria and uric acid excretion increase in pregnancy (predisposing to stone formation), so do urinary citrate and magnesium levels (protecting against stone formation). The incidence of ureteric colic is thus the same as in nonpregnant women. [1]

Ureteric stones occur in 1 in 1500–2500 pregnancies, mostly during the second and third trimesters. They are associated with a significant risk of preterm labor,[2] and the pain caused by ureteric stones can be difficult to distinguish from other causes.

The hydronephrosis of pregnancy

Ninety percent of pregnant women have bilateral hydronephrosis from weeks 6–10 of gestation and up to 2 months after birth (smooth muscle relaxant effect of progesterone and mechanical obstruction of ureter from the enlarging fetus and uterus). Hydronephrosis is taken as surrogate evidence of ureteric obstruction in nonpregnant individuals, but because it is a normal finding in the majority of pregnancies, its presence *cannot* be taken as a sign of a possible ureteric stone.

Ultrasound is unreliable for diagnosing the presence of stones in pregnant (and in nonpregnant) women (sensitivity, 34%—i.e., it misses 66% of stones; specificity, 86%—i.e., false-positive rate of 14%).[3]

Differential diagnosis of flank pain in pregnancy

This includes ureteric stone, placental abruption, appendicitis, pyelonephritis, and all the other (many) causes of flank pain in nonpregnant women.

Diagnostic imaging studies in pregnancy

Exposure of the fetus to ionizing radiation can cause fetal malformations, malignancies in later life (leukemia), and mutagenic effects (damage to genes causing inherited disease in the offspring of the fetus). Fetal radiation doses during various procedures are shown in Table 8.4.

While the recommended maximum radiation levels shown in Table 8.4 are well above those occurring during even CT scanning, and a dose of 50 mGy or less is regarded as safe, every effort should be made to limit exposure of the fetus to radiation. Pregnant women may be reassured that the risk to the unborn child as a consequence of radiation exposure is likely to be minimal.

---

1 Coe FL, Parks JH, Lindhermer MD (1978). Nephrolithiasis during pregnancy. *N Engl J Med* 298:324–326.

2 Hendricks SK (1991). An algorithm for diagnosis and therapy of urolithiasis during pregnancy *Surg Gyne Obst* 172:49–54.

3 Stothers L, Lee LM (1992). Renal colic in pregnancy. *J Urol* 148:1383–1387.

4 Hellawell GO, Cowan NC, Holt SJ, Mutch SJ (2002). A radiation perspective for treating loin pain in pregnancy by double-pigtail stents. *Br J Urol Int* 90:801–808.

Table 8.4 Fetal radiation dose after various radiological investigations

Procedure	Fetal dose (mGy) (mean)	Risk of inducing cancer (up to age 15 years)
KUB X-ray	1.4	—
IVP 6 shot	1.7	1 in 10,000
IVP 3 shot	—	—
CT: abdominal	8	—
CT: pelvic	25	—
Fluoroscopy for JJ stent insertion	0.4	1 in 42,000

Radiation doses of <100 mGy are very unlikely to have an adverse effect on the fetus.[4] In the United States, the National Council on Radiation Protection has stated that "fetal risk is considered to be negligible at <50 mGy when compared to the other risks of pregnancy, and the risk of malformations is significantly increased above control levels at doses >150 mGy."[5]

The American College of Obstetricians and Gynecologists has stated that "X-ray exposure to <50 mGy has not been associated with an increase in fetal anomalies or pregnancy loss."[6]

Plain radiography and IVP

These have limited usefulness (fetal skeleton and the enlarged uterus obscure ureteric stones; delayed excretion of contrast limits opacification of ureter; theoretical risk of fetal toxicity from the contrast material).

CTU

CTU is a very accurate method for detecting ureteric stones, but most radiologists and urologists are unhappy to recommend this form of imaging in pregnant women.

MRU

The American College of Obstetricians and Gynecologists and the U.S. National Council on Radiation Protection state that "although there is no evidence to suggest that the embryo is sensitive to magnetic and radiofrequency at the intensities encountered in MRI, it might be prudent to exclude pregnant women during the first trimester."[5,6]

MRU can thus potentially be used during the second and third trimesters, but not during the first trimester. It involves no ionizing radiation. It is

5 National Council on Radiation Protection and Measurement (1997). Medical radiation exposure of pregnant and potentially pregnant women. NCRP Report no. 54. Bethesda, MD: NCRPM.
6 American College of Obstetricians and Gynecologists Committee on Obstetric Practice (1995). Guidelines for Diagnostic Imaging During Pregnancy. ACOG Committee Opinion no. 158. Washington DC: ACOG.
7 Roy C (1996). Assessment of painful ureterohydronephrosis during pregnancy by MR urography. *Eur Radiol* 6:334–338.

very accurate (100% sensitivity for detecting ureteric stones[7]) but expensive, and not readily available in most hospitals, particularly after hours.

Management

Most (70–80%) stones will pass spontaneously. Pain relief is with opiate-based analgesics; avoid NSAIDs (can cause premature closure of the ductus arteriosus by blocking prostaglandin synthesis).

Indications for intervention are the same as in nonpregnant patients (pain refractory to analgesics, suspected urinary sepsis [high fever, high white count], high-grade obstruction and obstruction in a solitary kidney).

Options for intervention

Options depend on the stage of pregnancy and on local facilities' equipment and expertise:
- JJ stent urinary diversion
- Nephrostomy urinary diversion
- Ureteroscopic stone removal

Aim to minimize radiation exposure to the fetus and to minimize the risk of miscarriage and preterm labor.

General anesthesia can precipitate preterm labor, and many urologists and obstetricians will prefer temporizing options, such as nephrostomy tube drainage or JJ stent placement, over operative treatment in the form of ureteroscopic stone removal.

Upper tract obstruction, flank pain, hydronephrosis

Hydronephrosis 406
Management of ureteric strictures (other than UPJ
   obstruction) 410
Pathophysiology of urinary tract obstruction 414
Physiology of urine flow from kidneys to bladder 416
Ureter innervation 417

Hydronephrosis

Hydronephrosis is dilatation of the renal pelvis and calyces (Fig. 9.1). When combined with dilatation of the ureters it is known as *hydroureteronephrosis*.

Obstructive nephropathy is damage to the renal parenchyma resulting from obstruction to the flow of urine anywhere along the urinary tract.

Dilatation of the renal pelvis and calyces can occur without obstruction and thus hydronephrosis should not be taken to necessarily imply the presence of obstructive uropathy.

Ultrasound

- False negative (i.e., obstruction present, no hydronephrosis)—acute onset of obstruction; in the presence of an intrarenal collecting system; with dehydration; misdiagnosis of dilatation of the calyces as renal cortical cysts (in acute ureteric colic, ultrasonography fails to detect hydronephrosis in up to 35% of patients with proven acute obstruction on IVP)
- False positive (i.e., hydronephrosis, no obstruction)—capacious extrarenal pelvis; parapelvic cysts; vesicoureteric reflux; high urine flow

Diagnostic approach to the patient with hydronephrosis

Hydronephrosis may present either as an incidental finding on an ultrasound or CT done because of nonspecific symptoms or it may be identified in a patient with a raised creatinine or presenting with flank pain.

Symptoms, if present, will depend on the rapidity of onset of obstruction of the kidney (if that is the cause of the hydronephrosis); whether obstruction is complete or partial, unilateral or bilateral; and whether the obstruction to the ureter is extrinsic to the ureter or within its lumen. Causes of hydronephrosis are listed in Box 9.1.

History

- Severe flank pain suggests a more acute onset of obstruction and, if very sudden in onset, a ureteric stone may well be the cause. Pain induced by a diuresis (e.g., following consumption of alcohol) suggests a possible UPJ obstruction (See Chapter 7, p. 346).
- Anuria (the symptom of bilateral ureteric obstruction or complete obstruction of a solitary kidney)
- If renal function is impaired, symptoms of renal failure may be present (e.g., nausea, lethargy, anorexia).
- Extrinsic causes of obstruction (e.g., compression of the ureters by retroperitoneal malignancy) usually have a more insidious onset, whereas intrinsic obstruction (ureteric stone) is often present with severe pain of very sudden onset.
- An increase in urine output may be reported by the patient that is due to poor renal concentrating ability.
- Obstruction in the presence of bacterial urinary tract infection—signs and symptoms of pyelonephritis (flank pain and tenderness, fever) or sepsis

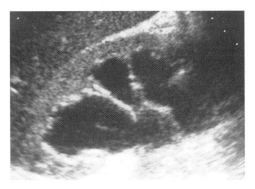

Figure 9.1 Hydronephrosis as seen on renal ultrasonography.

Examination
- Measure blood pressure—elevated in high-pressure chronic retention (HPCR) due to benign prostatic obstruction (caused by fluid overload).
- Bilateral edema (due to fluid overload)
- Abdominal examination—percuss and palpate for an enlarged bladder.
- In men, DRE (?prostate or rectal cancer), and in women, vaginal examination (?cervical cancer)
- Check serum creatinine to determine the functional effect of the hydronephrosis.
- Renal ultrasonography (if not already done)

IVP findings in renal obstruction
- An obstructive (dense) nephrogram
- A delay in filling of the collecting system with contrast material
- Dilatation of the collecting system
- An increase in renal size
- Rupture of fornices (junction between renal papilla and its calyx) with urinary extravasation
- Ureteric dilatation and tortuosity
- A standing column of contrast material in the ureter

Unilateral hydronephrosis
Obtain a KUB X-ray (a ureteric stone may be seen), or CTU (or IVP) if a stone is suspected.
- If no stone is seen, but hydronephrosis is confirmed and ureter is nondilated, the obstruction must be at the UPJ. In the absence of a ureteric stone visible on CTU, the diagnosis must be UPJ obstruction.
- If no stone is seen and the ureter is dilated as well as kidney, ureteric TCC is likely. Arrange for retrograde pyelography to identify site of obstruction, and ureteroscopy/ureteric biopsy.

Bilateral hydronephrosis
- If the patient is in retention or has a substantial post-void residual urine volume, pass a catheter. If the elevated creatinine falls (and the hydronephrosis improves), the diagnosis is bladder outlet obstruction (BOO), due, for example, to BPH, prostate cancer, urethral stricture, or detrusor-sphincter dyssynergia. If the creatinine remains elevated, the obstruction affecting both ureters is higher upstream.
- Obtain TRUS and prostatic biopsy if prostate cancer is suspected on DRE, and a CT scan to look for malignant bilateral ureteric obstruction or abdominal aortic aneurism (AAA).

Box 9.1 Causes of hydronephrosis

Unilateral
- Obstructing ureteric stone
- UPJ obstruction
- Obstructing clot in ureter
- Obstructing ureteric TCC
- Any of the causes listed below when the pathological process has not yet extended to involve both ureters

Bilateral
- Bladder outlet obstruction (BOO)
  - BPH
  - Prostate cancer
  - Urethral stricture
  - Detrusor-sphincter dyssynergia (DSD)
  - Posterior urethral valve
- Bilateral ureteric obstruction at their level of entry into the bladder
  - Locally advanced cervical cancer
  - Locally advanced prostate cancer
  - Locally advanced rectal cancer
  - Poor bladder compliance (often combined with DSD): neuropathic bladder (spinal cord injury, spina bifida); post-pelvic radiotherapy
- Periureteric inflammation
  - From adjacent bowel involved with inflammatory bowel disease (e.g., Crohn's, ulcerative colitis) or diverticular disease
- Retroperitoneal fibrosis
  - Idiopathic (diagnosed following exclusion of other causes)
  - Periarteritis—aortic aneurysm, iliac artery aneurysm
  - Post-irradiation
  - Drugs—methysergide, hydralazine, haloperidol, LSD, methyldopa, β-blockers, phenacetin, amphetamines
  - Malignant—retroperitoneal malignancy (lymphoma, metastatic disease from e.g., breast cancer), post-chemotherapy
  - Chemicals—talcum powder
  - Infection—TB, syphilis, gonorrhea, chronic UTI
  - Sarcoidosis
- Bilateral UPJ obstruction (uncommon)
- Hydronephrosis of pregnancy (partly due to smooth-muscle relaxant effect of progesterone, partly obstruction of ureters by fetus)
- Hydronephrosis in association with an ileal conduit (a substantial proportion of patients with ileal conduit urinary diversion have bilateral hydronephrosis, in the absence of obstruction)
- Bilateral ureteric stones (rare)

Management of ureteric strictures (other than UPJ obstruction)

Definition
A normal ureter undergoes peristalsis and therefore at any one moment at least one area of the ureter will be physiologically narrowed. A *ureteric stricture* is a segment of ureter that is narrowed *and remains so on several images* (i.e., it is a length of ureter that is constantly narrow).

Causes
Most ureteric strictures are benign and iatrogenic. Some follow impaction of a ureteric stone for a prolonged period. Malignant strictures are within the wall of the ureter (e.g., TCC ureter) or due to extrinsic compression from the outside wall of the ureter (e.g., lymphoma, malignant retroperitoneal lymphadenopathy). Retroperitoneal fibrosis (RPF) may be benign (idiopathic, aortic aneurysm, post-irradiation, analgesic abuse) or malignant (retroperitoneal malignancy, post-chemotherapy).

Mechanism of iatrogenic ureteric stricture formation
Normally it is ischemic:
- Usually injury at time of open or endoscopic surgery (e.g., damage to ureteric blood supply or direct damage to ureter at time of colorectal resection, AAA graft, hysterectomy); at ureteroscopy— mucosal trauma (from ureteroscope or electrohydraulic lithotripsy), perforation of ureter (urine extravasation leading to fibrosis)
- Radiotherapy in the vicinity of the ureter
- Stricture of ureteroneocystostomy of renal transplant

Investigations
The stricture may be diagnosed following investigation for symptoms (flank pain, upper tract infection) or may be an incidental finding on an investigation done for some other reason. The stricture may be diagnosed on a renal ultrasound (hydronephrosis), an IVP, or a CTU.

A MAG3 renogram will confirm the presence of obstruction (some minor strictures may cause no renal obstruction) and establish split renal function. Where ureteric TCC is possible, proceed with ureteroscopy and biopsy.

Treatment options
- Nothing (symptomless stricture in an older patient with significant comorbidity or <25% function in an otherwise healthy patient with a normally functioning contralateral kidney)
- Permanent JJ stent or nephrostomy, changed at regular intervals (symptomatic stricture in an older patient with significant comorbidity or <25% function in affected kidney with compromised overall renal function)
- Dilatation (balloon or graduated dilator) (see Figs. 9.2 and 9.3).

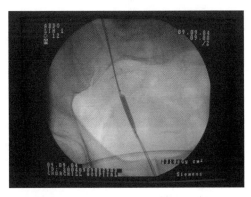

Figure 9.2 Balloon dilatation of a lower ureteric stricture.

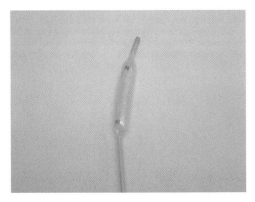

Figure 9.3 The catheter used for balloon dilatation.

- Incision + balloon dilatation (endoureterotomy by Acucise balloon; ureteroscopy or nephrostomy and incision e.g., by laser). Leave a 12Fr. stent in for 4 weeks.
- Excision of stricture and repair of ureter (open or laparoscopic approach)
- Nephrectomy

Factors associated with reduced likelihood of a good outcome after endoureterotomy are as follows:
- <25% function in kidney
- Stricture length >1 cm
- Ischemic stricture
- Mid-ureteric stricture (compared with upper and lower)—tenuous blood supply
- JJ stent size <12 Fr

Ureteroenteric strictures (ileal conduits, ureteric implantation into neobladder)

These are due to ischemia and/or periureteral urine leak in the immediate postoperative period, which leads to fibrosis in the tissues around the ureter.

In ileal conduits, the left ureter is affected more than the right ureter because greater mobilization is required to bring it to the right side and it may be compressed under the sigmoid mesocolon, both of which impair blood flow to the distal end of the ureter.

Pathophysiology of urinary tract obstruction

Effects of obstruction on renal blood flow and ureteric pressure

Acute unilateral obstruction of a ureter (UUO)

This leads to a triphasic relationship between renal blood flow (RBF) and ureteric pressure.

- **Phase 1** (up to 1.5 hours post-obstruction): ureteric pressure rises, RBF rises (afferent arteriole dilatation)
- **Phase 2** (1.5–5 hours post obstruction): ureteric pressure continues to rise, RBF falls (efferent arteriole vasoconstriction)
- **Phase 3** (beyond 5 hours): ureteric pressure falls, RBF continues to fall (afferent arteriole vasoconstriction)

Acute bilateral obstruction of a ureter (BUO) or obstruction of a solitary kidney

- **Phase 1** (up to 1.5 hours post-obstruction): ureteric pressure rises, RBF rises (afferent arteriole dilatation)
- **Phase 2** (1.5–5 hours post-obstruction): ureteric pressure continues to rise, RBF is significantly lower than that during unilateral ureteric obstruction
- **Phase 3** (beyond 5 hours): ureteric pressure remains elevated (in contrast to UUO). By 24 hours, RBF has declined to the same level as or both unilateral and bilateral ureteric obstruction.

In UUO, the decrease in urine flow through the nephron results in a greater degree of Na absorption, so Na excretion falls. Water loss from the obstructed kidney increases.

Release of BUO is followed by a marked natriuresis, increased K excretion, and a diuresis (a solute diuresis). This is due to the following:

- An appropriate (physiological) natriuresis, to excrete excessive Na that is a consequence of BUO
- A solute diuresis from the accumulation of urea in extracellular fluid
- A diminution of the corticomedullary concentration gradient, which is normally established by the countercurrent mechanism of the loop of Henle, and is dependent on maintenance of flow through the nephron. Reduction of flow, as occurs in BUO, reduces the efficiency of the countercurrent mechanism (effectively, the corticomedullary concentration gradient is washed out).

There may also be accumulation of natriuretic peptides (e.g., ANP) during BUO, which contributes to the natriuresis following release of the obstruction.

Likelihood of recovery of renal function after release of obstruction

In dogs with completely obstructed kidneys, full recovery of renal function after 7 days of UUO occurred within 2 weeks of relief of obstruction. After 14 days of obstruction there was a permanent reduction in renal function to 70% of control levels (recovery to this level taking 3–6 months after reversal of obstruction).

There is some recovery of function after 4 weeks of obstruction, but after 6 weeks of complete obstruction there is no recovery. In humans, there is no clear relationship between the duration of BUO and the degree of recovery of renal function after relief of obstruction.

Physiology of urine flow from kidneys to bladder

Urine production by the kidneys is a continuous process. Its transport from the kidneys, down the ureter, and into the bladder occurs intermittently, by waves of peristaltic contraction of the renal pelvis and ureter (*peristalsis* = wavelike contractions and relaxations). The renal pelvis delivers urine to the proximal ureter. As the proximal ureter receives a bolus of urine it is stretched, and this stimulates it to contract, while the segment of ureter just distal to the bolus of urine relaxes. Thus the bolus of urine is projected distally.

The origin of the peristaltic wave is from collections of pacemaker cells in the proximal-most regions of the renal calyces. In species with multiple calyces, such as humans, there are multiple pacemaker sites in the proximal calyces.

The frequency of contraction of the calyces is independent of urine flow rate (it is the same at high and low flow rates) and it occurs at a higher rate than that of the renal pelvis. Precisely how frequency of contraction of each calyx is integrated into a single contraction of the renal pelvis is not known.

All areas of the ureter are capable of acting as a pacemaker. Stimulation of the ureter at any site produces a contraction wave that propagates proximally and distally from the site of stimulation, but under normal conditions, electrical activity arises proximally and is conducted distally from one muscle cell to another (the proximal most pacemakers are dominant over these latent pacemakers).

Peristalsis persists after renal transplantation and denervation and does not therefore appear to require innervation. The ureter does, however, receive both parasympathetic and sympathetic innervation, and stimulation of these systems can influence the frequency of peristalsis and the volume of urine bolus transmitted.

At normal urine flow, the frequency of calyceal and renal pelvic contractions is greater than that in the upper ureter, and there is a relative block of electrical activity at the UPJ. The renal pelvis fills; the ureter below it is collapsed and empty. As renal pelvic pressure rises, urine is extruded into the upper ureter. The ureteric contractile pressures that move the bolus of urine are higher than renal pelvic pressures.

A closed UPJ may prevent back-pressure on the kidney. At higher urine flow rates, every pacemaker-induced renal pelvic contraction is transmitted to the ureter.

To propel a bolus of urine, the walls of the ureter must coapt (touch). Resting ureteric pressure is ~0–5 cmH$_2$O and ureteric contraction pressures range from 20 to 80 cmH$_2$O.

Ureteric peristaltic waves occur 2–6 times per minute. The VUJ acts as a one-way valve under normal conditions, allowing urine transport into the bladder and preventing reflux back into the ureter.

Ureter innervation

Autonomic

The ureter has a rich autonomic innervation.

- *Sympathetic*—preganglionic fibers from spinal segments T10 to L2; postganglionic fibers arise from the celiac, aorticorenal, mesenteric, superior and inferior hypogastric (pelvic) autonomic plexuses
- *Parasympathetic*—vagal fibers via celiac to upper ureter; fibers from S2–4 to lower ureter

The role of ureteric autonomic innervation is unclear. It is not required for ureteric peristalsis (though it may modulate this). Peristaltic waves originate from intrinsic smooth muscle pacemakers located in minor calyces of renal collecting system.

Afferent

- Upper ureter—afferents pass (alongside sympathetic nerves) to T10–L2
- Lower ureter—afferents pass (alongside sympathetic nerves and by way of pelvic plexus) to S2–4.

Afferents subserve stretch sensation from the renal capsule, collecting system of kidney (renal pelvis and calyces), and ureter. Stimulation of the mucosa of the renal pelvis, calyces, and ureter also stimulates nociceptors, the pain felt being referred in a somatic distribution to T8–L2 (kidney T8–L1, ureter T10–L2), in the distribution of the subcostal, iliohypogastric, ileoinguinal, or genitofemoral nerves.

Thus, ureteric pain can be felt in the flank, groin, scrotum or labia, and upper thigh, depending on the precise site in the ureter from which the pain arises.

Trauma to the urinary tract and other urological emergencies

Renal trauma: classification and grading 420
Renal trauma: clinical and radiological assessment 422
Renal trauma: treatment 426
Ureteral injuries: mechanisms and diagnosis 432
Ureteral injuries: management 434
Bladder and urethral injuries associated with pelvic fractures 440
Bladder injuries 444
Posterior urethral injuries in males and urethral injuries in females 448
Anterior urethral injuries 452
Testicular injuries 454
Penile injuries 456
Torsion of the testis and testicular appendages 460
Paraphimosis 462
Malignant ureteral obstruction 463
Spinal cord and cauda equina compression 464

Renal trauma: classification and grading

Classification

There are two categories of renal trauma—blunt and penetrating. At least 90% of renal injuries in the United States occur from blunt trauma, and most of these are trivial in nature (either superficial lacerations or contusions).

The mechanism of injury is important to consider because it predicts the likely need for surgical exploration to control bleeding. Experience from large series shows that 95% of blunt injuries can be managed conservatively. Penetrating renal injuries tend to be of greater severity; thus, roughly 50% of stab injuries and 75% of gunshot wounds require surgical exploration.

Blunt injures
- Direct blow to the kidney
- Rapid deceleration

A direct blow from a fall, assault, or sports injury is often associated with renal laceration. Rapid-deceleration injuries usually occur as a result of motor vehicle collisions. Because the renal pedicle is the site of attachment of kidney to other fixed retroperitoneal structures, renal vascular injuries (tears or thrombosis) or UPJ disruption may occur.

Penetrating injuries

Stab or gunshot injuries to the flank, lower chest, and anterior abdominal area may inflict renal damage; half of patients with penetrating trauma and hematuria have grade III, IV, or V renal injuries.

Penetrating injuries anterior to the anterior axillary line are more likely to injure the renal vessels and renal pelvis than are injuries posterior to this line, where less serious parenchymal injuries are more likely. Thus, renal injuries from stab wounds to the flank (i.e., posterior to anterior axillary line) can often be managed nonoperatively.

Wound profile of a low-velocity gunshot wound is similar to that of a stab wound. High-velocity gunshot wounds (>350 m/s) cause greater tissue damage due to a cavitation effect, which produces stretching and disruption of surrounding tissues.

Mechanism

Because the kidneys are retroperitoneal structures surrounded by perirenal fat, the vertebral column and spinal muscles, the lower ribs, and abdominal contents, they are relatively well protected from injury and a considerable degree of force is usually required to injure them—only 1.5–3% of trauma patients have renal injuries. Associated injuries are therefore common (e.g., spleen, liver, mesentery of bowel).

Renal trauma: clinical and radiological assessment

Renal injuries may not initially be obvious, hidden as they are by other structures. To confirm or exclude a renal injury, imaging studies are required. In children, there is proportionately less perirenal fat to cushion the kidneys against injury, thus renal injuries occur with lesser degrees of trauma. Staging of renal injuries is given in Box 10.1.

History includes mechanism of the trauma (blunt, penetrating).

Examination

Pulse rate, systolic blood pressure, respiratory rate, location of entry and exit wounds, flank bruising, and rib fractures need to be assessed. The *lowest recorded systolic blood pressure* is used to determine the presence of shock and thus the need for renal imaging.

Remember, in young adults and children, hypotension is a late manifestation of hypovolemia; blood pressure is maintained until there has been substantial blood loss, thus making shock a less reliable indicator.

Indications for renal imaging

- Gross hematuria
- Microscopic (>5 RBCs per high-powered field [hpf]) or dipstick hematuria in a hypotensive patient (systolic blood pressure of <90 mmHg recorded at any time since the injury[1])
- History of rapid deceleration with evidence of multisystem trauma (e..g., fall from a height, high-speed motor vehicle accident).
- Penetrating chest and abdominal wounds (knives, bullets) with any degree of hematuria or suspicion of renal injury based on wound location
- Any child with urinalysis showing ≥50 RBC/hpf after blunt trauma

Adult and pediatric patients with *isolated microhematuria* after blunt trauma need not have their kidneys imaged immediately as long as there is no history of rapid deceleration and no evidence of multisystem trauma or shock, since the chances of a significant renal injury are <0.2% in this setting.

Degree of hematuria

While deep renal lacerations may often be associated with obvious gross hematuria, in some cases of severe renal injury (renal vascular injury, UPJ avulsion) hematuria may be absent. Thus the relationship between the presence, absence, and degree of hematuria and the severity of renal injury is neither predictable nor reliable.

With blunt renal trauma in adults there is a chance of significant renal injury vs. degree of hematuria and systolic blood pressure (Table 10.1).

Box 10.1 Staging of the renal injury

Using CT, renal injuries are staged according to the American Association for the Surgery of Trauma (AAST) Organ Injury Severity Scale. Higher injury severity scales are associated with poorer outcomes.

Grade I	Contusion or subcapsular hematoma with no parenchymal laceration
Grade II	Parenchymal laceration of cortex <1 cm deep, no extravasation of urine (i.e., collecting system intact) (Fig. 10.1)
Grade III	Parenchymal laceration of cortex >1 cm deep, no extravasation of urine (i.e., collecting system intact)
Grade IV	Parenchymal laceration involving cortex, medulla, and collecting system OR segmental renal artery or renal vein injury with contained hemorrhage
Grade V	Completely shattered kidney OR avulsion of renal hilum

Table 10.1 Renal injury as indicated by hematuria and SBP

Degree of hematuria; systolic BP (mmHg)	Significant renal injury
Microhematuria;* SBP >90	0.2%
Gross hematuria; SBP >90	10%
Gross or microhematuria; SBP <90	10%

* Dipstick or microscopic hematuria

The hemodynamically unstable patient

While CT is always the preferred imaging method for stable patients with suspected renal injuries, hemodynamic instability may preclude its use. Such patients may need to be taken to the operating room immediately to control bleeding. In this situation, an intraoperative on-table IVP (see Table 10.1) is indicated if
• A retroperitoneal hematoma is found and/or
• A renal injury is found that is likely to require nephrectomy.

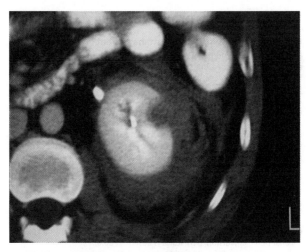

Figure 10.1 Renal CT with IV contrast in blunt trauma patent shows a superficial (grade 2) laceration amenable to nonoperative management.

Renal trauma: treatment

Conservative (nonoperative) management

Most blunt (95%) and many penetrating renal injuries (50% of stab injuries and 25% of gunshot wounds) can be managed nonoperatively.

Dipstick or microscopic hematuria: If systolic BP since injury has always been >90 mmHg and there is no history of deceleration, imaging and admission is not required. Outpatient follow-up of microhematuria should be considered.

Gross hematuria: In a hemodynamically stable patient whose injury has been staged with CT, admit for bed rest, antibiotics, serial labs, and observation until the hematuria resolves (cross-match in case blood pressure drops). High-grade injuries can be managed nonoperatively if they are cardiovascularly stable. However, grade IV and, especially, grade V injuries may require prompt nephrectomy to control bleeding (grade V injuries function poorly if repaired).

Surgical exploration (see Box 10.2)

This is indicated (whether blunt or penetrating injury) if
- Expanding, large, or pulsatile perirenal hematoma is present (suggests a renal pedicle avulsion; hematuria is absent in 20%).
- The patient develops shock that does not respond to resuscitation with fluids and/or blood transfusion.
- The hemoglobin decreases (there are no strict definitions of what represents a significant fall in hemoglobin).
- There is urinary extravasation and associated bowel or pancreatic injury.

Urinary extravasation

This is not an absolute indication for exploration. Almost 80–90% of these injuries will heal spontaneously. The threshold for operative repair is lower with associated bowel or pancreatic injury—bowel contents mixing with urine is a recipe for sepsis. In these situations, the renal repair should be well drained and omentum interposed between the kidney and bowel or pancreas.

If there is substantial contrast extravasation, consider placing a JJ stent and a Foley catheter.

Repeat CT imaging if the patient develops a prolonged ileus or a fever, since these signs may indicate development of a urinoma, which can be drained percutaneously. Renal exploration is needed for a persistent leak.

Devitalized segments

Exploration is usually not required for patients with devitalized segments of kidney (Fig. 10.2). If urinary extravasation is also present, these patients may be at higher risk for septic complications.

Box 10.2 Technique of renal exploration

Midline incision allows the following:
- Exposure of renal pedicle, for early control of renal artery and vein
- Inspection for injury to other organs

Lift the small bowel upward to allow access to the retroperitoneum. Incise the peritoneum over the aorta, above the inferior mesenteric artery. A large perirenal hematoma may obscure the correct site for this incision. If this is the case, look for the inferior mesenteric vein and make your incision medial to this. Once on the aorta, trace it upward toward the crossing of the left renal vein. Here, both renal arteries may be accessed and vessel loops passed around these vessels.

Expose kidney by reflecting the colon up off of the retroperitoneum. Bleeding may be reduced by applying pressure to vessels via a Rummel tourniquet. Control bleeding vessels within the kidney with 4-0 absorbable sutures. Close any defects in the collecting system similarly.

If your sutures cut out, place perirenal fat or a strip of gelatin or collagen over the site of bleeding, place your sutures through the renal capsule on either side of this, and tie them over the bolster. This will stop them from cutting through the friable renal parenchyma.

Finding a nonexpanding, nonpulsatile retroperitoneal hematoma at laparotomy

An expanding or pulsatile retroperitoneal hematoma found at laparotomy in an unstable patient often indicates renal pedicle avulsion or laceration. Nephrectomy may be required to stop life-threatening hemorrhage.

Controversy surrounds management of the nonexpanding, nonpulsatile retroperitoneal hematoma found at laparotomy. If the patient is stable, most can be left alone or treated with percutaneous angiographic embolization if needed postoperatively. In inexperienced hands, renal exploration may release retroperitoneal tamponade, thus increasing risk of bleeding that can be controlled only by nephrectomy.

Preoperative or intraoperative imaging	Action
Normal	Leave the hematoma alone.
Abnormal	Explore and repair kidney if major injury is suspected (especially for penetrating injury). Leave hematoma alone unless pulsatile and/or patient is unstable (especially blunt injuries).
None	Consider 1-shot IVP on table. Explore and repair renal injury if hematoma is pulsatile and patient is unstable.

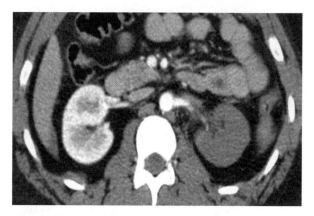

Figure 10.2 Left renal artery thrombosis after blunt trauma resulting in devitalized parenchyma successfully treated nonoperatively.

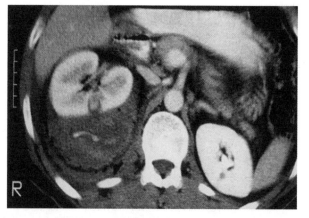

Figure 10.3 Contrast CT after abdominal stab wound shows deep central renal laceration and large perirenal hematoma with intravascular contrast extravasation. This patient remained unstable after 3 units of blood were transfused and thus underwent nephrectomy. Notice the normal contralateral kidney on this scan.

Nephrectomy

For severe renal injuries producing life-threatening bleeding, prompt nephrectomy is warranted. These are usually unstable patients who persist in shock despite multiple transfusions and have deep renal lacerations near the hilum (Fig. 10.3).

Hypertension and renal injury

Excess renin excretion occurs following renal ischemia from renal artery injury or thrombosis or renal compression by hematoma or fibrosis. This can lead to hypertension months or years after renal injury. The exact incidence of post-traumatic hypertension is uncertain but felt to be rare.

Iatrogenic renal injury: renal hemorrhage after percutaneous nephrolithotomy

Significant renal injuries can occur during percutaneous nephrolithotomy (PCNL) for kidney stones. This is the surgical equivalent of a stab wound and serious hemorrhage results in ~1% of cases.

Bleeding during or after PCNL can occur from vessels in the nephrostomy track itself, from an arteriovenous fistula, or from a pseudoaneurysm that has ruptured. Track bleeding will usually tamponade around a large-bore nephrostomy tube.

Traditionally, persistent bleeding through the nephrostomy tube is managed by clamping the nephrostomy tube and waiting for the clot to tamponade the bleeding. While this may control bleeding in some cases, in others a rising or persistently elevated pulse rate (with later hypotension) indicates the possibility of persistent bleeding and is an indication for renal arteriography and embolization of the arteriovenous fistula or pseudoaneurysm (Figs. 10.4 and 10.5). Failure to stop the bleeding by this technique is an indication for renal exploration.

Arteriovenous fistulae can sometimes occur following open renal surgery for stones or tumors, and arteriography with embolization can also be used to stop the bleeding in these cases. However, the bleeding usually occurs over a longer time course (days or even weeks), rather than as acute hemorrhage causing shock.

1 Martin X (2000). Severe bleeding after nephrolithotomy: results of hyperselective embolization. *Eur Urol* 37:136–139.

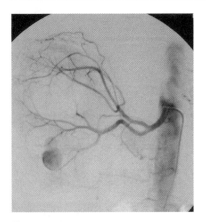

Figure 10.4 Renal arteriography after PCNL where severe bleeding was encountered. An arteriovenous fistula was found and embolized.

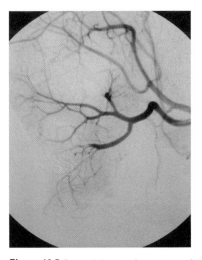

Figure 10.5 Post-embolization of arteriovenous fistula. Note the embolization coils in the lower pole.

Ureteral injuries: mechanisms and diagnosis

Types, causes, and mechanisms
- *External:* nearly always due to penetrating trauma (knife or gunshot wounds); only rarely due to blunt trauma
- *Iatrogenic:* during pelvic or abdominal surgery (e.g., hysterectomy, colectomy, appendectomy, AAA repair; repeated or traumatic ureteroscopy). The ureter may be divided, ligated, or angulated by a suture or damaged by diathermy.

External injury: diagnosis
Suspicion for possible ureteral injury is based on wound location or the above clinical scenarios. Hematuria may be absent in 30% of cases.

Imaging studies
In stable patients, contrasted CT with delayed cuts (10–20 minutes) is superior to IVP for clearly determining the presence of a ureteric injury (Fig. 10.6). If doubt remains regarding the integrity of the ureters, retrograde pyelography should be done.

Iatrogenic injury: diagnosis
The injury may be suspected at the time of surgery, but injury may not become apparent until some days or weeks postoperatively.

Intraoperative diagnosis
Direct inspection of the ureter
IVP is notoriously inaccurate for detecting ureteral injuries. Direct intraoperative inspection of the ureter is the best way to detect injury of the ureter. IV injection of methylene blue or indigo carmine may reveal a laceration. Direct injection into the ureter, either retrograde or antegrade, may also reveal extravasation from a laceration.

Ureteral contusion
Discoloration of the ureter observed during laparotomy suggests ischemic injury related to a blast effect after an abdominal gunshot wound. This may lead to a delayed slough and leak if not repaired and/or stented primarily.

Postoperative diagnosis
The diagnosis is usually apparent in the first few days following surgery (see Box 10.3), but it may be delayed by weeks, months, or years (presentation is flank pain; post-hysterectomy incontinence—continuous leak of urine suggests a ureterovaginal fistula).

Investigation
Ultrasonography may demonstrate hydronephrosis, but hydronephrosis may be absent when urine is leaking from a transected ureter into the retroperitoneum or peritoneal cavity.

IVP may show an obstructed ureter or possibly a contrast leak from the site of injury, but CT is more accurate and is thus preferred. Retrograde pyelogram is an accurate method of delineating the site of injury, but is best used in conjunction with attempted stent placement.

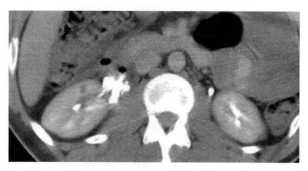

Figure 10.6 CT of patient with right ureteral injury after stab wound.

Box 10.3 Symptoms and signs of ureteral injury

These may include the following:
- Ileus (due to urine within the peritoneal cavity)
- Prolonged postoperative fever or overt urinary sepsis
- Drainage of fluid from drains, abdominal wound, or vagina. Send aliquot for creatinine estimation. Creatinine level higher than that of serum = urine (creatinine level will be at least 300 μmol/L [4.0 mg/dL]).
- Flank pain if the ureter has been ligated
- Abdominal mass, representing a urinoma
- Vague abdominal pain
- The pathology report on the organ that has been removed may note presence of segment of ureter.

Ureteral injuries: management

When to repair the ureteral injury

In general, the best time to repair the ureter is as soon as the injury has been diagnosed (if intraoperatively), or if the diagnosis is made within the first week after injury. If the diagnosis is made between days 7 and 14 after ureteric injury, caution is advised, since edema and inflammation at the site of repair often occur.

Percutaneous nephrostomy should be placed, the infection drained percutaneously, intravenous antibiotics given, and ureteric repair delayed until the patient is stable and afebrile.

Delay definitive ureteral repair when

- The patient is unable to tolerate a prolonged procedure under general anesthesia—(consider damage control: divert urine by placing a 90 cm single J stent through the defect into the kidney, suture into place, and bring out to abdominal wall in anticipation of later repair).
- There is evidence of active infection at the site of proposed ureteral repair (infected urinoma).
- Diagnosis is made more than 14 days after injury.

Definitive treatment of ureteral injuries

The options depend on the following:

- Whether the injury is recognized immediately
- The nature and level of injury
- Other associated problems

The options are as follows (see also Box 10.4):

- *JJ stenting* for 3–6 weeks (e.g., ligature injury from absorbable suture—may cut suture if recognized intraoperatively). Stent placement is also indicated for cases of ureterovaginal fistula.
- *Primary closure* of partial transection of the ureter and stent placement
- *Direct spatulated anastomosis* (primary ureteroureterostomy)—if the defect between the ends of the ureter is short (<2 cm) and a tension-free anastomosis is possible (usually performed for upper ureteral injuries in a setting of immediate laparotomy after a gunshot wound)
- *Reimplantation* of the ureter into the bladder (ureteroneocystostomy) either directly (for short traumatic lower ureteral injuries) or with psoas hitch and/or a Boari bladder flap (for longer injuries or those associated with extensive fibrosis; Figs. 10.7 and 10.8) may reach up to L4–5 level.
- *Transureteroureterostomy* (Fig. 10.9) is only used in a setting of advanced pelvic fibrosis, and is contraindicated if there is history of stone disease or pelvic malignancy (best used in delayed setting).
- *Replacement of the ureter* with ileum is used when the segment of damaged ureter is very long. It is used rarely, only if the urinary tract cannot be used (e.g., Boari bladder flap), in a delayed setting.
- *Autotransplantation* of the kidney into the pelvis is used when the segment of damaged ureter is very long.
- *Permanent cutaneous ureterostomy* is used when the patient's life expectancy is limited.

Nephrectomy is traditionally advocated for ureteral injury during vascular graft procedures (e.g., aortobifemoral graft for AAA), but the current trend is toward repair and renal preservation, reserving nephrectomy only when urine leak develops postoperatively.[1]

Nephrectomy is best used when ureteral injury is high and extensive, and the patient is not a candidate for ileal ureter or Boari flap reconstruction (e.g., hostile abdomen, older or debilitated patient).

Box 10.4 General principles of ureteric repair

- Optical magnification via 2.5x loupes is suggested.
- The ends of the ureter should be mobilized and débrided judiciously.
- The anastomosis must be tension free.
- For complete transection, the ends of the ureter should be spatulated, to allow a wide anastomosis to be done.
- A stent should be placed across the repair.
- Mucosa-to-mucosa anastomosis should be done, to achieve a watertight closure.
- Use fine sutures (4/0 or 5–0 absorbable suture material on RB-1 needle).
- A drain should be placed near the site of anastomosis.
- Repair should be covered with the peritoneal flap and/or retroperitoneal fat to exclude the site from the abdominal cavity.

1 McAninch JW (2002). In Walsh PC, Retik AB, Vaughan ED, Wein AJ (Eds.) *Campbell's Urology*, 8th edition. Philadelphia: W.B. Saunders, pp. 3703–3714.

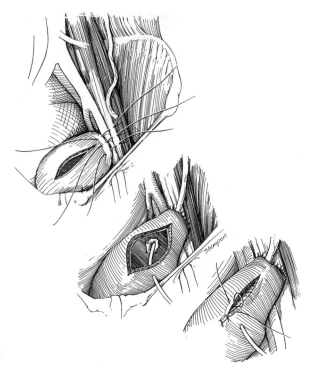

Figure 10.7 A psoas hitch. This figure was published in Walsh PC, et al. *Campbell's Urology*, 8th edition, pp. 3703–3714. Copyright Elsevier 2002.

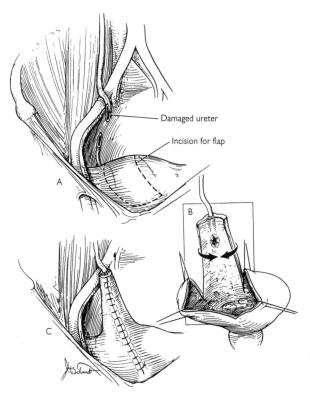

Figure 10.8 A Boari flap. This figure was published in Walsh PC, et al. *Campbell's Urology*, 8th edition, p. 3703–3714. Copyright Elsevier 2002.

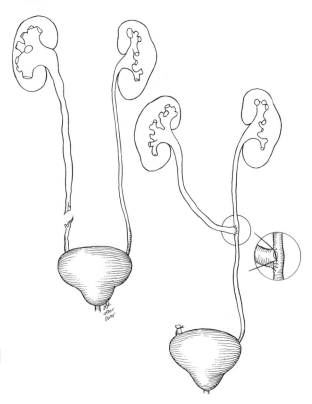

Figure 10.9 Transureteroureterostomy. This figure was published in Walsh PC, et al. *Campbell's Urology*, 8th edition, p. 3703–3714. Copyright Elsevier 2002.

Bladder and urethral injuries associated with pelvic fractures

Pelvic fractures are usually due to crush injuries, where massive force is applied to the pelvis. Associated head, chest, intra-abdominal (spleen, liver, mesentery of bowel), pelvic (bladder, urethra, vagina, rectum), and genital injuries are common and these injuries plus the massive blood loss from torn pelvic veins and arteries account for the substantial (20%) mortality after pelvic fracture.

Urologists must often work closely with orthopedists and/or trauma surgeons called to treat other associated injuries.

Abdominal and pelvic imaging in pelvic fracture

- Retrograde urethrography is performed to detect urethral injury when blood is present at the meatus.
- If the urethra appears intact, a Foley catheter is inserted. If gross hematuria is noted, a retrograde cystogram is done to assess integrity of the bladder.
- Abdominal/pelvic CT establishes presence/absence of associated pelvic (rectum, bladder) and abdominal organ injury (liver, bowel, spleen).

Is urethral catheterization of a pelvic fracture safe for the patient?

If there is no blood present at the meatus, a gentle attempt at urethral catheterization should be made. While it has traditionally been suggested that this could convert a partial urethral rupture into a complete rupture, recent evidence has not supported this concern.

If resistance is encountered, stop, and obtain a retrograde urethrogram. If the retrograde urethrogram demonstrates a normal urethra, proceed with another attempt at catheterization, using plenty of lubricant and a Coude' tip catheter or a flexible cystoscope. If there is a urethral rupture, insert a suprapubic catheter via a formal open approach, to allow inspection of the bladder (and repair of injuries if present).

If CT demonstrates marked bladder distension with no gross evidence of rupture, a percutaneous SP tube is reasonable.

Bladder injuries associated with pelvic fractures

All patients presenting with gross hematuria and pelvic fracture (Fig. 10.10) should undergo cystography—roughly 30% will be found to have bladder rupture. Most normal individuals with traumatic bladder ruptures are symptomatic and present with suprapubic pain.

- 10% of pelvic fractures are associated with bladder injury.
- 90% of bladder ruptures are associated with pelvic fracture.
- 60% of bladder ruptures are extraperitoneal.
- 30% are intraperitoneal.
- 10% are combined extraperitoneal and intraperitoneal.

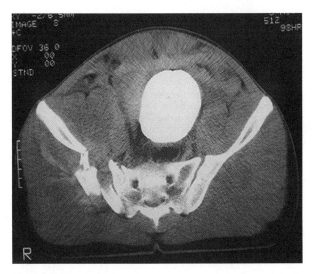

Figure 10.10 Normal CT cystogram in a patient with gross hematuria and right iliac wing fracture. Notice the large pelvic hematoma displacing the bladder and the complete visualization behind the distended bladder, thus obviating the need for additional post-drainage views or plain films.

Patients with (a) microhematuria and pelvic fracture or (b) gross hematuria without pelvic fracture are much less likely to have bladder rupture (<5%) and thus require bladder imaging only if they have significant suprapubic pain, low urine output, altered sensorium, or other clinical indicators suggestive of bladder rupture (e.g., free fluid on abdominal ultrasound or CT).

Urethral injuries associated with pelvic fractures
The posterior urethra is injured with roughly the same frequency as the bladder in subjects who sustain a pelvic fracture (roughly 10%). Ten percent of patients with a pelvic fracture and bladder rupture also have a posterior urethral rupture.

Symptoms and signs of bladder or urethral injury in pelvic fracture
- Blood at meatus—in 40–50% of patients (no blood at meatus in 50–60%)
- Gross hematuria
- Inability to void
- Perineal or scrotal bruising

- High-riding prostate
- Inability to pass a urethral catheter, or poor urinary drainage from previously placed catheter
- Altered sensorium—patients who are intoxicated or obtunded may not present with typical symptoms of bladder rupture

High-riding prostate

The prostate and bladder become detached from the membranous urethra and are pushed upward by the expanding pelvic hematoma. The high-riding prostate detected during DRE has traditionally been reported as a classic sign of posterior urethral rupture.

However, the presence of a high-riding prostate is an unreliable sign. The pelvic hematoma may make it impossible to feel the prostate, so the patient may be thought to have a high-riding prostate when, in fact, it is in a normal position. Conversely, what may be thought to be a normal prostate in a normal position may actually be the palpable pelvic hematoma.

Bladder injuries

Other situations in which the bladder may be injured

These include TURBT, cystoscopic bladder biopsy, TURP, cystolithopaxy, penetrating trauma to the lower abdomen or back, cesarean section (especially as an emergency), minor trauma in the inebriated patient, rapid deceleration injury (e.g., seat belt injury with full bladder in the absence of a pelvic fracture), and spontaneous rupture after bladder augmentation.

Types of perforation

- *Intraperitoneal perforation*—the peritoneum overlying the bladder is breached allowing urine to escape into the peritoneal cavity.
- *Extraperitoneal perforation*—the peritoneum is intact and urine escapes into the space around the bladder, but not into the peritoneal cavity (Fig. 10.11).

Making the diagnosis

During endoscopic urological operations (e.g., TURBT, cystolithopaxy), the diagnosis is usually obvious on visual inspection alone—a dark hole is seen in the bladder and loops of bowel may be seen on the other side. No further diagnostic tests are required.

In cases of trauma, the classic triad of symptoms and signs suggesting a bladder rupture is

- Gross hematuria
- Suprapubic pain and tenderness
- Difficulty or inability in passing urine

Additional signs are as follows:

- Abdominal distension
- Absent bowel sounds (indicating an ileus from urine in the peritoneal cavity)
- Free fluid on abdominal CT or ultrasound

These symptoms and signs are an indication for a retrograde cystogram.

Imaging studies

Either retrograde plain-film cystography or CT cystography are appropriate, depending on the patient's clinical status and associated injuries. CT cystography is usually more appropriate, since many trauma patients are already undergoing CT for other abdominal, chest, head, or pelvic injuries.

Plain-film cystography is usually reserved for stable patients in the trauma bay or intraoperatively in patients taken directly for surgery.

Ensure the bladder is adequately distended with dilute contrast. With inadequate distension a clot, omentum, or small bowel may plug the perforation, which may not therefore be diagnosed. Use at least 300 mL of dilute (25%) contrast in an adult and (age + 2) × 30 mL in children.

Clamping a urethral catheter and imaging the pelvis after IV contrast administration alone is usually nondiagnostic—repeat imaging with a distended bladder is required. For CT cystography, only a "full-bladder"

A

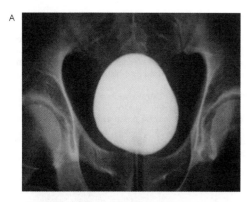

B

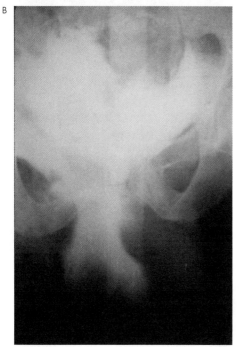

Figure 10.11 A) Normal-filling cystogram. B) Extraperitoneal perforation with extravasation of contrast.

phase is required—a post-drainage view is not required since the retro-vesical space is well visualized.

For plain-film imaging, obtain three views: a scout film, an anteropos-terior (AP) full-bladder film, and a post-drainage film, after the contrast has been completely drained from the bladder. Contrast drainage from a posterior perforation may be obscured by a bladder distended with con-trast in the AP view.

In extraperitoneal perforations, extravasation of contrast is limited to the immediate area surrounding the bladder—a dense "flame-shaped" collection of contrast. Contrast may be noted extending into the retro-peritoneum or scrotum, neither of which alters management.

In intraperitoneal perforations, loops of bowel or the peritoneal cavity may be outlined by the contrast.

Treatment

For treatment of bladder rupture, see Box. 10.5.

Box 10.5 Treatment of bladder rupture

Extraperitoneal

When conditions are ideal, use bladder drainage with a urethral catheter for ~2 weeks followed by a cystogram to confirm the perforation has healed. If extravasation is noted, replace the catheter for 2 more weeks and repeat imaging; some injuries may take up to 6 weeks to heal.

Indications for surgical repair of extraperitoneal bladder perforation:
- Associated rectal or vaginal perforation
- When the patient is undergoing open fixation of a pelvic fracture, the bladder should be simultaneously repaired to prevent infection of the orthopedic hardware.
- If the bladder was opened to place a suprapubic catheter for a urethral injury
- Bone spike protruding into the bladder on CT
- Injuries discovered intraoperatively during nonurological surgery
- Injuries occurring as a result of penetrating trauma
- Poor urinary drainage due to clot obstruction

Intraperitoneal

When resulting from external trauma, surgical repair is required to prevent complications from leakage of urine into the peritoneal cavity. Selected patients with small iatrogenic perforations occurring during urological procedures (e.g., TURBT) may be treated nonoperatively under close observation with large-bore urethral catheter drainage and antibiotics alone.

Spontaneous rupture after bladder augmentation

Spontaneous bladder rupture occasionally occurs months or years after bladder augmentation and usually with no history of trauma. If the patient has spina bifida or a spinal cord injury, they usually have limited awareness of bladder fullness and pelvic pain. Their abdominal pain may therefore be mild and vague in onset and nature. Fever or other signs of sepsis may be present.

Have a high index of suspicion in patients with augmentation who present with nonspecific signs of illness. A cystogram usually, though not always, confirms the diagnosis. If doubt exists, consider exploratory laparotomy.

Posterior urethral injuries in males and urethral injuries in females

Male posterior urethral injuries

The great majority of posterior urethral injuries are associated with pelvic fracture, usually involving a diastasis or crush injury of the pubis. The prostate is tightly bound to the back of the pubis via the dense puboprostatic ligaments and also intimately associated with the sphincter mechanism. With distortion of the pubic symphysis, the prostate and membranous urethra are avulsed as a unit off of the proximal bulb.

The result is a bulbomembranous urethral disruption, often erroneously termed *prostatomembranous*. Retrograde urethrogram will reveal gross extravasation of contrast without bladder filling (Fig. 10.12)

Prompt suprapubic urinary diversion is required for complete injuries. Primary urethral realignment may be briefly attempted, but prolonged attempts may lead to pelvic abscess and thus must be avoided. Even if the injured posterior urethra is realigned primarily, concomitant suprapubic diversion is also prudent since many of these patients will stenose rapidly upon removal of the urethral catheter, even after 4 weeks of urethral stenting.

Immediate (within 48 hours) open repair of posterior urethral injuries is to be avoided, since this practice is associated with a high incidence of urethral stenosis (70%), incontinence (20%), and impotence (40%). The surrounding hematoma and tissue swelling make it difficult to identify structures and to mobilize the two ends of the urethra to allow tension-free anastomosis.

In the majority of male posterior urethral injuries, treatment should be deferred for 3 months to allow the edema and hematoma to completely resolve (Fig. 10.13). As this occurs, the two distracted ends of the urethra settle closer together, usually resulting in a gap <3 cm in length.

This defect is an obliterative stenosis, not a stricture, and the prostatic urethra may often be displaced posteriorly or laterally. Most such injuries can be repaired by a delayed anastomotic urethroplasty with a success rate of >90% in referral centers.

The key to successful posterior urethral reconstruction is complete scar excision with wide-bore, tension-free, mucosa-to-mucosa anastomosis. Optical urethrotomy (division of the stricture using an endoscopic knife or laser, via a cystoscope inserted into the urethra) is generally not recommended initially since the lumen is usually obliterated but may be useful for recurrent stenosis after open surgery (when continuity is established and spongiofibrosis is decreased).

Urethral injuries in females

These are rare, because the female urethra is short and its attachments to the pubic bone are weak, such that it is less prone to tearing during pubic bone fracture.

When they do occur, such injuries are usually associated with vaginal and/or rectal injuries. Immediate closure of the vaginal laceration is performed in conjunction with suprapubic drainage. Urethral stenting is also recommended whenever possible to prevent obliteration of the bladder neck.

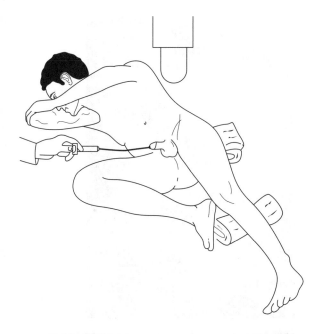

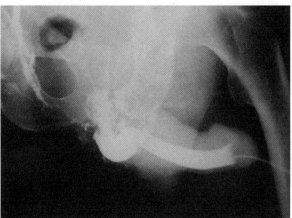

Figure 10.12 Top: Technique of retrograde urethrogram. Bottom: Complete posterior urethral disruption after pelvic fracture.

A

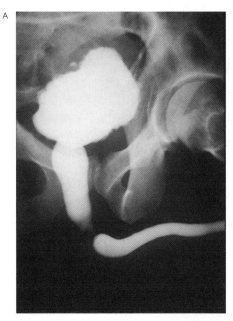

B

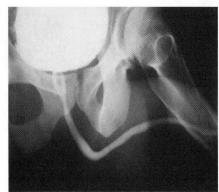

Figure 10.13 A) Following posterior urethral disruption, after 3 months of suprapubic urinary drainage, a short obliterative stenosis is observed on this combined antegrade/retrograde urethrogram. B) Postoperative appearance after delayed posterior urethral reconstruction—wide urethral patency is observed.

Anterior urethral injuries

History and examination

Anterior urethral injuries typically occur as a result of straddle injury to the perineum. Other causes include iatrogenic (e.g., traumatic catheterization), penile fracture, or penetrating trauma. Gunshot wounds affecting the anterior urethra also typically involve the thigh, groin, or buttock.

The patient usually presents with blood at the meatus, difficulty in passing urine, and/or gross hematuria. If Buck fascia (the deep layer of fascia surrounding the penis) has been ruptured, urine and blood coalesce in the scrotum and perineum in a classic "butterfly" pattern of bruising, reflecting the lateral attachments of Colle fascia—the superficial fascia of the groin and perineum (see Fig. 10.14 and Box 10.6).

Confirming the diagnosis and subsequent management

Retrograde urethrography delineates the presence and extent of urethral injury. Extravasation of contrast around the urethra indicates the need for urinary diversion via either urethral or suprapubic catheter to prevent further extravasation of urine and infectious complications. It is helpful to determine whether the injury is partial or complete.

Partial rupture of anterior urethra

There is contrast leak from the urethra with retrograde flow into the bladder preserved. Most cases (70%) heal without stricture formation when managed by a period of urinary diversion alone. Flexible cystoscopy may be used to place a guide wire into the bladder under direct vision, followed by placement of a Councill tip catheter. Alternatively, passage of a 16 Fr Coude tip catheter may be performed to stent the injury.

Broad-spectrum antibiotics are given to prevent infection of extravasated urine and blood. If a voiding cystogram 2 weeks later confirms urethral healing, remove the catheter. If contrast still extravasates, leave it in place a little longer. Suprapubic catheterization (percutaneously) should be performed if urethral catheterization is not easily accomplished.

Complete rupture of anterior urethra

Leak of contrast from the urethra on retrograde urethrogram without filling of the posterior urethra or bladder indicates a greater magnitude of injury. Suprapubic urinary diversion should be performed promptly to prevent complications. A short, dense urethral stricture will likely result, which is easily repaired with a high degree of success at most referral centers.

Several recent studies have shown that realignment of such injuries acutely, followed by repeated instrumentation to maintain patency, actually leads to longer strictures and more complex repairs.

Penetrating anterior urethral injuries

Urethral injuries due to gunshot or knife wounds should be treated via immediate primary suture repair using optical magnification and fine absorbable suture over a 16 Fr catheter. Voiding cystourethrography should be done in 2 weeks to confirm healing.

Immediate surgical repair of anterior urethral injuries is also done in the context of penile fracture or where there is an open wound.

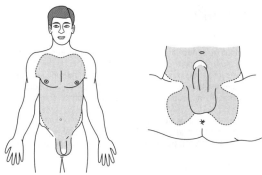

Figure 10.14 Butterfly bruising following rupture of Buck fascia.

Box 10.6 Anatomical explanation for "butterfly" pattern of bruising in anterior urethral rupture

Fascial layers of penis from superficial to deep:
- Penile skin
- Superficial fascia of the penis (Dartos fascia)—continuous with the superficial fascia of the groin and perineum (Colles fascia) and abdomen (Scarpa fascia)
- Buck fascia (deep layer of superficial fascia that envelopes penis)
- Deep fascia of the penis (tunica albuginea)—dense tissue lining containing the erectile tissue within the corpora cavernosa and the corpus spongiosum

If Buck fascia is intact, bruising from a urethral rupture is confined in a sleeve-like configuration, along the length of the penis. If Buck fascia has ruptured, the extravasation of blood, and thus the subsequent bruising, extends to the lateral attachments of Colles fascia, which forms a butterfly-like pattern in the perineum.

How to perform a retrograde urethrogram
- Use aseptic technique.
- Position patient with the pelvis at an oblique angle (bottom leg flexed at the hip and knee).
- A 16 Fr unlubricated catheter is placed in the fossa navicularis of the penis 1–2 cm from the external meatus, with the catheter balloon filled with 3 mL of water to hold the catheter in place.
- Slowly inject 30 cc of dilute contrast.
- Continuous screening (fluoroscopy) is done as contrast is instilled until the entire length of the urethra is demonstrated. Remember, as the urethra passes through the pelvic floor and membranous urethra (located at the lower portion of the obturator foramen), there is a normal narrowing, and similarly, the prostatic urethra is narrower than the bulbar urethra.
- Take film during contrast injection.

Testicular injuries

Mechanisms

These can be blunt or penetrating. Most testicular injuries in civilian practice are blunt, a blow forcing the testicle against the pubis or the thigh.

Bleeding occurs into the parenchyma of the testis, and if sufficient force is applied, the tunica albuginea of the testis (the tough fibrous coat surrounding the parenchyma) ruptures, allowing extrusion of seminiferous tubules.

Penetrating injuries occur as a consequence of gunshot or knife wounds and from explosive blasts; associated limb (e.g., femoral vessel), perineal (penis, urethra, rectum), pelvic, abdominal, and chest wounds often occur.

Usually, the force is sufficient to rupture the tunica albuginea and the tunica vaginalis, and seminiferous tubules and blood extrude into the layers of the scrotum. This is a *hematoma*.

Where bleeding is confined by the tunica vaginalis, a *hematocele* is said to exist. Intraparenchymal (intratesticular) hemorrhage and bleeding beneath the parietal layer of tunica vaginalis will cause the testis to enlarge slightly. The testis may be under great pressure as a consequence of the intratesticular hemorrhage confined by the tunica vaginalis. This can lead to ischemia, pain, necrosis, and atrophy of the testis.

History and examination

Severe pain is common, as are nausea and vomiting. As a result, bimanual physical exam is notoriously difficult. If the testis is surrounded by a hematoma it will not be palpable. If it is possible to palpate the testis, it is usually very tender.

The resulting scrotal hematoma can be very large and the bruising and swelling caused may spread into the inguinal region and lower abdomen.

Testicular ultrasound in cases of blunt trauma

Scrotal ultrasound is the imaging test of choice for evaluating suspected testicular rupture. A normal, homogenous intratesticular parenchymal echo pattern suggests there is no significant testicular injury (i.e., no testicular rupture).

Hypoechoic areas within the testis (indicating intraparenchymal hemorrhage) suggest testicular rupture (Fig. 10.15).

Indications for exploration in scrotal trauma

- Testicular rupture. Exploration allows evacuation of the hematoma, excision of extruded seminiferous tubules, and repair of the tear in the tunica albuginea.
- Penetrating trauma. Exploration allows repair to damaged structures (e.g., the vas deferens or spermatic cord vessels may have been severed and can be repaired).
- In roughly 75% of cases, testicular injuries can and should be repaired primarily in lieu of orchiectomy.

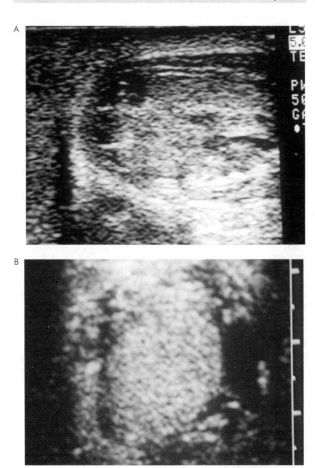

Figure 10.15 Scrotal ultrasound after blunt trauma shows A) multiple intraparenchymal hypoechoic areas consistent with rupture, and B) normal contralateral testis.

Penile injuries

Penile fracture

This involves rupture of the tunica albuginea of the erect penis (i.e., rupture of one or both corpora cavernosa and/or rupture of the corpus spongiosum and urethra). The tunica albuginea is 2 mm thick in the flaccid penis and thins to 0.25 mm during erection, which makes it vulnerable to rupture if the penis is forcibly bent (e.g., during vigorous sexual intercourse).

In general, the diagnosis of penile fracture is straightforward and based on the presence of classic history and physical findings. Delay in diagnosis is common, as many men are initially too embarrassed, ashamed, or frightened to present immediately for medical attention. Penile imaging is not needed to diagnose penile fracture, although MRI has been reported to be accurate in equivocal cases.

The patient usually reports a sudden "snapping" sound or "popping" sensation, with sudden penile pain and detumescence of the erection. The penis immediately becomes markedly swollen and bruised, a classic appearance known as the "eggplant" deformity (Fig. 10.16).

A tender, palpable defect may be felt over the site of the tear in the tunica albuginea. If Buck fascia has ruptured, bruising extends onto the lower abdominal wall and into the perineum and scrotum; otherwise, the discoloration is contained along the penile shaft.

If the urethra is damaged, there may be blood at the meatus or hematuria (dipstick/microscopic or macroscopic) and pain on voiding or urinary retention. Arrange a retrograde urethrogram or flexible cystoscopy in such cases. Immediate primary urethral repair is warranted for concomitant urethral injuries.

Treatment

Immediate surgical repair has been repeatedly associated with a lower complication rate (e.g., reduced impotence, penile deformity and scar tissue formation, prolonged penile pain) than that of conservative treatment of penile fracture.

The fracture site in the tunica albuginea is exposed via a circumcision incision, the hematoma evacuated, and the defect in the tunica closed with interrupted 2–0 absorbable sutures. Deep stitches in the underlying erectile tissue are unnecessary and possibly harmful; only tunical closure is warranted.

A self-adhesive compressive bandage, application of cold compresses to the penis, analgesics and anti-inflammatory drugs, and abstinence from sexual activity for 6–8 weeks are prudent adjunct measures to promote optimal healing.

Surgical repair of penile fracture

Expose the fracture site by degloving the penis via a circumcising incision around the subcoronal sulcus or by an incision directly over the defect if palpable. A degloving incision allows better exposure of the urethra for associated urethral injuries.

Alternatively, use a midline incision extending distally from the midline raphe of the scrotum, along the shaft of the penis. This latter incision,

A

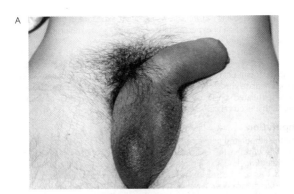

B

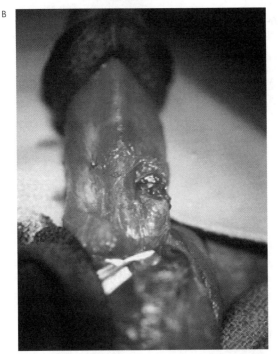

Figure 10.16 A) Typical "eggplant deformity" appearance of fractured penis.
B) Intraoperative appearance of penile fracture—a transverse defect in the tunica
albuginea in the midshaft.

along with a degloving incision, allows excellent exposure of both corpora cavernosa so that an unexpected bilateral injury can be repaired easily, as can a urethral injury should this have occurred.

Close the defect in the tunica albuginea with absorbable 2–0 sutures. Cover the knots with Buck fascia or bury them so that the patient is unable to palpate them. Leave a urethral catheter overnight (voiding can be difficult immediately postoperatively). Repair a urethral rupture, if present, with a spatulated single or two-layer urethral anastomosis, and splint repair with a urethral catheter for 2 weeks.

Amputation

Place the amputated penile remnant, if found, in a wet gauze pad inside a plastic bag, which is then placed inside another bag containing ice (bag in a bag). It can survive for 24 hours.

Blood loss can be severe; resuscitate the shocked patient and cross-match blood. Consider psychiatric consultation if the wound was self-inflicted.

Knife and gunshot wounds

Associated injuries are common (e.g., scrotum, major vessels of the lower limb). Most corporal injuries, other than minor ones, should undergo primary repair to prevent long-term disturbance of erectile function.

Remove debris from wound (e.g., particles of clothing) and débride necrotic tissue sparingly. Repair as for penile fractures (see Box 10.7).

Box 10.7 Treatment of penile injuries

Surgical reimplantation of amputated penis

Repair the urethra first, over a catheter, to provide a stable base for subsequent neurovascular repair. Concomitant suprapubic urinary diversion is usually recommended. Close the tunica albuginea of the corpora with 2–0 absorbable sutures.

Cavernosal artery repair is not recommended, since it is technically very difficult and does not improve penile viability.

Microsurgical anastomosis (via plastic surgical consultation) is then performed on the dorsal artery of the penis, the dorsal vein to provide venous drainage, and, finally, the dorsal penile nerve and skin. In the absence of microsurgical expertise availability, a "macroreplantation" of the urethra, corpora, and skin is acceptable.

Penile bites and skin loss injuries

Clean the wound copiously. Give broad-spectrum antibiotics (e.g., cephalosporin and amoxycillin). If skin loss has occurred via degloving injury, a loose primary closure with 3–0 chromic is recommended.

Zipper injuries

If the penis is still caught in the zipper, use lubricant jelly and gently attempt to open it. The zipper bar may have to be cut with orthopedic cutters or pried apart with a pair of surgical clamps on either side of the zipper.

Torsion of the testis and testicular appendages

Definition

Testicular torsion is a twist of the spermatic cord, resulting in strangulation of the blood supply to the testis and epididymis. Testicular torsion occurs most frequently between the ages of 10 and 30 (peak incidence 13–15 years of age), but any age group may be affected.

History and examination

There is a sudden onset of severe pain in the hemiscrotum, sometimes waking the patient from sleep. It may radiate to the groin, flank, or epigastrium (reflecting its origin from the dorsal abdominal wall of the embryo and its nerve supply from T10/11) and is often associated with nausea.

There is sometimes a history of minor trauma to the testis. Some patients report previous episodes with spontaneous resolution of the pain (suggesting previous torsion with spontaneous detorsion).

The patient is often writhing on the exam table, unable to find a comfortable position. The torsed testis is usually moderately swollen and very tender to the touch. It may be high riding compared to the contralateral testis and may lie in a horizontal position due to twisting of the cord.

The cremasteric reflex is nearly always absent in the event of true testicular torsion—if a prompt bilateral reflex elevation of the testes is noted when lightly scratching the inner thigh (cremasteric reflex), the diagnosis is unlikely. Elevation of the scrotum and supporting may relieve the pain of epididymitis but not in torsion.

Differential diagnosis and investigations

Common diagnoses that may masquerade as torsion include epididymo-orchitis, torsion of a testicular appendage, and causes of flank pain with radiation into the groin and testis (e.g., a ureteric stone). The diagnosis of epididymitis should be made intraoperatively in an adolescent with an acute scrotum.

Radiographic studies are generally used to confirm the absence of torsion. If torsion is suspected clinically, arrangements should immediately be made for surgical exploration and detorsion.

Color Doppler ultrasound (reduced arterial blood flow in the testicular artery) and radionuclide scanning (decreased radioisotope uptake) can be used to diagnose testicular torsion. In many hospitals these tests are not readily available and the diagnosis is based on symptoms and signs.

Surgical management

Scrotal exploration should be undertaken as a matter of urgency since delay in relieving the twisted testis results in permanent ischemic damage to the testis, causing atrophy, loss of hormone and sperm production, and, as the testis undergoes necrosis and the blood–testis barrier breaks down, an autoimmune reaction against the contralateral testis (sympathetic orchidopathy).

Bilateral testicular fixation should always be performed since the bell-clapper abnormality that predisposes to torsion often occurs bilaterally. A soft, braided, permanent suture is recommended with fixation at two or three sites.

Manual detorsion may be attempted in the emergency room while awaiting surgery. Occasionally, the induction of anesthesia will reduce spasm and promote spontaneous detorsion—in both of these instances, bilateral orchiopexy should still be performed to prevent recurrence.

Infarction of testicular appendages

The appendix testis (remnant of the Müllerian duct) and the appendix epididymis (remnant of a cranial mesonephric tubule of the Wolffian duct) can undergo infarction, causing pain that mimics a testicular torsion. The "blue dot" sign is the typical physical finding for appendix testis infarction. At scrotal exploration they are easily removed with scissors or electrocautery.

If these diagnoses are confirmed radiographically, analgesics may be given and surgical exploration is unnecessary.

Paraphimosis

Definition and presentation

Paraphimosis is when the uncircumcised foreskin is retracted under the glans penis and the foreskin becomes edematous, and cannot be pulled back over the glans into its normal anatomical position. It occurs most commonly in teenagers or young men and also in elderly men (who have had the foreskin retracted during catheterization, but where it has not been returned to its normal position).

Paraphimosis is usually painful. The foreskin is edematous and a small area of ulceration of the foreskin may have developed.

Treatment

The best initial maneuver for manually reducing paraphimosis is to forcefully squeeze the edematous prepuce for several minutes. Then the skin may be manipulated distally with the fingers of both hands as the glans is pressed down with the thumbs.

If this fails, the traditional surgical treatment is a dorsal slit under general anesthetic or ring block. A longitudinal incision is made in the tight band of constricting tissue and the foreskin pulled back over the glans. Close the incision transversely with chromic sutures to widen the circumference of the foreskin and prevent recurrences. Many patients subsequently require elective circumcision.

Malignant ureteral obstruction

Locally advanced prostate cancer, bladder or ureteral cancer may cause unilateral or bilateral ureteral obstruction. Locally advanced nonurological malignancies can also obstruct the ureters (e.g., cervical cancer, rectal cancer, lymphoma).

Unilateral obstruction

This is often asymptomatic and an incidental ultrasound finding that requires no specific treatment in the presence of a normal contralateral kidney in a patient with limited life expectancy.

Occasionally, flank pain and systemic symptoms may develop due to infection of the obstructed upper urinary tract. In this circumstance, drainage by nephrostomy or stenting is required.

Bilateral ureteric obstruction

This is a urological emergency. The patient either presents with symptoms and signs of renal failure or is anuric without a palpable bladder. A mass will probably be palpable on rectal examination.

Investigations

Renal ultrasound will demonstrate bilateral hydronephrosis and an empty bladder. Noncontrasted CT will confirm the presence of dilated ureters down to a mass at the bladder base.

Immediate treatment of bilateral ureteric obstruction

After treating any life-threatening hyperkalemia, options include bilateral percutaneous nephrostomy or ureteric stenting. Serum coagulation studies are required prior to nephrostomy insertion. Insertion of retrograde ureteric stents in this setting is usually unsuccessful because tumor involving the trigone obscures the location of the ureteric orifices.

More successful is antegrade ureteric stenting following nephrostomy insertion, both of which are performed under IV sedation. The double-J silicone or polyurethane ureteric stents require periodic (4–6 monthly) changes to prevent calcification or blockage.

In the case of prostate cancer, rapid reduction in testosterone through hormone therapy should be started if not previously used.

Spinal cord and cauda equina compression

Spinal cord compression due to spinal metastases from urological cancers

This is a urological oncological emergency; failure to diagnose and treat promptly can lead to permanent paraplegia and autonomic dysfunction (failure of bladder and bowel emptying; inability to achieve an erection).

Due to epidural compression arising from vertebral body metastasis in the majority of cases, 95% of patients will complain of back pain and have a positive bone scan. Ten percent of cases do not exhibit these features because their disease is paravertebral.

Patients with back pain should be examined neurologically and evaluated radiologically. Pain usually precedes cord compression by about 4 months. Other clinical features include sensory changes and muscle weakness in the lower limbs and bladder and bowel dysfunction, and these can progress rapidly to become irreversible.

If cord compression is suspected, the investigation of choice is spinal MRI, which will reveal the deposits (multiple in 20% of cases).

Treatment

Initial treatment is with high-dose intravenous corticosteroids (e.g., dexamethasone 10 mg followed by 4 mg q6h for 2–3 weeks). If the patient has prostate cancer but has not had prior androgen deprivation therapy, ketoconazole should be started to lower circulating androgen levels.

Without delay, further treatment with direct spinal radiotherapy or, less frequently, neurosurgical decompression is carried out. Surgery should be considered preferable if there is a pathological fracture, unknown tissue diagnosis, or previous history of radiotherapy.

Cauda equina compression

The adult spinal cord tapers below L2 vertebral level into the conus medullaris. The cauda equina consists of nerve roots of spinal cord segments below L2, as they run in the subarachnoid space to their exit levels in the lower lumbar and sacral spines.

Pathophysiology

The cauda equina may be compressed by a central intervertebral disc prolapse, spinal stenosis, or a benign or malignant tumor within the lower lumbar or sacral vertebral canal.

Symptoms

The diagnosis should be considered in any female or young male presenting with difficulty voiding or in urinary retention. There may be back pain.

Signs

These include palpable bladder, loss of perianal (S2–4) and lateral foot sensation (S1–2), reduced anal tone, and priapism.

Treatment is intermittent self-catheterization.

Infertility

Male reproductive physiology 466
Etiology and evaluation of male infertility 470
Lab investigation of male infertility 472
Oligospermia and azoospermia 476
Varicocele 478
Treatment options for male factor infertility 480

Male reproductive physiology

Hypothalamic–pituitary–testicular axis

The hypothalamus secretes luteinizing hormone–releasing hormone (LHRH), also known as gonadotrophin-releasing hormone (GnRH). This causes pulsatile release of anterior pituitary gonadotrophins, called follicle-stimulating hormone (FSH) and luteinizing hormone (LH), which act on the testis.

FSH stimulates the seminiferous tubules to secrete inhibin and produce sperm; LH acts on Leydig cells to produce testosterone (Fig. 11.1).

Testosterone

Testosterone is secreted by the interstitial **Leydig cells**, which lie adjacent to the seminiferous tubules in the testis. It promotes development of the male reproductive system and secondary sexual characteristics.

Steroidogenesis is stimulated by a cAMP-protein kinase C mechanism, which converts cholesterol to pregnenolone. Further steps in the biosynthesis pathway produce intermediary substances (dehydroepiandrosterone and androstenedione) prior to producing testosterone.

In the blood, testosterone is attached to sex hormone–binding globulin (SHBG) and albumin. At androgen-responsive target tissues, testosterone is converted into a potent androgen, dihydrotestosterone (DHT), by intracellular 5α-reductase (see p. 64).

Spermatogenesis

Seminiferous tubules are lined with **Sertoli cells**, which surround developing germ cells (spermatogonia) providing nutrients and stimulating factors, as well as secreting androgen-binding factor and inhibin (Fig. 11.2).

Primordial germ cells (spermatogonia) divide via mitosis to form primary spermatocytes. These undergo a first meiotic division to create secondary spermatocytes (46 chromosomes), followed by a second meiotic division to form spermatids (23 chromosomes). Finally, these differentiate into spermatozoa.

Spermatogenesis takes 74 days. The nonmotile spermatozoa leave the seminiferous tubules and pass to the epididymis, where they undergo maturation (gain motility and the ability to fertilized). Ductal transit time takes another 2 weeks, so the total time from beginning of spermatogenesis to ejaculation is 3 months.

Motile sperm are stored in the globus minor of the epididymis until ejaculation. Spermatozoa that are not released are reabsorbed by phagocytosis.

Mature sperm

Mature sperm have a head, middle piece, and tail (Fig. 11.3). The head is composed of a nucleus covered by an acrosome cap, containing vesicles filled with lytic enzymes that break down the outer layer of the female ovum. The middle piece contains mitochondria and contractile filaments, which extend into the tail to aid motility.

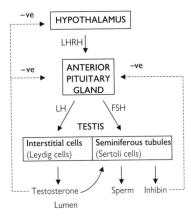

Figure 11.1 Hypothalamic–pituitary–testicular axis.

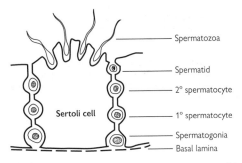

Figure 11.2 Spermatogenesis in the seminiferous tubules of the testis.

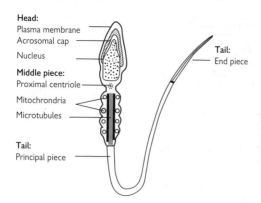

Head:
Plasma membrane
Acrosomal cap
Nucleus

Tail:
End piece

Middle piece:
Proximal centriole
Mitochrondria
Microtubules

Tail:
Principal piece

Figure 11.3 A spermatozoon.

After deposition at the cervix, sperm penetrate cervical mucus and travel through the uterus to the site of fertilization in the fallopian tube. Along the way, within the female reproductive tract, they undergo capacitation—a further activation of their ability to fertilize marked by an increase in their motility.

When a sperm penetrates the oocyte, it binds to the zona pellucida, which alters its permeability so that other sperm cannot penetrate the ovum, leading to enzyme release, penetration into the cytoplasm of the oocyte, fusion, and fertilization.

Etiology and evaluation of male infertility

Definition of infertility

Infertility is failure of conception after at least 12 months of unprotected intercourse. The chance of a normal couple conceiving is estimated at 20–25% per month, 75% by 6 months, and 90% at 1 year. Up to 50% of infertility is due to male factors. Up to 25% of couples may be affected at some point in their reproductive years.

Pathophysiology

Failure of fertilization of the normal ovum is due to defective sperm development, function, or inadequate numbers. There may be abnormalities of morphology (teratospermia) or motility (asthenospermia), low sperm numbers (oligospermia), combined disorders (oligoasthenospermia), or absent sperm (azoospermia).

Abnormal epididymal function may result in defective spermatozoa maturation or transport, or induce cell death.

Etiology

- **Idiopathic** (25%)
- **Varicocele** (present in 40%)
- **Cryptorchidism** (undescended testes)
- **Functional sperm disorders:** immunological infertility (sperm antibodies); head or tail defects; Kartagener's syndrome (immotile cilia); dyskinetic cilia syndrome
- **Erectile or ejaculatory problems**
- **Testicular injury:** orchitis (postpubertal, bilateral mumps orchitis); testicular torsion; trauma; radiotherapy
- **Endocrine disorders:** Kallmann's syndrome (isolated gonadotrophin deficiency causing hypogonadism and anosmia); Prader–Willi syndrome (hypogonadism, short stature, hyperphagia, obesity); pituitary gland adenoma, radiation, or infection
- **Hormone excess:** excess prolactin (pituitary tumor); excess androgen (adrenal tumor, congenital adrenal hyperplasia, anabolic steroids); excess estrogens
- **Genetic disorders:** Kleinfelter's syndrome (47XXY) involves azoospermia, ↑FSH/LH AND ↓testosterone; XX male; XYY syndrome
- **Male genital tract obstruction:** congenital absence of vas deferens; epididymal obstruction or infection; Müllerian prostatic cysts; groin or scrotal surgery
- **Systemic disease:** renal failure; liver cirrhosis; cystic fibrosis
- **Drugs:** chemotherapy; alcohol; marijuana; sulfasalazine; smoking
- **Environmental factors:** pesticides; heavy metals; hot baths

History

- **Sexual:** duration of problem; frequency and timing of intercourse; previous successful conceptions; previous birth control; erectile or ejaculatory dysfunction
- **Developmental:** age at puberty; history of cryptorchidism; gynecomastia
- **Medical and surgical:** detailed assessment for risk factors—recent febrile illness; postpubertal mumps orchitis; varicocele; testicular torsion, trauma, or tumor; sexually transmitted diseases; genitourinary surgery; radiotherapy; respiratory diseases associated with ciliary dysfunction; diabetes
- **Drugs and environmental:** previous chemotherapy; exposure to substances that impair spermatogenesis or erectile function; alcohol consumption; smoking habits; hot baths
- **Family:** hypogonadism; cryptorchidism

Examination

Perform a full assessment of all systems, with attention to general appearance (evidence of secondary sexual development; signs of hypogonadism; gynecomastia).

Urogenital examination should include assessment of the penis (Peyronie's plaque, phimosis, hypospadias); measurement of testicular consistency, tenderness, and volume with a Prader orchidometer (normal >20 mL; varies with race); palpation of epididymis (tenderness, swelling) and spermatic cord (vas deferens present or absent, varicocele); and digital rectal examination of the prostate.

Lab investigation of male infertility

Basic investigations

Semen analysis

Obtain 2 or 3 specimens over several weeks, collected after 2–7 days of sexual abstinence. Deliver specimens to the laboratory within 1 hour. Ejaculate volume, liquefaction time, and pH are noted (Table 11.1).

Microscopy techniques measure sperm concentration, total numbers, morphology, and motility (Table 11.2).

The mixed agglutination reaction (MAR test) is used to detect anti-sperm antibodies. The presence of leukocytes or round cells in the ejaculate ($>1 \times 10^6$/mL of semen) suggests infection, and cultures should be requested.

Hormone measurement

Obtain serum FSH, LH, and testosterone (Table 11.3). Elevated serum FSH levels (2 x normal) suggest irreversible testicular failure. In cases of isolated low testosterone level, it is recommended that morning and free testosterone levels be tested.

Elevated prolactin is associated with sexual dysfunction and low serum testosterone levels, and usually indicates the presence of a pituitary adenoma.

Special investigations

- *Chromosome analysis* is indicated for clinical suspicion of an abnormality (azoospermia or oligospermia, small atrophic testes with ↑FSH).
- *Fructose* is produced in the seminal vescle and is a major source of energy for sperm metabolism. If semen fructose is low, an ejaculatory duct obstruction or seminal vesical abnormality should be suspected.
- *Testicular biopsy* is performed for azoospermic patients with normal FSH levels, to differentiate between idiopathic (e.g., maturation arrest, Sertoli cell only syndrome) and obstructive causes. It may also be used for sperm retrieval.

Sperm function tests

Postcoital test

Cervical mucus is taken just before ovulation and within 8 hours of inter-course, and microscopy is performed. Normal results shows >10 sperm per high-powered field, the majority demonstrating progressive motility. Abnormal results indicate inappropriate timing of the test; cervical mucus antisperm antibodies; abnormal semen; or inappropriately performed coitus.

Sperm penetration test

A sample of semen is placed directly onto preovulatory cervical mucus on a slide and the penetrative ability of spermatozoa is observed.

Sperm-cervical mucus test

A specimen of semen (control) and one mixed with cervical mucus are placed separately on a slide and observed for 30 minutes. More than 25% exhibiting jerking movements in the mixed sample (but not the control) is a positive test for antisperm antibodies.

Table 11.1 Semen analysis: normal parameters*

Semen analysis	Normal values
Semen volume	>2.0 mL
pH	7.2–7.8
Total sperm count	>40 × 10⁶/ejaculate
Sperm concentration	>20 × 10⁶/mL
Sperm motility	>50% with progressive motility (grades >2); or >25% grade 4
Sperm morphology	>15% normal forms
Viability	>75% viable sperm
Time to liquefy	5–25 minutes
White blood cells	<1 × 10⁶ WBC/mL
MAR test (for antisperm Ab)	Negative (<10% with adherent particles)
Zinc	>2.4 mol/ejaculate
Semen fructose	120–145 mg/dL

*Adapted from World Health Organization (WHO) reference values for semen analysis.

Table 11.2 Grading of sperm motility

Grade	Type of sperm motility
0	No motility
1	Sluggish; no progressive movement
2	Slow, meandering forward progression
3	Moving in a straight line with moderate speed
4	Moving in a straight line at high speed

Table 11.3 Clinical diagnosis on hormone assay

FSH*	LH**	Testosterone	Diagnosis
↑	Normal	Normal	Seminiferous tubule damage (defective spermatogenesis)
Normal	Normal	Normal	Normal; or bilateral genital tract obstruction
↑	↑	Normal/↓	Testicular failure
↓	↓	↓	Hypogonadotrophism

* Follicle stimulation hormone.
** Luteinizing hormone.

Imaging

Scrotal ultrasound

This is used to confirm a varicocele and assess testicular abnormalities.

Transrectal ultrasound

TRUS is indicated for low ejaculate volumes, to investigate seminal vesicle obstruction (>1.5 cm width) or absence and ejaculatory duct obstruction (>2 .3 mm).

Vasography

Vas deferens is punctured at the level of the scrotum and injected with contrast toward the prostate, never toward the epdidymis. Vasography is performed at the time of planned reconstruction.

A normal test shows the passage of contrast along the vas deferens, seminal vesicles, ejaculatory duct, and into the bladder, which rules out obstruction—indigo carmine is commonly used to confirm patency.

Formal radiographic vasography is only indicated to localize obstructions proximal to the inguinal ring.

Venography

This is used to diagnose and treat varicoceles (embolization).

Oligospermia and azoospermia

Oligospermia
Oligospermia is defined as a sperm concentration of <20 million/mL of ejaculate.

Etiology
It is often idiopathic. It is identified in ~60% of patients presenting with testicular cancer or lymphoma.

Associated disorders
It is often associated with abnormalities of morphology and motility (oligoasthenoteratospermia). Common causes include varicoceles, cryptorchidism, idiopathic, drug and toxin exposure, and febrile illness.

Investigations
Semen analysis: Severely low sperm counts (<5–10 million/mL) require hormone investigation, including FSH and testosterone. Severe oligospermia is associated with seminiferous tubular failure, small soft testes, and ↑FSH.

Treatment
Correct the underlying cause. Idiopathic cases may respond to empirical medical therapy. Clomiphene and tamoxifen are mild antiestrogens that work best for men with low to normal testosterone and FSH levels.

Consider assisted reproductive techniques, such as intrauterine insemination (IUI) or intracytoplasmic sperm injection (ICSI).

Azoospermia
This is defined as a complete absence of sperm in the ejaculate fluid.

Etiology
- *Obstructive:* absent or obstructed vas deferens; epididymal or ejaculatory duct obstruction. The cystic fibrosis gene is located on chromosome 7 and the condition is associated with congenital absence of the vas deferens (CAVD).
- *Nonobstructive:* hypogonadotrophism (Kallmann's syndrome, pituitary tumour); abnormalities of spermatogenesis (chromosomal anomalies, toxins, idiopathic, varicocele, orchitis, testicular torsion)

Investigations
Hormone assay
Elevated FSH indicates a nonobstructive cause; normal FSH with normal testes indicates an increased likelihood of obstruction. Low levels of FSH, LH, and testosterone indicate Kallmann's syndrome (hypogonadotropic hypogonadism) due to hypothalamic dysfunction and absence of GnRH secretion.

Prader-Willi syndrome also has absent GnRH secretion. It is associated with obesity, mental retardation, and short stature, whereas Kallman's syndrome is associated with anosmia.

Chromosomal analysis

This may be used to exclude Kleinfelter's syndrome in patients presenting with azoospermia, small soft testes, gynecomastia, ↑FSH/LH, and ↓testosterone.

Testicular biopsy

This is best performed as an open procedure. It is performed to assess if normal sperm maturation is occurring and for sperm retrieval (for later therapeutic use).

Diagnostic biopsy is indicated in azoospermic men with testes of normal size and consistency, palpable vasa deferentia, and normal FSH levels. Biospy may also be therapeutic, since sperm can be retrieved on testis biopsy from 25–50% of patients with Sertoli cell only syndrome, and 50–75% of men with maturation arrest. Multiple sample sites are performed if sperm are not immediately obtained.

Transrectal ultrasound

This is indicated for low semen volume to assess for ejaculatory duct obstruction. Men with ejaculatory duct obstruction will tend to have low semen volume and fructose, and semen pH <7.

Management

Treatment will depend on the underlying etiology.

- *Transurethral resection of ejaculatory ducts (TURED)* is associated with improved semen quality in 52%.
- *Bilateral absence or agenesis of vas deferens:* microsurgical epididymal sperm aspiration (MESA), or consider artificial insemination using donor (AID).
- *Primary testicular failure with testicular atrophy:* testicular sperm extraction (TESE); in vitro fertilization (IVF); or consider AID.
- *Primary testicular failure with normal testis:* TESE; IVF; AID
- *Obstructive cause with normal testis:* epididymovasostomy; vasovasostomy

Varicocele

Definition
Varicocele is dilatation of the veins of the pampiniform plexus of the spermatic cord.

Prevalence
This is the most common correctable cause of male infertility. Varicocele is found in 15% of men in the general population and 40% of males presenting with infertility. Bilateral or unilateral (left side affected in 90%).

Etiology
Incompetent values in the internal spermatic veins lead to retrograde blood flow, vessel dilatation, and tortuosity of the pampiniform plexus. The left internal spermatic vein enters the renal vein at a right angle, creating a column of blood that is under a higher pressure than that in the right vein, which enters the vena cava obliquely at a lower level. As a consequence, the left side is more likely to develop a varicocele.

Pathophysiology
Testicular venous drainage is via the pampiniform plexus, a meshwork of veins encircling the testicular arteries. This arrangement normally provides a countercurrent heat exchange mechanism that cools arterial blood as it reaches the testis. Varicoceles adversely affect this mechanism, resulting in elevated scrotal temperatures and consequent deleterious effects on spermatogenesis (± loss of testicular volume).

Varicocele grading system

Grade	Size	Definition
1	Small	Palpable only with Valsalva maneuver
2	Moderate	Palpable in a standing position
3	Large	Visible through the scrotal skin

Presentation
The majority of varicoceles are asymptomatic, although large varicoceles may cause pain or a heavy feeling in the scrotal area. Examine patient both lying and standing, and ask patient to perform Valsalva maneuver (strain down).

A varicocele is identified as a mass of dilated and tortuous veins above the testicle (described as feeling like a "bag of worms"), which decompress on lying supine. Examine for testicular atrophy, which is often associated with chronic testicular injury.

Investigation
• *Scrotal Doppler ultrasound scan* is diagnostic.
• *Semen analysis:* Varicoceles are associated with reduced sperm counts and motility, and abnormal morphology, either alone or in combination (oligoasthenoteratospermia).

Management

Surgical ligation

- **Retroperitoneal approach:** A muscle-splitting incision is made near the anterior superior iliac spine, and the spermatic vessels are ligated at that level.
- **Inguinal approach:** The inguinal canal is incised to access the spermatic cord, and the veins are tied off as they exit the internal ring.
- **Subinguinal approach:** Veins are accessed and ligated via a small transverse incision below the external ring.
- **Laparoscopic:** Veins are occluded high in the retroperitoneum.

Surgical complications include varicocele recurrence, hydrocele formation, and testicular infarction and atrophy.

Surgical outcome

There is a 95% success rate; 70% of men have improvement of sperm parameters—most often motility, followed by count and then morphology. Testicular growth is often impaired in adolescents with varicoceles, but surgical repair may result in catch-up growth.

Embolization

In this interventional radiological technique, the femoral vein is used to access the spermatic vein for venography and embolization (with coils or other sclerosing agents).

Treatment options for male factor infertility

General treatment includes modification of lifestyle factors (reduce alcohol consumption; avoid hot baths).

Medical treatment

Correct any reversible causative factors.

Hormonal

- **Antiestrogens** (clomiphene citrate 25 mg qd) are often used empirically to increase LHRH, which stimulates endogenous gonadotrophin secretion.
- **Secondary hypogonadism** (pituitary intact) may respond to human chorionic gonadotrophin (hCG) 2000 IU subcutaneously 3 times a week, which stimulates an increase in testosterone and testicular size.
- **Testosterone deficiency** requires testosterone replacement therapy.
- **Hyperprolactinemia** is treated with dopamine agonists.

Erectile and ejaculatory dysfunction

Erectile dysfunction may be treated conventionally (oral, intraurethral, intracavernosal drugs; vacuum devices or prostheses). Ejaculatory failure may respond to sympathomimetic drugs (desipramine) or electroejaculation (used in spinal cord injury), where an electrical stimulus is delivered via a rectal probe to the postganglionic sympathetic nerves that innervate the prostate and seminal vesicles.

Antisperm antibodies

Corticosteroids have been used, but assisted conception methods are usually required.

Surgical treatment

Genital tract obstruction

- **Epididymal obstruction** can be overcome by microsurgical anastomosis between the epididymal tubule and vas (epididymovasovasostomy).
- **Vas deferens obstruction** is treated by microsurgical reanastomosis of ends of the vas, and is used for vasectomy reversal. Highest success rates for finding viable sperm occur in the first 8 years post-vasectomy (80–90%).
- **Ejaculatory duct obstruction** requires transurethral resection of the ducts.

Varicocele

This is repaired by embolization or open/laparoscopic surgical ligation.

Assisted reproductive techniques (ART)

Sperm extraction

This is used for obstructive azoospermia. Sperm are removed directly from the epididymis by microsurgical epididymal sperm aspiration (MESA) or by percutaneous retrieval (PESA). If these methods fail, testicular sperm extraction (TESE) or aspiration (TESA) may be tried.

Sperm undergo cryopreservation until required. Later, they are separated from seminal fluid by dilution and centrifuge methods, with further selection of motile sperm and normal forms using Percoll gradient techniques.

Assisted conception

- *Intrauterine insemination (IUI):* Following ovarian stimulation, sperm are placed directly into the uterus.
- *In vitro fertilization (IVF):* Controlled ovarian stimulation produces oocytes that are then retrieved under transvaginal ultrasound guidance. Oocytes and sperm are placed in a Petri dish for fertilization to occur. Embryos are transferred to the uterine cavity. Pregnancy rates are 20–30% per cycle.
- *Gamete intrafallopian transfer (GIFT):* Oocytes and sperm are mixed and deposited into the fallopian tubes via laparoscopy. Variations include zygote intrafallopian transfer (ZIFT) and tubal embryo transfer (TET).
- *Intracytoplasmic sperm injection (ICSI):* A single spermatozoon is injected directly into the oocyte cytoplasm (through the intact zona pellucida). Pregnancy rates are 15–22% per cycle.

Chapter 12

Disorders of erectile function, ejaculation, and seminal vesicles

Physiology of erection and ejaculation *484*
Impotence: evaluation *488*
Impotence: treatment *490*
Retrograde ejaculation *492*
Peyronie's disease *494*
Priapism *496*

Physiology of erection and ejaculation

Innervation

Autonomic

Autonomic sympathetic nerves originating from T11–L2, and parasympathetic nerves originating from S2–4 join to form the pelvic plexus. The cavernosal nerves are branches of pelvic plexus (i.e., parasympathetic) that innervate the penis.

Parasympathetic stimulation causes erection; sympathetic activity causes ejaculation and detumescence (loss of erection).

Somatic

Somatosensory (afferent) information travels via the dorsal penile and pudendal nerves and enters the spinal cord at S2–4. Onuf nucleus (segments S2–4) is the somatic center for efferent (i.e., somatomotor) innervation of the ischiocavernosus and bulbocavernosus muscles of the penis.

Central

The medial preoptic area (MPOA) and paraventricular nucleus (PVN) in the hypothalamus are important centers for sexual function and penile erection.

Mechanism of erection

Neuroendocrine signals from the brain, created by audiovisual or tactile stimuli, activate the autonomic nuclei of the spinal erection center (T11–L2 and S2–4). Signals are relayed via the cavernosal nerve to the erectile tissue of the corpora cavernosa, where nitric oxide (the principle neurotransmitter for penile erection) is released from nonadrenergic, noncholinergic (NANC) nerve terminals and from endothelium in the penis.

Cyclic GMP is then secondarily released via guanlyl cyclase, lowering intracellular calcium concentration within the endothelial cells, causing smooth muscle relaxation and increased arterial blood flow into the cavernosal sinuses of the penis.

A *veno-occlusive mechanism* (Table 12.1) is created by expansion of the sinusoidal spaces against the tunica albuginea, which compresses the subtunical venous plexuses, decreasing venous outflow and thus allowing "trapping" of blood within the erect penis. Maximal stretching of the tunica albuginea acts to compress the emissary veins that lie within its inner circular and outer longitudinal layers, reducing venous flow even further. Rising intracavernosal pressure and contraction of the ischiocavernosus muscles produces a rigid erection.

Following orgasm and ejaculation, vasoconstriction due to increased sympathetic activity and breakdown of cGMP via phophodiesterase type 5 produces detumescence (Figs. 12.1 and 12.2).

Ejaculation

Tactile stimulation of the penis causes sensory information to travel (via the pudendal nerve) to the lumbar spinal sympathetic nuclei. Sympathetic efferent signals (traveling in the hypogastric nerve) cause contraction of smooth muscle of the epididymis, vas deferens, and secretory glands, propelling spermatozoa and glandular secretions into the prostatic urethra.

There is simultaneous closure of the internal urethral sphincter and relaxation of the extrinsic sphincter, directing sperm into the bulbourethra (emission), but preventing sperm from entering the bladder. Rhythmic contraction of the bulbocavernosus muscle (somatomotor innervation) leads to the pulsatile emission of the ejaculate from the urethra.

During ejaculation, the alkaline prostatic secretion is discharged first, followed by spermatozoa and, finally, seminal vesicle secretions (ejaculate volume 2–5 mL). Ejaculatory latency of less than 2 minutes suggests a diagnosis of premature ejaculation.

Table 12.1 Phases of erectile process

Phase	Term	Description
0	Flaccid phase	Cavernosal smooth muscle contracted; sinusoids empty; minimal arterial flow
1	Latent (filling) phase	Increased pudendal artery flow; penile elongation
2	Tumescent phase	Rising intracavernosal pressure; erection forming
3	Full erection phase	Increased cavernosal pressure causes penis to become fully erect
4	Rigid erection phase	Further increases in pressure + ischiocavernosal muscle contraction
5	Detumescence phase	Following ejaculation, sympathetic discharge resumes; there is smooth muscle contraction and vasoconstriction; reduced arterial flow; blood is expelled from sinusoidal spaces

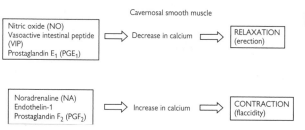

Figure 12.1 Factors influencing cavernosal smooth muscle.

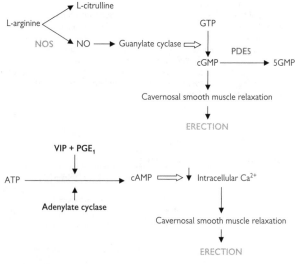

Figure 12.2 Secondary messenger pathways involved in erection.

Impotence: evaluation

Impotence (also called *erectile dysfunction* or *ED*) describes the persistent inability to achieve or maintain a penile erection sufficient for sexual intercourse.

Epidemiology

Moderate to severe ED is found in ~10% of men aged 40–70 years. Prevalence increases with age.

Etiology

ED is generally divided into psychogenic and organic causes (Table 12.2), although most cases are multifactorial.

History

- *Sexual:* onset of ED (sudden or gradual); duration of problem; presence of erections (nocturnal, early morning, spontaneous); ability to maintain erections (early collapse, not fully rigid); loss of libido; relationship issues (frequency of intercourse and sexual desire, relationship problems).
- *Medical and surgical:* hypertension; cardiac disease; peripheral vascular disease; diabetes mellitus; endocrine or neurological disorders; pelvic surgery, radiotherapy, or trauma (damaging innervation and blood supply to the pelvis and penis).
- *Drugs:* inquire about current medications and ED treatments already tried (and outcome).
- *Social:* smoking, alcohol consumption.

An organic cause is more likely with gradual onset (unless associated with an obvious cause such as surgery, where onset is acute); loss of spontaneous erections; intact libido and ejaculatory function; existing medical risk factors; and older age groups. The International Index of Erectile Function (IIEF) can be used to quantify severity.

Examination

Full physical examination (CVS, abdomen, neurological); digital rectal examination to assess prostate; external genitalia assessment to document foreskin phimosis and penile lesions (Peyronie's plaques); confirm presence, size, and location of testicles.

The bulbocavernosus reflex can be performed to test integrity of spinal segments S2–4 (squeezing the glans causes anal sphincter and bulbocavernosal muscle contraction).

Investigation

- *Blood tests:* fasting glucose; PSA; serum testosterone; sex hormone binding globulin; LH/FSH; prolactin; thyroid function test; fasting lipid profile
- *Nocturnal penile tumescence testing:* Rigiscan device contains two rings that are placed around the base and distal penile shaft to measure tumescence and number, duration, and rigidity of nocturnal erections. Erections occur most frequently during REM sleep—80%.

- *Color Doppler US* measures arterial peak systolic and end diastolic velocities,[1] pre- and post-intracavernosal injection of PGE.[1]
- *Cavernosometry:* intracavernosal injection of vasoactive drug followed by saline infusion, the rate of which is proportional to the degree of any venous leaking
- *Cavernosography:* imaging and measurement of blood flow of the penis after intracavernosal injection of contrast and induction of artificial erection. It is used to identify venous leaks.
- *Penile arteriography* is only indicated in young, otherwise healthy patients with a history of trauma-related impotence in whom vascular reconstruction is being contemplated.

Table 12.2 Causes of erectile dysfunction: "IMPOTENCE"*

Inflammatory	Prostatitis
Mechanical	Peyronie's disease
Psychological	Depression; anxiety; relationship difficulties; lack of attraction; stress
Occlusive vascular factors	**Arteriogenic:** hypertension; smoking; hyperlipidemia; diabetes mellitus; peripheral vascular disease
	Venogenic: impairment of veno-occlusive mechanism (due to anatomical or degenerative changes)
Trauma	Pelvic fracture; spinal cord injury; penile trauma
Extra factors	**Iatrogenic:** pelvic surgery; prostatectomy **Other:** increasing age; chronic renal failure; cirrhosis
Neurogenic	**CNS:** multiple sclerosis (MS); Parkinson disease; multisystem atrophy; tumor
	Spinal cord: spina bifida; MS; syringomyelia; tumor
	PNS: pelvic surgery or radiotherapy; peripheral neuropathy (diabetes, alcohol-related)
Chemical	Antihypertensives (β-blockers, thiazides, ACE inhibitors)
	Antiarrhythmics (amiodarone)
	Antidepressants (tricyclics, MAOIs, SSRIs)
	Anxiolytics (benzodiazepine)
	Antiandrogens (finasteride, cyproterone acetate)
	LHRH analogues
	Anticonvulsants (phenytoin, carbamazepine)
	Anti-Parkinson drugs (levodopa)
	Statins (atorvastatin)
	Alcohol
Endocrine	Hypogonadism; hyperprolactinemia; hypo and hyperthyroidism; diabetes mellitus

* Note that this list of causes of impotence is not in the order of frequency.
MAOIs, monoamine-oxidase inhibitors; SSRIs, serotonin reuptake inhibitors.

Impotence: treatment

A summary of treatment options is given in Table 12.3.

Psychosexual therapy

The aim is to understand and address underlying psychological issues and provide information and treatment in the form of sex education, instruction on improving partner communication skills, cognitive therapy, and behavioral therapy (programmed relearning of couple's sexual relationship).

Oral medication

Phosphodiesterase type-5 (PDE5) inhibitors

These include sildenafil (Viagra), tadalafil (Cialis), and vardenafil (Levitra). PDE5 inhibitors enhance cavernosal smooth muscle relaxation and erection by blocking the breakdown of cGMP. Sildenafil and vardenafil cross-react slightly with PDE-6, which may explain visual disturbances; Tadalafil cross-reacts with PDE-11, but the consequences of this are unknown. Sexual stimulus is still required to initiate events.

Side effects include headache, flushing, and visual disturbance.

Contraindications are patients taking nitrates; recent myocardial infarction; recent stroke; hypotension; and unstable angina.

Androgen replacement therapy

Testosterone replacement is indicated for hypogonadism. It is available in oral, intramuscular, pellet, patch, and gel forms. In older men, it is recommended that PSA be checked before and during treatment.

Intraurethral therapy

Alprostadil (MUSE) is used. A synthetic prostaglandin E_1 (PGE_1) pellet is administered into the urethra via a specialized applicator. Once inserted, the penis is gently rolled to encourage the pellet to dissolve into the urethral mucosa, from where it enters the corpora.

Prostaglandin E_1 produces an increase in intracellular cAMP, which leads to decreased calcium concentrations and thus smooth muscle relaxation and increased blood flow to the penis.

Side effects include penile pain, priapism, and local reactions.

Intracavernosal therapy

This involves alprostadil/Caverject™ (synthetic PGE_1), and papaverine (smooth muscle relaxant) ± phentolamine (α-adrenoceptor agonist). Training of technique and first dose is given by a health professional. The needle is inserted at right angles into the corpus cavernosum on the lateral aspects of mid-penile shaft.

Adverse effects include pain, priapism, and hematoma.

Vacuum erection device

The device contains three components: a vacuum chamber, pump, and constriction band. The penis is placed in the chamber and the vacuum created by the pump increases blood flow to the corpora cavernosa to induce an erection. The constriction band is placed onto the base of the penis to retain blood in the corpora and maintain rigidity.

Adverse effects include penile coldness and bruising.

Penile prosthesis

Malleable and inflatable penile prostheses are available for surgical implantation into the corpora to provide penile rigidity sufficient for sexual intercourse.

Side effects include mechanical failure, erosions, and infections.

Table 12.3 Treatment options for erectile dysfunction

Organic	Psychogenic
Eliminate underlying risk factors	Psychosexual counseling ± partner
Oral medication	Oral medication
Androgen replacement	Intraurethral therapy
Intraurethral therapy	Intracavernosal therapy
Intracavernosal therapy	
Vacuum devices	
Penile prosthesis	

Retrograde ejaculation

Definition
This is a failure of adequate bladder neck contraction, resulting in the propulsion of sperm back into the bladder on ejaculation.

Etiology
It is secondary to damage or dysfunction of the bladder neck sphincter mechanism.

Underlying causes may be **neurological** (spinal cord injury; neuropathy associated with diabetes mellitus; nerve damage after retroperitoneal surgery) or **anatomical disruption** following transurethral resection of ejaculatory ducts (for obstruction), bladder neck incision (BNI), transurethral resection of the prostate (TURP), or open prostatectomy.

It may also occur as a result of selective α-blocker therapy for BPH (particularly tamsulosin).

Incidence
Retrograde ejaculation following TURP or open prostatectomy occurs in 9 out of 10 men and after BNI in 1–5 in 10 men.

Presentation
Dry ejaculation (failure to expel ejaculate fluid from the urethral meatus) and cloudy urine (containing sperm) in the first void after intercourse are the presenting symptoms.

Investigation
The presence of >10–15 sperm per high-powered field in a post-ejaculate mid-stream urine specimen confirms the diagnosis of retrograde ejaculation.

Treatment
Medical therapy is initiated in men wishing to preserve fertility and is only effective in patients who have not had bladder neck surgery. Oral adrenergic drugs may be used to increase the sympathetic tone of the bladder neck smooth muscle sphincter mechanism. Drugs include ephedrine sulfate (25–50 mg qid), pseudoephedrine (60 mg qid), or imipramine (25 mg bid).

Therapy is often given for 7–10 days prior to a planned ejaculation (coordinated with the partner's ovulation). Alternatively, sperm retrieval may be attempted. Oral sodium bicarbonate and adjustment of fluid intake are initiated to optimize urine osmolarity and pH and to enhance sperm survival.

Sperm are collected by gentle urine centrifuge and washed in insemination media in preparation for intrauterine insemination (IUI) or in vitro fertilization (IVF) treatments.

Peyronie's disease

Definition
This is a benign penile condition characterized by curvature of the penile shaft secondary to the formation of fibrous tissue plaques within the tunica albuginea. It is also called "a disease of aging tissue in a patient with a youthful libido."

Epidemiology
Prevalence is ~1%, predominantly affecting men aged 40–60 years (average age, 53 years).

Pathophysiology
Scar formation in the tunica albuginea known as plaque is believed to arise as a result of buckling trauma. Dorsal penile plaques are most common (66%).

The corpus cavernosum underlying the lesion cannot lengthen fully on erection, resulting in penile curvature. It may be associated with distal flaccidity or an unstable penis (due to cavernosal fibrosis). The disorder has two phases:
- **Active phase** (1–6 months): painful erections and changing penile deformity
- **Quiescent phase** (9–12 months): disease "burns out." Pain disappears with resolution of inflammation, and there is stabilization of the penile deformity.

Etiology
The exact cause is unknown. It is likely that repeated minor trauma during intercourse causes microvascular injury and bleeding into the tunica, resulting in inflammation and fibrosis (exacerbated by transforming growth factor-β [TGF-β]).

Autoimmune disease processes have also been suggested, and there is a reported familial predisposition.

Presentation
Patients experience pain and curvature of the erect penis. There is a hard area (plaque) on the penis, as well as erectile dysfunction (30–40%) and penile shortening.

Associated disorders
These include Dupuytren's contractures (40%), plantar fascial contracture, tympanosclerosis, previous trauma, diabetes mellitus, and arterial disease.

Evaluation
A full medical and sexual history is taken. Patient's photographs of the curvature are useful. Assess the location and size of the plaque (is it tender?).

Color Doppler US is used to assess vascular abnormalities, whereas contrast-enhanced **MRI** is indicated for complex and extensive cavernosal fibrosis.

Management

Early disease with active inflammation (<3 months, penile pain, changing deformity) benefits most from medical therapy. Surgery is indicated for a stable, significant deformity (preventing intercourse).

Concomitant erectile dysfunction can be treated conventionally (oral or intracavernosal medications; vacuum device; penile implant).

Medical treatments

These consist of vitamin E (200 mg tid) for 3 months; tamoxifen (20 mg bid) for 3 months; or colchicine (500 mg tid) for 6 weeks.

Nesbit procedure

The penis is degloved via a circumglandular incision. An artificial erection is induced by intracavernosal saline injection. On the opposite side of maximal deformity, an ellipse is excised (a width of 1 mm is taken for every 10° of penile curvature) and then closed with sutures.

Success rates are 88–94%. Warn the patient that penile shortening of 2–3 cm frequently occurs.

Penile plication

This involves placement of soft permanent sutures in parallel rows along the convex side of the penile shaft. Penile shortening of 0.4–1.5 cm is reported in 40% of patients.

Pain at the site of tunical suture placement is reported in roughly 12%.

Plaque incision and grafting

This involves incision of plaque with venous patch insertion to lengthen the affected side (and minimize penile shortening). Other grafts reported include nonautologous grafts of dermis, porcine small intestinal submucosa (SIS) or pericardium, or autografts of dermis or rectus abdominis fascia.

Success rates are 75–96%.

Adverse effects include erectile dysfunction in 5–12% of patients.

Penile implant

When significant deformity is coupled with resistant or worsening impotence, placement of an inflatable penile prosthesis with intraoperative "molding" of the deformity is an effective way of treating both problems.

Priapism

Priapism is prolonged and often painful erection in the absence of a sexual stimulus, lasting >4–6 hours, which predominantly affects the corpus cavernosa.

Epidemiology
It peaks in incidence at ages 5–10 and 20–50 years.

Classification
Low-flow (ischemic) priapism
This is due to veno-occlusion (intracavernosal pressures of 80–120 mmHg). It is more common than high-flow priapism.

It manifests as a painful, rigid erection, with absent or low cavernosal blood flow. Ischemic priapism beyond 4 hours requires emergency intervention.

Blood gas analysis shows hypoxia and acidosis.

High-flow (nonischemic) priapism
This is usually post-traumatic in nature and does not require emergent intervention. It is due to unregulated arterial blood flow, presenting with a semi-rigid, painless erection.

Blood gas analysis shows similar results to arterial blood.

Etiology
Causes are primary (idiopathic) or secondary (see Tables 12.4 and 12.5):
- **Intracavernosal injection therapy**—PGE_1; papaverine
- **Drugs** β-blockers; antidepressants; antipsychotics; psychotropics; tranquilizers; anxiolytics; anticoagulants; recreational drugs; alcohol excess; total parenteral nutrition
- **Thromboembolic**—sickle cell disease (roughly one-third develop stuttering/recurrent priapism); leukemia; thalassemia; fat emboli
- **Malignant infiltration of the corpora cavernosa** (e.g., advanced bladder cancer)
- **Neurogenic**—spinal cord lesion; autonomic neuropathy; anesthesia
- **Trauma**—penile or perineal injury resulting in cavernosal artery laceration or arteriovenous fistula formation
- **Infection**—malaria; rabies; scorpion sting

Pathophysiology
Priapism lasting for 12 hours causes trabecular interstitial edema, followed by destruction of sinusoidal endothelium and exposure of the basement membrane at 24 hours, and sinusoidal thrombi, smooth muscle cell necrosis, and fibrosis at 48 hours.

Evaluation
- **CBC** to exclude sickle cell and leukemia.
- **Cavernous arterial blood samples** to determine the type of priapism (high or low flow). Ischemic priapism is typically associated with a PO_2

Table 12.4 Causes of low- and high-flow priapism

Low-flow priapism	High-flow priapism
Intracorporeal drug injection	Arteriovenous fistula (secondary penile or perineal trauma)
Oral medications (anticoagulants)	
Sickle cells disease (recurrent priapism)	
Leukemia	
Fat embolus	
Spinal cord lesion	
Autonomic neuropathy	
Malignant penile inflammation	

Table 12.5 Examples of drugs that may cause priapism

β-blockers	Prazosin; hydralazine
Antidepressants	Sertraline; fluoxetine; lithium
Antipsychotics	Clozapine
Psychotropics	Chlorpromazine
Tranquilizers	Mesoridazine
Anxiolytics	Hydroxyzine
Anticoagulants	Warfarin; heparin
Recreational drugs	Cocaine

of <30 mmHg, PCO_2 >60 mmHg, and pH <7.25. Nonischemic priapism commonly shows a PO_2 of > 90 mmHg, PCO_2 <40 mmHg, and pH 7.4. Normal flaccid penile cavernous blood gas levels are roughly equal to those of normal mixed venous blood (PO_2 40 mmHg, PCO_2 50 mmHg, pH 7.35).

- **Color Doppler ultrasound scan** of cavernosal artery and corpora cavernosa. Reduced blood flow in ischemic priapism; ruptured artery with pooling of blood around injured area in nonischemic priapism

Management

Low-flow priapism
Ischemic priapism of >4 hours implies a compartment syndrome and requires decompression of the corpora cavernosa. Aspiration of blood from corpora (50 mL portions using a 18–20 gauge butterfly needle) ± intracavernosal injection of α_1-adrenergic selective agonist (phenylephrine 100–200 µg (0.5–1 mL of a 200 µg/mL solution to a maximum of 1 mg) are performed every 5–10 minutes until detumescence occurs.

Monitor blood pressure and pulse during drug administration. Oral terbutaline may be effective for intracavernosal injection-related cases.

Sickle cell disease requires, in addition, aggressive rehydration, oxygenation, analgesia, and hematological input (consider exchange transfusion). Repeated aspirations or irrigations and sympathomimetic injections during several hours are often necessary and should be performed before initiation of surgical therapy.

High-flow priapism

Early stages may respond to a cool bath or icepack (causing vasospasm ± arterial thrombosis). Delayed presentations require arteriography and selective embolization of the internal pudendal artery.

Complications

These include fibrosis and impotence.

Neuropathic bladder

Innervation of the lower urinary tract (LUT) 500
Physiology of urine storage and micturition 504
Bladder and sphincter behavior in the patient with
    neurological disease 506
The neuropathic lower urinary tract: clinical consequences
    of storage and emptying problems 508
Bladder management techniques for the neuropathic
    patient 510
Catheters and sheaths and the neuropathic patient 516
Management of incontinence in the neuropathic patient 518
Management of recurrent urinary tract infections (UTIs) in
    the neuropathic patient 520
Management of hydronephrosis in the neuropathic
    patient 522
Management of autonomic dysreflexia in the neuropathic
    patient 523
Bladder dysfunction in multiple sclerosis, in Parkinson
    disease, after stroke, and in other neurological
    disease 524
Neuromodulation in lower urinary tract dysfunction 528

Innervation of the lower urinary tract (LUT)

Motor innervation of the bladder

Parasympathetic motor innervation of the bladder

This neural pathway is primarily responsible for stimulating detrusor contractions, and to a lesser degree, relaxation of the bladder outflow region (bladder neck and urethra).

Preganglionic, parasympathetic nerve cell bodies are located in the intermediolateral column of spinal segments S2–4. These preganglionic, parasympathetic fibers pass out of the spinal cord through the anterior primary rami of S2, S3, and S4 and, contained within nerves called the nervi erigentes, they head toward the pelvic plexus. In the pelvic plexus (in front of the piriformis muscle) the preganglionic, parasympathetic fibers synapse, within ganglia, with the cell bodies of the postganglionic parasympathetic nerves, which then run to the bladder and urethra.

Half of the ganglia of the pelvic plexus lie in the adventitia of the bladder and bladder base (the connective tissue surrounding the bladder), and 50% are within the bladder wall. The postganglionic axons provide cholinergic excitatory input to stimulate contraction of the smooth muscle of the bladder.

Sympathetic motor innervation of the bladder

The primary role of the sympathetic innervation is to contract the bladder base and the urethra.

In the male, preganglionic sympathetic nerve fibers arise from the intermediolateral column of T10–12 and L1–2. These preganglionic neurons synapse in the sympathetic chain, and postganglionic sympathetic nerve fibers travel as the hypogastric nerves to innervate the trigone, blood vessels of the bladder and the smooth muscle of the prostate and preprostatic sphincter (i.e., the bladder neck).

In the female, there is sparse sympathetic innervation of the bladder neck and urethra, with the major continence mechanism being the external sphincter.

In both sexes, some postganglionic sympathetic nerves also terminate in parasympathetic ganglia (in the adventitia surrounding the bladder and within the bladder wall) and exert an inhibitory effect on bladder smooth muscle contraction.

Afferent innervation of the bladder

Afferent nerves from receptors throughout the bladder ascend with parasympathetic neurons back to the cord and from there up to the pontine storage and micturition centers or to the cerebral cortex. They sense bladder filling.

Other receptors are located in the trigone, and afferent neurons from these neurons ascend with sympathetic neurons up to the thoracolumbar cord and from there to the pons and cerebral cortex.

Additionally, afferent receptors are located in the urethra. The afferent neurons pass through the pudendal nerve and again ascend to the pons and cerebral cortex. All these neurons have local relays in the cord.

Somatic motor innervation of the urethral sphincter: the distal urethral sphincter mechanism

Anatomically, this is located slightly distal to the apex of the prostate in the male (between the verumontanum and proximal bulbar urethra) and in the mid-urethra in the female. It has three components:

- *Extrinsic skeletal muscle*. This is the outermost layer, the pubourethral sling (part of levator ani). It is composed of striated muscle and innervated by the pudendal nerve (spinal segments S2–4, somatic nerve fibers). It is activated under conditions of stress and augments urethral occlusion pressure.
- *Smooth muscle within the wall of the urethra*. Cholinergic innervation. This is tonically active and relaxed by nitric oxide.
- *Intrinsic striated muscle* (i.e., skeletal muscle *within* the wall of the urethra, hence known as the *intrinsic rhabdosphincter*). It forms a U shape around the urethra, around the anterior and lateral aspects of the membranous urethra, and is absent posteriorly (i.e., it does not completely encircle the membranous urethra). It may produce urethral occlusion by kinking the urethra rather than by circumferential compression.

Preganglionic *somatic* nerve fibers (i.e., neurons that innervate *striated* muscle) are, along with *parasympathetic* nerve fibers (which innervate the bladder), derived from spinal segments S2–4, specifically from Onuf nucleus (also known as *spinal nucleus X*), which lies in the medial part of the anterior horn of the spinal cord.

Onuf nucleus is the location of the cell bodies of somatic motoneurons that provide motor input to the *striated* muscle of the pelvic floor—the external urethral and anal sphincters. These somatomotor nerves travel to the rhabdosphincter via the perineal branch of the pudendal nerve (documented by direct stimulation studies and horseradish peroxidase [HRP] tracing, which accumulates in Onuf nucleus following injection into either the pudendal or pelvic nerves).

There also seems to be some innervation to the rhabdosphincter from branches of the pelvic plexus (specifically the inferior hypogastric plexus) via pelvic nerves. In dogs, complete silence of the rhabdosphincter is seen only if both the pudendal and pelvic efferents are sectioned. Thus, pudendal nerve block or pudendal neurectomy does not cause incontinence.

The nerve fibers that pass distally to the distal sphincter mechanism are located in a dorsolateral position (5 and 7 o'clock). More distally, they move to a more lateral position.

Consequences of damage to the nerves innervating the LUT are provided in Box 13.1.

Box 13.1 Clinical consequences of damage to the nerves innervating the LUT

Clinical focal neurological examination for nerve pathways
- Motor function
  - Tibialis anterior (L4–S1): controls dorsiflexion of foot
  - Gastrocnemius (L5–S2): controls plantarflexion of foot
  - Toe extensors (L5–S2): controls toe extension
- Sensory function: perianal/perineal sensation S2/S3

Reflexes
- Anal reflex (S2–5)
  - Gently stroke mucocutaneous junction of circumanal skin
  - If visible contraction (anal "wink") absent, suggests peripheral nerve or sacral (conus medullaris) abnormality
- Bulbocavernosus reflex (BCR) (S2–4)
  - Elicited by squeezing glans to cause reflex contraction of anal sphincter
  - Absence of BCR suggests sacral nerve damage

Bladder neck function in the female
Approximately 75% of continent young women and 50% of perimenopausal continent women have a closed bladder neck during the bladder-filling phase. 25% of continent young women and 50% of perimenopausal continent women have an open bladder neck and yet they remain continent (because of their functioning distal sphincter mechanism, the external sphincter).[1,2]

Presacral neurectomy (to destroy afferent pain pathways) does not lead to incontinence because of maintenance of the somatic innervation of the external sphincter.

Sympathetic motor innervation of the bladder
Division of the hypogastric plexus of nerves during procedures such as a retroperitoneal lymph node dissection for metastatic testis tumors results in paralysis of the bladder neck. This is of significance during ejaculation, where normally sympathetic activity results in seminal emission and closure of the bladder neck so that the ejaculate is directed distally into the posterior and then anterior urethra.

If there is failure of emission or the bladder neck is incompetent, the patient develops retrograde ejaculation. They remain continent of urine because the distal urethral sphincter remains functional, being innervated by somatic neurons from S2–4.

During pelvic fracture, the external sphincter and/or its somatic motor innervation may be damaged, such that it is incompetent and unable to maintain urinary continence. Preservation of bladder neck function (the sympathetic innervation of the bladder neck usually remains intact) can preserve continence. However, if in later life the patient undergoes a TURP or bladder neck incision for symptomatic prostatic obstruction, they may well be rendered incontinent because their one remaining sphincter mechanism (the bladder neck) will be divided during these operations.

Sensory innervation of the urethra

Afferent neurons from the urethra travel in the pudendal nerve. Their cell bodies lie in the dorsal root ganglia, and they terminate in the dorsal horn of the spinal cord at S2–4, connecting with neurons that relay somatic sensory information to the brainstem and cerebral cortex.

The pudendal nerve—a somatic nerve derived from spinal segments S2–4—innervates striated muscle of the pelvic floor (levator ani—i.e., the pubourethral sling). Bilateral pudendal nerve block[1] does not lead to incontinence because of maintenance of internal (sympathetic innervation) and external sphincter function (somatic innervation, S2–4, nerve fibers traveling to the external sphincter alongside parasympathetic neurons in the nervi erigentes).

1 Chapple CR, et al. (1989). Asymptomatic bladder neck incompetence in nulliparous females. *Br J Urol* 64:357–359.
2 Versi E, et al. (1990). Distal urethral compensatory mechanisms in women with an incompetent bladder neck who remain continent and the effect of the menopause. *Neurourol Urodyn* 9:579–590.

Physiology of urine storage and micturition

Urine storage

During bladder filling, bladder pressure remains low despite a substantial increase in volume. The bladder is thus highly *compliant*. Its high compliance is partly due to elastic properties (viscoelasticity) of the connective tissues of the bladder and partly due to the ability of detrusor smooth muscle cells to increase their length without any change in tension.

The detrusor is able to do this as a consequence of prevention of transmission of activity from preganglionic parasympathetic neurons to postganglionic efferent neurons—a so-called gating mechanism within the parasympathetic ganglia. In addition, inhibitory interneuron activity in the spinal cord prevents transmission of afferent activity from sensors of bladder filling.

Micturition

A spinobulbar-spinal reflex, coordinated in the pontine micturition center in the brainstem (also known as Barrington's nucleus or the M region), results in simultaneous detrusor contraction, urethral relaxation, and subsequent micturition. Receptors located in the bladder wall sense increasing *tension* as the bladder fills (rather than stretch). This information is relayed, by afferent neurons, to the dorsal horn of the sacral cord. Neurons project from here to the periaqueductal gray matter (PAG) in the pons.

The PAG is thus informed about the state of bladder filling. The PAG and other areas of the brain (limbic system, orbitofrontal cortex) input into the pontine micturition center (PMC) and determine whether it is appropriate to start micturition.

At times when it is appropriate to void, micturition is initiated by relaxation of the external urethral sphincter and pelvic floor. Urine enters the posterior urethra and this, combined with pelvic floor relaxation, activates afferent neurons, which results in stimulation of the PMC, located in the brainstem.

Activation of the PMC switches on a detrusor contraction via a direct communication between neurons of the PMC and the cell bodies of parasympathetic, preganglionic motoneurons located in the sacral intermediolateral cell column of S2–4. At the same time that the detrusor contracts, the urethra (the external sphincter) relaxes.

The PMC inhibits the somatic motoneurons located in Onuf nucleus (the activation of which causes external sphincter contraction) by exciting GABA and glycine-containing, inhibitory neurons in the intermediolateral cell column of the sacral cord, which in turn project to the motoneurons in Onuf nucleus. In this way, the PMC relaxes the external sphincter.

Micturition is an example of a positive feedback loop, the aim being to maintain bladder contraction until the bladder is empty. As the detrusor contracts, tension in the bladder wall rises. The bladder wall tension receptors are stimulated and the detrusor contraction is driven harder.

One of the problems of positive feedback loops is their instability. Several inhibitory pathways exist to stabilize the storage–micturition loop.

- Tension receptors activate bladder afferents, which, via the pudendal and hypogastric nerves, inhibit S2–4 parasympathetic motor nerve output. An ongoing detrusor contraction cannot be overridden.
- Afferents in the anal and genital regions and in the distribution of the posterior tibial nerve stimulate inhibitory neurons in the sacral cord, and these neurons inhibit S2–4 parasympathetic motor nerve output. This pathway can override an ongoing detrusor contraction. It is hypothesized that this system prevents involuntary detrusor contraction during sexual activity, defecation, and while walking, running, and jumping.

Excitatory neurotransmission in the normal detrusor is exclusively cholinergic, and reciprocal relaxation of the urethral sphincter and bladder neck is mediated by nitrous oxide (NO), released from postganglionic parasympathetic neurons.

Bladder and sphincter behavior in the patient with neurological disease

A variety of neurological conditions are associated with abnormal bladder and sphincter function (e.g., spinal cord injury [SCI], spina bifida (myelomeningocele), MS). The bladder and sphincters of such patients are described as *neuropathic*. A discussion of bladder and sphincter problems and urinary incontinence in the patient without neurological disease can be found in Chapter 4.

Patients with neurological disease may have abnormal bladder function or abnormal sphincter function or, more commonly, both. The bladder may be overactive or underactive, as may the sphincter, and any combination of bladder and sphincter over or underactivity may coexist. "Activity" here means bladder and sphincter pressure.

In the normal lower urinary tract during bladder filling, the detrusor muscle is inactive and the sphincter pressure is high. Bladder pressure is therefore low and the high sphincter pressure maintains continence.

During voiding, the sphincter relaxes and the detrusor contracts. This leads to a short-lived increase in bladder pressure, sustained until the bladder is completely empty. The detrusor and sphincter thus function in synergy—when the sphincter is active, the detrusor is relaxed (storage phase), and when the detrusor contracts, the sphincter relaxes (voiding phase).

An *overactive bladder* (OAB) is a recently defined clinical disorder during which patients experience urgency with or without urge incontinence, usually accompanied by frequency and/or nocturia in the absence of causative infection or identified pathological conditions.

The bladder intermittently contracts during bladder filling, thus developing high pressures when normally bladder pressure should be low. In between these waves of contraction, bladder pressure returns to normal or near normal levels.

In a patient with an underlying neurological problem, bladder overactivity is commonly called *detrusor hyperreflexia* (DH) or *neurogenic detrusor overactivity* (NDO). *Detrusor overactivity* (DO) is a urodynamic observation characterized by involuntary detrusor (bladder muscle) contractions during bladder filling.

In other patients the bladder wall is stiffer than normal, a condition known as *poor compliance*. Bladder pressure rises progressively during filling; such bladders are unable to store urine at low pressures.

Some patients have a combination of DH and poor compliance. The opposite end of the spectrum of bladder behavior is the underactive bladder, which is low pressure during filling and voiding. This is called *detrusor areflexia*.

An overactive sphincter generates high pressure during bladder filling, but it also does so during voiding, when normally it should relax. This pathologic condition is known as detrusor-external sphincter dyssynergia (DESD, or detrusor sphincter dyssynergia [DSD]). DSD is always associated with detrusor overactivity, although NDO may occur with synergic sphincter function (i.e., without DSD).

Pontine mesencephalic reticular formation is responsible for coordinating sphincter relaxation with detrusor contraction. Spinal cord lesions impair the transmission of coordinating influences from the pons during reflex detrusor contraction, and the uninhibited detrusor contraction stimulates a reflex sphincter contraction, resulting in bladder outflow obstruction.

See Fig. 13.1. During electromyographic (EMG) recording, necessary to diagnose DSD, activity in the external sphincter increases during attempted voiding (the external sphincter should normally be "quiet" during voiding). An underactive sphincter is unable to maintain enough pressure, in the face of normal bladder pressures, to prevent leakage of urine.

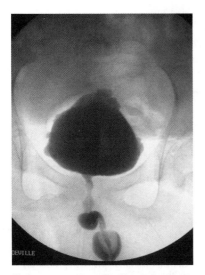

Figure 13.1 Detrusor-external sphincter dyssynergia (DSD) seen during videocystourethrography.

The neuropathic lower urinary tract: clinical consequences of storage and emptying problems

Neuropathic patients experience two broad categories of problems—bladder filling and emptying—depending on the *balance* between bladder and sphincter pressures during filling and emptying. The effects of these bladder filling and emptying problems include incontinence, retention, recurrent UTIs, and renal failure.

High-pressure sphincter

High-pressure bladder

If the bladder is overactive (detrusor hyperreflexia) or poorly compliant, bladder pressures during filling are high. The kidneys have to function against these chronically high pressures. Hydronephrosis can develop and ultimately cause renal failure.

At times the bladder pressure overcomes the sphincter pressure and the patient leaks urine (incontinence). If the sphincter pressure is higher than the bladder pressure during voiding, as in DSD, bladder emptying is inefficient (leading to retention, recurrent UTIs, or bladder calculi).

Low-pressure bladder

If the bladder is underactive (detrusor areflexia), pressure during filling is low. The bladder simply fills up—it is unable to generate enough pressure to empty causing retention and stasis of urine.

Urine leaks at times if the bladder pressure becomes higher than the sphincter pressure (incontinence), but this may occur only at very high bladder volumes or not at all.

Low-pressure sphincter

High-pressure bladder

If the detrusor is hyperreflexic or poorly compliant, the bladder will only be able to hold low volumes of urine before leaking (incontinence).

Low-pressure bladder

If the detrusor is areflexic, such that it cannot develop high pressures, the patient may be dry for much of the time. They may, however, leak urine (incontinence) when abdominal pressure rises (e.g., when coughing, rising from a seated position, or when transferring to or from a wheelchair). Their low bladder pressure may compromise bladder emptying, causing recurrent UTIs.

Bladder management techniques for the neuropathic patient

A variety of techniques and procedures are used to treat retention, incontinence, recurrent UTIs, and hydronephrosis in the patient with a neuropathic bladder. A variety of neurological diseases, injury, congenital malformations, and medical conditions can result in a neuropathic bladder and variable degrees of voiding dysfunction. The incidence of voiding dysfunction with some common disorders is as follows:

* Cerebrovascular accident: 20–50%
* Parkinson disease: 35–70%
* Multiple sclerosis: 50–90%
* Diabetes mellitus; 5–59%

Each of the techniques described below can be used for a variety of clinical problems. Most patients require formal urodynamic evaluation (assessment of bladder filling, sensation, capacity, and compliance), urethral evaluation, voiding studies, and external sphincter electromyography to fully document the nature of the problem and identify the best clinical management.[1]

Thus, a patient with a high-pressure, hyperreflexic bladder that is causing incontinence can be managed with intermittent self-catheterization, sometimes supplemented with intravesical botulinum toxin injections, or a suprapubic catheter, or by sphincterotomy with condom sheath drainage, or by deafferentation combined with a sacral anterior root stimulator (SARS). Precisely which option to choose will depend on the individual patient's clinical problem, their hand function, their lifestyle, resources available, and other personal factors, such as body image and sexual function.

Some patients will opt for a suprapubic catheter as a simple, generally safe, generally very convenient and effective form of bladder drainage. Others wish to be free of external appliances and devices because of an understandable desire to look and feel normal. They might opt for deafferentation with a SARS. The general principles of the management of the patient with neuropathic bladder dysfunction are as follows:

* Urodynamics are essential to plan urological management.
* Control intravesical pressure (prevent high pressure to protect upper tracts).
* Spontaneous voiding with continence is possible with NDO controlled medically.
* Urinary drainage: use intermittent catheterization or an external collection appliance.
  * Indwelling catheterization is to be avoided long term because of complications (UTI, urethral erosion, calculi).
  * Intermittent self-catheterization is the most effective treatment for most with detrusor areflexia, but requires low storage pressure.

1 Abrams P. Cardozo L. Fall M. et al. (2002). The standardization of terminology of lower urinary tract function: report from the Standardization Sub-committee of the International Continence Society. *Neurourol Urodynam* 21(2):167–178.

Medical therapy
Give anticholinergics to improve urinary storage pressure and decrease involuntary contraction. Use agents such as the following:
- Oxybutynin 5 mg PO tid–qid
- Hyoscyamine 0.125 mg PO qid
- Tolterodine LA 4 mg PO qd

α-Adrenergic blockers are used to decrease internal sphincter resistance and lower voiding pressure; they are ineffective for DSD. They may help control symptoms of autonomic dysreflexia. Medications include:
- Doxazosin 2 to 8 mg PO qd
- Terazosin 2 to 5 mg PO qd–bid
- Tamsulosin 0.4 mg PO qd
- Silodosin 8 mg PO qd

Botulinum toxin injection into the detrusor for detrusor overactivity is being used. The toxin selectively blocks acetylcholine release from nerve endings but is not FDA approved for bladder use.

Typical bladder regimens reported 10–30 individual endoscopic injections of 10 units/1 mL/site (posterior wall in midline, right and left lateral walls and dome), with sparing of the trigone.

Intermittent self-catheterization (ISC)
See p. 516.

Indwelling catheters, including suprapubic tubes
See p. 132.

External sphincterotomy
Deliberate ablation or stenting of the external sphincter is used to convert the high-pressure, poorly emptying bladder due to DSD to a low-pressure, efficiently emptying bladder. This is only for males with DSD; it requires a condom catheter afterward. *Indications* are retention, recurrent UTIs, recurrent bladder calculi, hydronephrosis, and renal insufficiency.

Techniques
- *Surgical* (with an electrically heated knife or vaporizing laser). Disadvantages are irreversibility, postoperative bleeding, septicemia, and stricture formation.[2]
- *Intrasphincteric botulinum toxin.* This technique is minimally invasive and reversible. Its disadvantage is that repeated injection is required every 3–9 months. It is not FDA approved for this use.
- *Stenting* (e.g., UroLume, AMS Minnetonka, MN). This is a 1.5–3 cm nonmetallic mesh alloy that expands to 42 F to keep the external sphincter open.[3]

2 JM Reynard (2003). Sphincterotomy and the treatment of detrusor–sphincter dyssynergia: current status, future prospects. *Spinal Cord* 41:1–11.
3 Chancellor M, Gajewski J, Ackman CFD, et al. (1999). Long-term follow-up of the North American Multicenter UroLume Trial for the treatment of external detrusor-sphincter dyssynergia. *J Urol* 161:1545–1550.

Sacral neuromodulation

Sacral and nonsacral neuromodulation using the InterStim can be attempted in cases of detrusor hyperactivity (see p. 528).

Bladder augmentation

This technique involves increasing bladder volume to lower pressure by implanting detubularized small bowel into the bivalved bladder ("clam" ileocystoplasty) (Fig. 13.2) or by removing a disc of muscle from the dome of the bladder (autoaugmentation or detrusor myectomy) and allowing the mucosa to balloon outward.

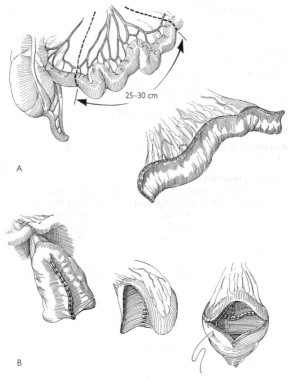

25–30 cm

A

B

Figure 13.2 A "clam" ileocystoplasty. This figure was published in McAninch JW, *Traumatic and Reconstructive Urology*, p. 2287. Copyright Elsevier 1996.

An autologous tissue-engineered bladder substitute for autoaugmentation is under study.[4]

Indications include refractory incontinence and hydronephrosis.

Urinary diversion

In the most extreme cases, permanent urinary diversion may be necessary.

• Cystectomy with continent urinary reservoir
• Ileal or colon pouch; continent catheterizable stoma (appendix or tapered ileum) on abdomen
• Cystectomy with ileal conduit

Deafferentation

This involves division of dorsal spinal nerve roots of S2–4 (sacral rhizotomy) to convert the hyperreflexic, high-pressure bladder into an areflexic, low-pressure one. Deafferentation can be used when the hyperreflexic bladder is the cause of incontinence or hydronephrosis.

Bladder emptying can subsequently be achieved by ISC or implantation of a nerve stimulator placed on ventral roots (efferent nerves) of S2–4 to drive micturition when the patient wants to void (a pager-sized externally applied radio transmitter activates micturition) (Figs. 13.3 and 13.4).

This technique is also useful for DSD/incomplete bladder emptying causing recurrent UTIs and retention.

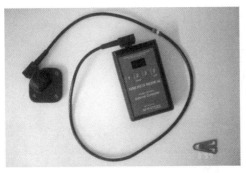

Figure 13.3 A sacral anterior root stimulator, used to drive micturition following a deafferentation (external components).

4 Atala A, Bauer SB, Soker S, Yoo JJ, Retik AB (2006). Tissue-engineered autologous bladders for patients needing cystoplasty. *Lancet* 367(9518):1241–1246.

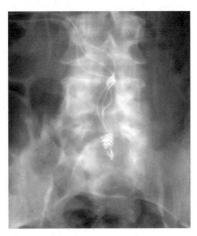

Figure 13.4 KUB X-ray showing the sacral electrodes positioned on the ventral roots of S2, 3, and 4.

Catheters and sheaths and the neuropathic patient

Many patients manage their bladders by intermittent catheterization (IC) done by themselves (intermittent self-catheterization, ISC) or by a caregiver if their hand function is inadequate, as is the case with most tetraplegics. Many others manage their bladders with an indwelling catheter (urethral or suprapubic). Both methods can be effective for managing incontinence, recurrent UTIs, and bladder outlet obstruction causing hydronephrosis.

Intermittent catheterization

IC requires adequate hand function. The technique is a clean one (simple handwashing prior to catheterization) rather than a sterile one.

Gel-coated catheters become slippery when in contact with water, thus providing lubrication. IC is usually done every 3–4 hours.

Problems

- Recurrent UTIs
- Recurrent incontinence: check technique (adequate drainage of last few drops of urine): Suggest increasing frequency of ISC to minimize volume of urine in the bladder (reduces bacterial colonization and minimizes bladder pressure). If incontinence persists, consider intravesical botulinum toxin.

Long-term catheterization

Some patients and clinicians prefer the convenience of a long-term catheter. Others regard it properly as a last resort when other methods of bladder drainage have failed.

The suprapubic route (suprapubic catheter [SPC]) is preferred over the urethral because of pressure necrosis of the ventral surface of the distal penile urethra in men (acquired hypospadias—"kippering" of the penis) and pressure necrosis of the bladder neck in women, which becomes so wide that urine leaks around the catheter ("patulous" urethra) or frequent expulsion of the catheter occurs with the balloon inflated.

Problems and complications of long-term catheters

Recurrent UTIs: colonization with bacteria provides a potential source of recurrent infection.

Catheter blockages are common due to encrustation of the lumen of the catheter with bacterial biofilm. *Proteus mirabilis, Morganella*, and *Providencia* species secrete a polysaccharide matrix. Within this, urease-producing bacteria generate ammonia from nitrogen in urine, raising the urine pH and precipitating magnesium and calcium phosphate crystals. The matrix–crystal complex blocks the catheter.

Bladder distension can cause autonomic dysreflexia. Regular bladder washouts and increased catheter size sometimes help. Impregnation of catheters with silver alloy particles can reduce the incidence of infection.[1]

Bladder stones develop in 1 in 4 patients over 5 years.

Chronic inflammation (from bladder stones, recurrent UTIs, long-term catheterization) may increase the risk of squamous cell carcinoma in SCI patients. Some studies report a higher incidence of bladder cancer (whether chronically catheterized or not); others do not.[2]

Condom catheter sheaths

These are an externally worn urine collection device consisting of a tubular sheath applied over the glans and shaft of the penis (just like a contraceptive condom only without the lubrication to prevent it from slipping off). Sheaths are usually made of silicone rubber with a tube attached to the distal end to allow urine drainage into a leg bag.

They are used as a convenient way of preventing leakage of urine, but are obviously only suitable for men. Detachment of the condom sheath from the penis is prevented by use of adhesive gels and tapes.

They are used for patients with reflex voiding (where the hyperreflexic bladder spontaneously empties, and where bladder pressure between voids never reaches a high enough level to compromise kidney function).

They are also used as a urine collection device for patients after external sphincterotomy (for combined detrusor hyperreflexia and sphincter dyssynergia where incomplete bladder emptying leads to recurrent UTIs and/or hydronephrosis).

Problems

The principal problem experienced by some patients is sheath detachment. This can be a major problem and, in some cases, requires a complete change of bladder management.

Skin reactions sometimes occur.

1 Seymour C (2006). Audit of catheter-associated UTI using silver alloy-coated Foley catheters. *Br J Nurs* 15(11):598–603.
2 Subramonian K, et al. (2004) Bladder cancer in patients with spinal cord injuries. *Br J Urol Int* 93:739–43.

Management of incontinence in the neuropathic patient

Causes
These include high-pressure bladder (detrusor hyperreflexia, reduced bladder compliance); sphincter weakness; UTI; bladder stones; and rarely, bladder cancer (ask about UTI symptoms and hematuria).

Hyperreflexic peripheral reflexes suggest that the bladder may be hyperreflexic (increased ankle jerk reflexes, S1–2 and a positive bulbocavernosus reflex indicating an intact sacral reflex arc—i.e., S2–4 intact).

Absent peripheral reflexes suggest that the bladder and sphincter may be areflexic (i.e., sphincter is unable to generate pressures adequate for maintaining continence).

Initial investigations
These include urine culture (for infection); KUB X-ray for bladder stones; bladder and renal ultrasound for residual urine volume and to detect hydronephrosis; cytology and cystoscopy if bladder cancer is suspected.

Empirical treatment
Start with simple treatments. If the bladder residual volume is large, regular ISC may lower bladder pressure and achieve continence. Try an anticholinergic drug (see p. 511).

Many SCI patients are already doing ISC and simply increasing ISC frequency to every 3–4 hours may achieve continence. ISC more frequently than every 3 hours is usually impractical, particularly for paraplegic women who usually have to transfer from their wheelchair onto a toilet and then back onto their wheelchair. See Table 13.1.

Management of failed empirical treatment
This is determined by cystometrogram, sphincter EMG, and VCUG to assess bladder and sphincter behavior.

Detrusor hyperreflexia or poor compliance
High-pressure sphincter (i.e., DSD)
Treating the high-pressure bladder is usually enough to achieve continence.
- Bladder treatments—intravesical botulinum toxin, detrusor myectomy (autoaugmentation), bladder augmentation (ileocystoplasty). All of these will usually require ISC for bladder emptying.
- Long-term suprapubic catheter
- Sacral deafferentation + ISC or Brindley implant (SARS—sacral anterior root stimulator)

Low-pressure sphincter
Treat the bladder first (as above). If bladder treatment alone fails, consider a urethral bulking agent, urethral sling procedure, or bladder neck closure in women (last resort) or an artificial urinary sphincter in either sex (Fig. 13.5).

Detrusor areflexia + low pressure sphincter
- Urethral bulking agents
- URETHRAL SLING PROCEDURE
- Bladder neck closure in women
- Artificial urinary sphincter

Table 13.1 Summary of treatment for incontinence

	High bladder pressure	Low bladder pressure
High sphincter pressure	Lower bladder pressure by anticholinergics +/– ISC or botulinum toxin or augmentation	ISC*
Low sphincter pressure	Lower bladder pressure by (anticholinergics +/– or botulinum toxin or augmentation) + urethral bulking agent, urethral sling procedure or bladder neck closure or artificial urinary sphincter	Urethral bulking agent Urethral sling procedure Bladder neck closure (women only) Artificial urinary sphincter

* High sphincter pressure is usually enough to keep the patient dry.

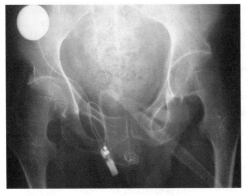

Figure 13.5 Artificial urinary sphincter implanted around the bulbar urethra.

Management of recurrent urinary tract infections (UTIs) in the neuropathic patient

Causes of recurrent UTIs
- Incomplete bladder emptying
- Kidney stones including staghorn calculi
- Bladder stones
- Vesicourethral reflux
- Presence of an indwelling catheter (urethral or suprapubic)

History
What the spinal cord–injured patient interprets as a UTI may be different from the UTI in a noninjured patient. The neuropathic bladder is frequently colonized with bacteria and the urine often contains white blood cells (pyuria). From time to time, it becomes cloudy from precipitation of calcium, magnesium, and phosphate salts in the absence of active infection.

The presence of bacteria, pus cells, or cloudy urine in the presence of nonspecific symptoms (abdominal pain, tiredness, headaches, feeling under the weather) is often suggestive of a UTI.

Indications for treatment of UTI in the neuropathic patient
It is impossible to eradicate bacteria or pus cells from the urine in the presence of a foreign body (e.g., a catheter). In the absence of fever and cloudy, foul-smelling urine, we do not prescribe antibiotics; the indiscriminate use of these encourages growth of antibiotic-resistant organisms.

We prescribe antibiotics to the chronically catheterized patient when there is a combination of fever, cloudy, and foul-smelling urine, and when the patient feels unwell. Culture urine and immediately start empirical antibiotic therapy with a quinolone (such as ciprofloxacin based on local sensitivity patterns), changing to a more specific antibiotic if the organism is resistant to the prescribed one.

Investigations
For recurrent UTIs, such as frequent episodes of fever, cloudy, smelly urine, and feeling unwell, the following are helpful:
- KUB X-ray for kidney and bladder stones. Some consider this to be standard annual screening in patients with chronically indwelling catheters.
- Renal and bladder ultrasound to determine the presence or absence of hydronephrosis and to measure pre-void bladder volume and post-void residual urine volume and to localize any stones.

Treatment
In the presence of fever and cloudy, foul-smelling urine, culture the urine and start antibiotics empirically (e.g., trimethoprim, amoxicillin, ciprofloxacin), changing the antibiotic if the culture result suggests resistance to

your empirical choice. Response to treatment is suggested by the patient feeling better and the urine clearing and becoming nonoffensive to smell.

Persistent fever, with constitutional symptoms (malaise, rigors) despite treatment with a specific oral antibiotic in an adequate dose is an indication for admission for treatment with intravenous antibiotics.

If the patient appears to have pyelonephritis or is manifesting signs of sepsis, hospitalization and empiric IV antibiotics (such as ampicillin and gentamicin or third-generation cephalosporin) is indicated with change to oral antibiotics when the patient is afebrile for 24 hours.

Management of recurrent UTIs (see Table 13.2)

If there is residual urine present, optimize bladder emptying by intermittent catheterization (males, females) or external sphincterotomy for DSD (males). Intermittent catheterization can be done by the patient (intermittent self-catheterization, ISC) if hand function is good (paraplegic), or by a caregiver if tetraplegic.

An indwelling catheter (IDC) is an option, but the presence of a foreign body in the bladder may itself cause recurrent UTIs (though in some it seems to reduce UTI frequency).

Table 13.2 Summary of treatment for recurrent UTI's

Low bladder pressure	High bladder pressure + DSD
ISC	ISC
IDC	IDC
	External sphincterotomy—surgical, botulinum toxin, sphincter stent
	Deafferentation/SARS

Remove stones if present—cystolitholapaxy for bladder stones, PCNL for staghorn stones.

Management of hydronephrosis in the neuropathic patient

An overactive bladder (detrusor hyperreflexia) or poorly compliant bladder is frequently combined with a high-pressure sphincter (detrusor-sphincter dyssynergia [DSD]). Bladder pressures during both filling and voiding are high.

At times the bladder pressure may overcome the sphincter pressure and the patient leaks small quantities of urine. For much of the time, however, the sphincter pressures are higher than the bladder pressures and the kidneys are chronically exposed to these high pressures. They are hydronephrotic on ultrasound, and renal function slowly, but inexorably, deteriorates.

Treatment options for hydronephrosis

Bypass the external sphincter
- IDC (indwelling catheter)
- ISC (intermittent self-catheterization) + anticholinergics

Treat the external sphincter
- Sphincterotomy: surgical incision via a cystoscope inserted down the urethra (electrically heated knife or laser), botulinum toxin injections into sphincter, urethral stent
- Deafferentation* + ISC or SARS

Treat the bladder
- Intravesical botulinum toxin + ISC
- Augmentation + ISC
- Deafferentation* + ISC or SARS

* Deafferentation converts the high-pressure sphincter into a low-pressure sphincter and the high-pressure bladder into low-pressure bladder.

Management of autonomic dysreflexia in the neuropathic patient

Autonomic dysreflexia (AD) is a unique and potentially life-threatening condition in spinal cord–injured patients. AD can cause rapid, extreme blood pressure elevation, headache, diaphoresis, bradycardia, sweating, nausea, and piloerection in patients with spinal cord lesions at and above the sixth thoracic level (T6).

Approximately 85% of quadriplegic and high paraplegic individuals are prone to AD in response to noxious stimuli. AD is more common in men than in women because of increased bladder outlet resistance. Stimuli, such as bladder distention, bowel distention, or pain, activate sympathetic neurons in the lateral horn of the spinal cord, causing unopposed reflex sympathetic activity.

Primary therapy should always be to remove the triggering stimulus (i.e., empty distended bladder or clear obstruction in Foley catheter). Rarely, acute episodes must be managed with intravenous nitrates or arterial dilators under closely monitored conditions. Chronic treatment with α-blockers may improve some symptoms of AD.

1 Vaidyanathan S, Soni BM, Sett P, et al. (1998). Pathophysiology of autonomic dysreflexia: long-term treatment with terazosin in adult and pediatric spinal cord injury patients manifesting recurrent dysreflexic episodes. *Spinal Cord* 36:761–770.

Bladder dysfunction in multiple sclerosis, in Parkinson disease, after stroke, and in other neurological disease

Multiple sclerosis (MS)

MS is a neurological disease caused by focal demyelination of white matter in the brain and spinal cord. Urological manifestations are the presenting complaint in about 2.5% of MS patients.

Three-quarters of patients with MS have spinal cord involvement and, in these patients, bladder dysfunction is common. Detrusor hyperreflexia with urge incontinence is the most common GU symptom present in 78% of patients with voiding dysfunction.

DSD is present in 30% to 65% of patients, leading to poor emptying and possible upper tract damage.

Parkinson disease (PD)

PD is a cause of Parkinsonism, a clinical complex of tremor, rigidity, and bradykinesis, and is due to degeneration of dopaminergic neurons in the substantia nigra in the basal ganglia. Mild intellectual deterioration may occur, and frequency, urgency, and urge incontinence are common.[1]

The most common urodynamic abnormality is DH (the basal ganglia may have an inhibitory effect on the micturition reflex). L-dopa seems to have a variable effect on these symptoms and DH, improving symptoms in some and making them worse in others.

LUTS in Parkinson disease may simply be due to benign prostatic obstruction or to the PD itself. Many PD patients have coexisting detrusor overactivity with impaired bladder contractility.

Consider combining intermittent catheterization with antimuscarinic drugs initially (e.g., oxybutynin 5 mg PO tid or tolterodine LA 4 mg PO qd). Second-line medical therapy can include tricyclic antidepressants such as imipramine 10–25 mg PO bid/tid.

Traditionally, patients with PD have had a poorer outcome after TURP than those without PD, but if the patient has urodynamically proven BOO, TURP is a treatment option.

Multiple system atrophy (MSA; formerly Shy–Drager syndrome)

MSA is a cause of Parkinsonism characterized clinically by postural hypotension and detrusor areflexia. Loss of cells in the pons leads to DH (symptoms of bladder overactivity). Loss of parasympathetic neurons due to cell loss in the intermediolateral cell column of the sacral cord causes poor bladder emptying, and loss of neurons in Onuf nucleus in the sacral anterior horns leads to denervation of the striated sphincter causing incontinence.

1 Winge K. Skau AM. Stimpel H, et al. (2006). Prevalence of bladder dysfunction in Parkinson's disease. *Neurourol Urodyn* 25(2):116–122.

The presentation is usually with DH (i.e., symptoms of bladder over-activity), followed over the course of several years by worsening bladder emptying.

Cerebrovascular accidents (CVAs)

DH occurs in 70%, DSD in 15% of patients. Detrusor areflexia can occur.[2] Frequency, nocturia, urgency, and urge incontinence are common. Retention occurs in 5% in the acute phase.

Incontinence within the first 7 days after a CVA predicts poor survival.[3] Common urodynamic findings with CVA include the following:[4,5]

- Normal bladder and normal sphincter
- Bladder overactivity and a normal sphincter
- Detrusor-sphincter dyssynergia is rare after a CVA.
- Diminished bladder contractility (often due to preexisting conditions)

Initial goals are adequate bladder drainage by CIC or Foley catheter until the patient resumes voiding. Long term, attain adequate bladder drainage and maintain urinary continence while preventing complications.

Anticholinergic/antimuscarinics may be used as needed in an attempt to decrease the frequency and force of involuntary bladder contractions. There are many medication choices and individual response is idiosyn-cratic, so several medications often have to be tried.

Botulism toxin and sacral neuromodulation have been used in this popu-lation with promising results.

Other neurological disease

Frontal lobe lesions (e.g., tumors, AVMs)

These may cause severe frequency and urgency (frontal lobe has inhibitory input to the pons).

Brainstem lesions (e.g., posterior fossa tumors)

These can cause urinary retention or bladder overactivity.

Transverse myelitis

Also known as *acute inflammatory demyelinating polyneuropathy*, this is an inflammatory demyelinating disorder of the autonomic and peripheral nervous system. It is thought to be immune related triggered by a bacterial or viral infection.

Symptoms may include muscle weakness, respiratory difficulties, auto-nomic neuropathy, cardiac, bowel, bladder, and sexual dysfunction. Lower urinary tract dysfunction can range from urge and stress incontinence to

2 Sakakibara R, et al. (1996). Micturitional disturbance after acute hemispheric stroke: analysis of the lesion site by CT and MRI. *J Neurol Sci* 137:47–56.

3 Wade D, et al. (1985). Outlook after an acute stroke: urinary incontinence and loss of conscious-ness compared in 532 patients. *Quart Med J* 56:601–608.

4 Pettersen R, Stien R, Wyller TB (2007). Post-stroke urinary incontinence with impaired aware-ness of the need to void: clinical and urodynamic features. *BJU Int* 99(5):1073–1077.

5 Chandiramani VA, Palace J, Fowler CJ (1997). How to recognise patients with prostatism who should not have urological surgery. *Br J Urol* 80:100–104.

urinary retention. There is severe tetraparesis and bladder dysfunction, which often recovers to a substantial degree as the other neurological symptoms resolve.

Manage transient acute lower urinary tract dysfunction with CIC, anticholinergics, etc.[6]

Peripheral neuropathies

The autonomic innervation of the bladder makes it vulnerable to the effects of peripheral neuropathies such as those occurring in diabetes mellitus and amyloidosis. The picture is usually one of reduced bladder contractility (poor bladder emptying—i.e., chronic low pressure retention).

6 Ganesan V, Borzyskowski M (2001). Characteristics and course of urinary tract dysfunction after acute transverse myelitis. *Dev Med Child Neurol* 43(7):473–475.

Neuromodulation in lower urinary tract dysfunction

Neuromodulation is the electrical activation of *afferent* nerve fibers to modulate their function. To treat urinary tract conditions, sacral and non-sacral neuromodulation can be employed.

Electrical stimulation applied anywhere in the body preferentially depolarizes nerves (higher current amplitudes are required to directly depolarize muscle). In patients with LUT dysfunction, the relevant spinal segments are the sacral nerves S2–4.

Neuromodulation is a second-line treatment for refractory lower urinary tract dysfunction, such as nonobstructive chronic urinary retention, urgency–frequency syndrome (overactive bladder), and urgency incontinence, when behavioral and drug therapy has failed.

Several sites of stimulation are available, with the electrical stimulus being applied directly to nerves, or as close as possible:
• Sacral nerve stimulation (SNS) is most widely studied.
• Pudendal nerve—direct pelvic floor electrical stimulation (of bladder, vagina, anus, pelvic floor muscles) or via stimulation of dorsal penile or clitoral nerve (DPN, DCN)
• Posterior tibial nerve stimulation (PTNS)

SNS

Sacral nerve stimulation, also known as *sacral neuromodulation* (SNM), uses continuous or cycling mode of electrical pulses to activate or inhibit neural reflexes associated with lower urinary tract function via stimulation of the sacral nerves.

The mechanism of action is not conclusive. One theory is that indirect stimulation of the pudendal nerve and direct inhibition of the preganglionic neurons suppress detrusor overactivity and therefore improve symptoms.

An alternate theory is that stimulation may inhibit involuntary reflex voiding by altering the transmission of sensory input from the bladder to the pontine micturition center, inhibiting ascending afferent pathways but not the descending pathways. In the patient with nonobstructive urinary retention, SNM most likely causes an inhibition of the guarding reflex, with a reduction in sphincteric overactivity that may reduce bladder outlet and urethral resistance.

Patients should have failed conservative management with medications and or behavioral therapies and should undergo extensive evaluation including urodynamics. The procedure involves implanting a programmable device that delivers a pulse low-amplitude stimulation to the sacral nerves (InterStim, Medtronic).

The procedure is typically performed in two stages. Percutaneous placement of the electrode is performed under fluoroscopic guidance near the S3 foramina. Position is tested by either verbal response from the patient or motor responses (tightening of the levators, bellows response in the anal area, plantar flexion of the great toe).

During a several-week trial, the electrode is connected to an external generator and the patient maintains a log of their voiding pattern. If improvement is noted (usually > 50%), a permanent generator can be implanted.

PTNS

Posterior tibial nerve stimulation is a type of nonsacral neuromodulation. The posterior tibial nerve (PTN) (L4,5; S1–3) shares common nerve roots with those innervating the bladder. PTNS can be applied transcutaneously (stick-on surface electrodes) or percutaneously (needle electrodes) that delivers "retrograde" access to the sacral nerve plexus.

The Urgent PC (Uroplasty, Minnetonka, MN) system is available with reports of up to 75% response rates for urinary tract symptoms as well as in fecal incontinence. Stimulation is applied via an acupuncture needle inserted just above the medial malleolus with a reference (or return) electrode—30 minutes of stimulation per week, over 12 weeks.

Thereafter, 30 minutes of treatment every 2–3 weeks can be used to maintain the treatment effect in those who respond. A study of PTNS compared with pharmacotherapy for overactive bladder demonstrated effectiveness comparable to that of pharmacotherapy.[1]

Further reading

Leng W, Morrisroe S (2006). Sacral nerve stimulation for the overactive bladder. *Urol Clin North Am* 33(4):491–501.

1 Peters KM, MacDiarmid SA, Wooldridge LS, et al. (2009). Randomized trial of percutaneous tibial nerve stimulation versus extended-release tolterodine: results from the overactive bladder innovative therapy trial. *J Urol* 182(3):1055–1061.

Chapter 14

Urological problems in pregnancy

Physiological and anatomical changes in the urinary tract *532*
Urinary tract infection (UTI) *534*
Hydronephrosis *536*

Physiological and anatomical changes in the urinary tract

Kidney

- **Renal size enlarges** by 1 cm, secondary to increased interstitial volume and increased renal vasculature.
- **Renal plasma flow rate (RPF)** increases early in the first trimester (up to 75% by term).
- **Glomerular filtration rate (GFR)** increases by 50%, related to an increased cardiac output.
- **Renal function and biochemical parameters** are affected by changes in RPF and GFR. Creatinine clearance increases, and serum levels of creatinine, urea, and urate fall in normal pregnancy (see Table 15.1). Raised GFR causes an increased glucose load at the renal tubules and results in glucose excretion (glycosuria) in most pregnancies. 24-hour protein excretion remains unchanged. Urine output increases.
- **Salt and water handling:** A reduction in serum sodium causes reduced plasma osmolality. The kidney compensates by increasing renal tubular reabsorption of sodium. Plasma renin activity is increased 10-fold, and levels of angiotensinogen and angiotensin are increased 5-fold. Osmotic thresholds for antidiuretic hormone (ADH) and thirst decrease.
- **Acid–base metabolism** Serum bicarbonate is reduced. Increased progesterone stimulates the respiratory center resulting in reduced PCO_2.

Bladder

- **Bladder displacement** occurs (superiorly and anteriorly) due to the enlarging uterus. The bladder becomes hyperemic, and raised estrogen levels cause hyperplasia of muscle and connective tissues. Bladder pressures can increase over pregnancy (from 8 to 20 cmH$_2$O), with associated rises in absolute and functional urethral length and pressures.
- **Lower urinary tract symptoms:** Urinary frequency (>7 voids during the day) and nocturia (>1 void at night) increases over the duration of gestation (incidence of 80–90% in third trimester). Urgency and urge incontinence also increase secondary to pressure effects from the enlarging uterus.
- **Stress urinary incontinence** occurs in 22%, and increases with parity (pregnancies that result in delivery beyond 28 weeks' gestation). It is partly caused by placental production of peptide hormones (relaxin), which induces collagen remodeling and consequent softening of tissues of the birth canal. Infant weight, duration of first and second stages of labor (vaginal delivery), and instrumental delivery (ventouse extraction or forceps delivery) increase risks of postpartum (after delivery of the child) stress incontinence.

Table 14.1 Biochemistry reference intervals

Substance	Nonpregnant	Pregnant
Sodium (mmol/L)	135–145	132–141
Urea (mmol/L)	2.5–6.7	2.0–4.2
Urate (µmol/L)	150–390	100–270
Creatinine (µmol/L)	70–150	24–68
Creatinine clearance (mL/min)	90–110	150–200
Bicarbonate (mmol/L)	24–30	20–25

Urinary tract infection (UTI)

Definition

UTI describes a bacterial infection of the urine with $>10^5$ colony forming units (CFU)/mL (or $>10^2$ CFU/mL if the patient is systemically unwell).

Incidence

Pregnancy does not alter the incidence of UTI, which remains at 4% for women of reproductive age. However, physiological and anatomical changes associated with pregnancy alter the course of infection, causing an increased risk of recurrent UTI and progression to acute pyelonephritis (up to 28%).

Risk factors

These include previous history of recurrent UTIs and pre-existing vesico-ureteric reflux. Physiological changes in pregnancy include hydronephrosis with decreased ureteral peristalsis causing urinary stasis. Up to 75% of pyelonephritis cases occur in the third trimester, when these changes are most prominent.

Pathogenesis

A common causative organism is *Escherichia coli*. An increased risk of gestational pyelonephritis is associated with *E. coli* containing the virulence factor Dr adhesin.

Complications

UTI increases the risk of preterm delivery, low fetal birth weight, and maternal anemia.

Screening tests

Midstream urine specimen (MSU)

MSU should be obtained at the first antenatal visit and sent for urinalysis and culture to look for bacteria, protein, and blood. A second MSU investigation is recommended at later visits (week 16) to examine for bacteria, protein, and glucose.

Treatment

All proven episodes of UTI should be treated (asymptomatic or symptomatic), guided by urine culture sensitivities. Antibiotics that are safe to use during pregnancy include **penicillins** (i.e., ampicillin, amoxicillin, penicillin V) and **cephalosporins** (i.e., cefaclor, cefalexin, cefotaxime, ceftriaxone, cefuroxime). Nitrofurantoin may be used in first and second trimesters only. See Table 14.2 for antibiotics that are not safe to use.

Repeat urine cultures after treatment to check that bacteria have been eliminated.

Acute pyelonephritis requires hospital admission for intravenous antibiotics (cephalosporin or aminopenicillin) until apyrexial, followed by oral antibiotics for 14 days, and repeated cultures for the duration of pregnancy.

Table 14.2 Antibiotics to avoid in pregnancy*

Trimester	Antibiotic	Risk in pregnancy
1,2,3	Tetracyclines	Fetal malformation; maternal hepatotoxicity; dental discoloration
	Quinolones	Arthropathy
1	Trimethoprim	Teratogenic risk (folate antagonist)
2,3	Aminoglycosides	Auditory or vestibular nerve damage
3	Chloramphenicol	Neonatal gray syndrome
	Sulfonamides	Neonatal hemolysis; methemoglobinemia
	Nitrofurantoin	Maternal or neonatal hemolysis (if used at term), in subjects with G6PD deficiency

* See Krieger JN (1986). Complications and treatment of urinary tract infection during pregnancy. *Urol Clin North Am* 13:685.

Hydronephrosis

Hydronephrosis develops from ~week 6 to week 10 of gestation. By week 28 of gestation, 90% of pregnant women have hydronephrosis. It has usually resolved within 2 months of birth.

It is due to a combination of the smooth muscle relaxant effect of progesterone and mechanical obstruction from the enlarging fetus and uterus, which compresses the ureter. (Hydronephrosis does not occur in pelvic kidneys or those transplanted into ileal conduits, nor does it occur in quadripeds such as dogs and cats, where the uterus is dependent and thus falls away from the ureter.)

The hydronephrosis of pregnancy poses diagnostic difficulties in women presenting with flank pain thought to be due to a renal or ureteral stone. To avoid using ionizing radiation in pregnant women, renal ultrasonography is often used as the initial imaging technique in those presenting with flank pain.

In the nonpregnant patient, the presence of hydronephrosis is taken as surrogate evidence of ureteral obstruction.

Because hydronephrosis is a normal finding in the majority of pregnancies, its presence *cannot* be taken as a sign of a possible ureteral stone. Ultrasound is an unreliable way of diagnosing the presence of stones in pregnant (and in nonpregnant) women.

In a series of pregnant women, ultrasound had a sensitivity of 34% (i.e. it misses 66% of stones) and a specificity of 86% for detecting an abnormality in the presence of a stone (i.e., false-positive rate of 14%).[1]

1 Stothers L, Lee LM (1992). Renal colic in pregnancy. *J Urol* 148:1383–1387.

Pediatric urology

Embryology: urinary tract 538
Undescended testes 540
Urinary tract infection (UTI) 542
Vesicoureteric reflux (VUR) 544
Ectopic ureter 546
Ureterocele 548
Ureteropelvic junction (UPJ) obstruction 549
Hypospadias 550
Normal sexual differentiation 552
Abnormal sexual differentiation 554
Cystic kidney disease 558
Exstrophy 560
Epispadias 562
Posterior urethral valves 564
Non-neurogenic voiding dysfunction 566
Nocturnal enuresis 568

Embryology: urinary tract

Following fertilization, a blastocyte (sphere of cells) is created, which implants into the uterine endometrium on day 6. The early embryonic disc of tissue develops a yolk sac and amniotic cavity, from which are derived ectoderm, endoderm, and mesoderm.

Organ formation occurs between 3 and 10 weeks' gestation. Most of the genitourinary tract is derived from mesoderm.

Upper urinary tract

The pronephros (precursor kidney; *pro* = (Gk) before), derived from an intermediate plate of mesoderm, is present at weeks 1–4. It then regresses.

The mesonephros (*meso* = (Gk) middle) functions at weeks 4–8 and is also associated with two duct systems—the mesonephric duct and, adjacent to this, the paramesonephric duct (*para* = (Gk) beside) (Fig. 15.1). The mesonephric (Wolffian) ducts develop laterally and advance downward to fuse with the primitive cloaca (hindgut). By week 5, a ureteric bud grows from the distal part of the mesonephric ducts and induces formation of the metanephros in the overlying mesoderm (permanent kidney; *meta* = (Gk) after).

Branching of the ureteric bud forms the renal pelvis, calyces, and collecting ducts. Glomeruli and nephrons are created from metanephric mesenchyme.

During weeks 6–10, the caudal end of the fetus grows rapidly and the fetal kidney effectively moves up the posterior abdominal wall to the lumbar region. Urine production starts at week 10.

Thus, in both males and females, the mesonephric duct forms the ureters and renal collecting system. The paramesonephric essentially forms the female genital system (fallopian tubes, uterus, upper vagina); in males, it regresses. The mesonephric duct forms the male genital duct system (epididymis, vas deferens, seminal vesicles, central zone of prostate); in the female, it regresses.

Lower urinary tract

The mesonephric ducts and ureters drain into the cloaca (Latin = sewer), which is later subdivided into the urogenital sinus (anteriorly) and the anorectal canal (posteriorly) during weeks 4–6 (see Fig. 15.1).

The bladder is formed by the upper part of the urogenital sinus. The lower part forms the urethra in females. In males, the mesonephric ducts form the posterior urethra, and closure of the urogenital groove creates the anterior urethra.

Upper urinary tract

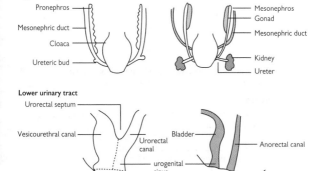

Figure 15.1 Development of the upper and lower parts of the urinary tract (weeks 4–6).

Undescended testes

The testes descend into the scrotum in the third trimester (passing through the inguinal canal at 24–28 weeks). Failure of testicular descent results in cryptorchidism (or undescended testes).

Incidence

Incidence is 3% at birth (unilateral > bilateral). Approximately 80% will spontaneously descend by 3 months. The incidence at 1 year is 1%.

Classification

- **Retractile**: an intermittent active cremasteric reflex causes the testis to retract up and out of the scrotum.
- **Ectopic** (<5%): abnormal testis migration below the external ring of the inguinal canal (to perineum, base of penis, or femoral areas)
- **Incomplete descent** (~95%): testis may be intra-abdominal, inguinal, or prescrotal
- **Atrophic/absent**

Risk factors

These include preterm infants, low birth weight, small for gestational age, and twins.

Etiology

This includes abnormal testis or gubernaculum (tissue that guides the testis into the scrotum during development); endocrine abnormalities (low level of androgens, human chorionic gonadotrophin [hCG], luteinizing hormone (LH), calcitonin gene–related peptide); and decreased intra-abdominal pressure (prune-belly syndrome, gastroschisis).

Pathology

There is degeneration of Sertoli cells, loss of Leydig cells, and atrophy and abnormal spermatogenesis.

Long-term complications

- Relative risk of cancer is 40-fold higher in the undescended testis. Most are seminomas; carcinoma in situ represents a small percentage (~2%). There is a slightly increased risk of cancer in the contralateral, normally descended testis.
- Reduced fertility
- Increased risk of testicular torsion
- Increased risk of direct inguinal hernias (due to a patent processus vaginalis)

Management

Full examination is required to elucidate if the testis is palpable and to identify location. Assess for associated congenital defects. If neither testis is palpable, consider chromosome analysis (to exclude an androgenized female) and hormone testing (high LH and FSH with a low testosterone indicates anorchia).

Treatment should be performed within the first year. Hormone therapy (hCG, LHRH) stimulates testosterone production. Surgery consists of inguinal exploration, mobilization of spermatic cord, ligation of processus vaginalis, and securing the testis into a dartos pouch in the scrotal wall (orchidopexy). Laparoscopy can be used in planning surgery and for treatment.

Intra-abdominal testes may require division of spermatic vessels to provide extra length (Fowler-Stevens procedure, relying on collateral blood flow from vas), two-stage procedures, or microvascular autotransplantation.

Urinary tract infection (UTI)

Definitions

UTI is a bacterial infection of the urine ($>10^5$ colony-forming units/ mL of urine), which may involve the bladder (cystitis) or kidney (pyelonephritis).

Classification

Children may be asymptomatic or symptomatic. It may be the first (initial) infection, recurrent UTI due to persistence of the causative organism and reinfection, or an unresolved infection due to inadequate treatment.

Incidence

Up to age 1 year, the incidence in boys is higher than in girls (males 2.7%: females 0.7%). Thereafter, the incidence in girls becomes greater (school age: males 1%; females 1–3%).

Pathology

Common bacterial pathogens are *Escherichia coli* (*E. coli*), *Enterococcus, Pseudomonas, Klebsiella, Proteus*, and *Staphylococcus epidermis*. Bacteria enter via the urethra to cause cystitis, and ascending infection causes pyelonephritis.

Alternatively, there can be hematogenous spread from other systemic infections.

Risk factors

- Age: Neonates and infants have increased bacterial colonization of the periurethral area and an immature immune system.
- Vesicoureteric reflux (VUR).
- Genitourinary abnormalities (UPJ obstruction; ureterocele; posterior urethral valves)
- Voiding dysfunction (abnormal bladder activity, compliance, or emptying).
- Gender (female > male after 1 year old)
- Foreskin: Uncircumcised boys have a 10-fold higher risk of UTI in the first year from bacterial colonization of the glans and foreskin.
- Fecal colonization (contributes to perineal bacterial colonization)

Presentation

UTI patients present with fever, irritability, vomiting, diarrhea, poor feeding, suprapubic pain, dysuria, voiding difficulties, incontinence, and flank pain.

Investigation

Diagnosis is made on urinalysis and culture. In young children, a catheterized urine specimen or a suprapubic aspirate is most accurate (bag specimens are less reliable because of skin flora contamination).

In toilet-trained children, a mid-stream specimen can be collected.

Imaging

UTI in children <5 years, febrile UTI, infection in non–sexually active boys, and girls (>5 years) with two or more episodes of cystitis require renal tract imaging.

- **Ultrasound** identifies bladder and kidney abnormalities.
- **Voiding cystourethrogram (VCUG)** demonstrates urethral and bladder anomalies, VUR, and ureteroceles.
- **DMSA** (dimercaptosuccinic acid) renogram can demonstrate and monitor renal scarring.

Management

Empirical treatment should be started if infection is suspected. Children <3 months old with severe infection or pyelonephritis should receive broad-spectrum intravenous antibiotics (gentamicin and ampicillin) until antibiotic sensitivities are available.

Older children, and infants tolerating feeds can be given oral antibiotics (cephalosporins, or nitrofurantoin and trimethoprim-sulfamethoxide after 2 months old).

Complications

Neonates and young children have an increased risk of associated renal involvement and subsequent renal scarring, which can result in hypertension and renal failure.

Vesicoureteric reflux (VUR)

Definition
VUR results from abnormal retrograde flow of urine from the bladder into the upper urinary tract.

Epidemiology
Overall incidence in children is >10%, with younger children affected more than older children, girls more than boys (female–male ratio 5:1). VUR occurs more often in Caucasian than in Afro-Caribbean children.

Siblings of an affected child have a 40% risk of reflux, and routine screening of siblings is recommended.

Pathogenesis
The ureter passes obliquely through the bladder wall (1–2 cm), where it is supported by muscular attachments that prevent urine reflux during bladder filling and voiding. The normal ratio of intramural ureteric length to ureteric diameter is 5:1.

Reflux occurs when the intramural length of ureter is too short (ratio <5:1). The degree of reflux is graded I–V (see Fig. 7.1, p. 345). The appearance of the ureteric orifice changes with increasing severity of reflux, classically described as stadium, horseshoe, golf-hole, or patulous.

Classification
- **Primary reflux** (1%) results from a congenital abnormality of the ureterovesical junction.
- **Secondary reflux** results from urinary tract dysfunction associated with elevated intravesical pressures. *Causes* include posterior urethral valves (reflux seen in 50%), urethral stenosis, neuropathic bladder, and detrusor sphincter dyssynergia (DSD).
- VUR is also seen with duplex ureters. The Weigert–Meyer rule states that the lower-pole ureter enters the bladder proximally and laterally, resulting in a shorter intramural tunnel, which predisposes to reflux.

Complications
VUR associated with UTI can result in reflux nephropathy with hypertension and progressive renal failure.

Presentation
Patients have symptoms of UTI, fever, dysuria, suprapubic or abdominal pain, failure to thrive, vomiting, and diarrhea.

Investigation
- Urinalysis and culture to diagnose UTI
- Urinary tract ultrasound scan and VCUG to diagnose and grade reflux and establish reversible causes (Fig. 15.2)
- Urodynamic assessment if suspicious of voiding dysfunction
- DMSA scan to detect and monitor associated renal cortical scarring.

Management

Correct problems contributing to secondary reflux. Most primary VUR grade I–II cases will resolve spontaneously (~85%), with 50% resolution in grade III. Observation and medical treatment are initially recommended.

Medical treatment

Low-dose antibiotic prophylaxis should be given to keep the urine sterile and lower the risk of renal damage until reflux resolves. Anticholinergic drugs are given to treat bladder overactivity.

Surgery is indicated for severe reflux, breakthrough UTIs, evidence of progressive renal scarring, and VUR that persists after puberty. Techniques of ureteral re-implantation include the following:

• **Intravesical** methods involve mobilizing the ureter and advancing it across the trigone (Cohen repair) or reinsertion into a higher, medial position in the bladder (Politano–Leadbetter repair).
• **Extravesical** techniques involve attaching the ureter into the bladder base and suturing muscle around it (Lich–Gregoir procedure).
• Alternatively, endoscopic **subtrigonal injection** of Deflux into the ureteral orifice has 70% success, and 95% with repeated treatments.

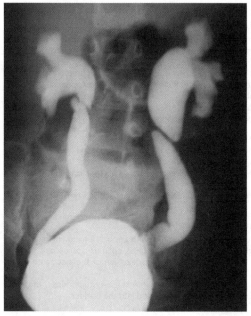

Figure 15.2 Massive bilateral reflux is seen on cystogram in young child.

Ectopic ureter

Definition
The ureteric orifice is situated below the normal anatomical insertion on the trigone of the bladder.

Pathogenesis
The ureteric bud arises from an abnormal position on the mesonephric duct during embryological development. Females are affected more than males (female–male ratio is 3:1). 80% of cases are associated with a duplicated collecting system (which predominantly affects females).

A duplex kidney has an upper pole and a lower pole, each with its own renal pelvis and ureter. The two ureters may join to form a single ureter, or they may pass down individually to the bladder (complete duplication). In this case, the upper pole ureter always opens onto the bladder below and medial to the lower pole ureter (Weigert–Meyer rule), predisposing to ectopic placement of the ureteric orifice.

Sites of ectopic ureters
- **Females**: bladder neck, urethra, vagina
- **Males**: posterior urethra, seminal vesicles, ejaculatory duct, vas deferens, epididymis, bladder neck

Presentation
Acute or recurrent UTI is common in both sexes. Obstruction of the ectopic ureter can lead to hydronephrosis and hydroureter, which may present as an abdominal mass.
- **Females**: When the ureteric opening is below the urethral sphincter, girls present with persistent vaginal discharge or incontinence, despite successful toilet training.
- **Males**: The ureter is always sited above the external urethral sphincter, so boys do not develop incontinence. UTIs may trigger epididymitis.

Investigation of urinary tract
- **US** demonstrates ureteric duplication, dilatation, and hydronephrosis.
- **VCUG** is used to assess reflux in lower pole ureters (Fig. 15.3).
- **Cystourethroscopy** can directly identify a ureteric opening in the urethra.
- **Isotope renogram** (^{99m}**Tc-DMSA**) is used to assess renal function to help plan surgery.

Treatment
An ectopic ureter is often associated with a poorly functioning renal upper pole or single-system kidney. In such cases, open or laparoscopic heminephrectomy or total nephrectomy with excision of the associated ureter is indicated.

When some function is retained in a single-system kidney, the distal ureter can be resected and reimplanted into the bladder.

A

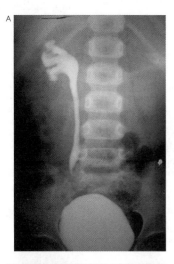

B

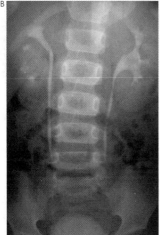

Figure 15.3 A) VCUG shows high-grade reflux into the lower pole of the duplicated right kidney. B) Intravenous pyelogram (IVP) in same patient shows upper-pole right renal moiety and normal left ureter.

Ureterocele

Definition
This is a cystic dilatation of the distal ureter as it drains into the bladder.

Incidence
Females are affected more than males (female–male ratio is 4:1). They predominantly affect Caucasians. 80% of cases are associated with the upper pole of a duplex system, although they can be found in single systems (more commonly in adults); 10% are bilateral.

Classification
- **Intravesical**: confined within the bladder
- **Ectopic**: if any part extends to the bladder neck or urethra
- **Stenotic**: intravesical ureterocele with a narrow opening
- **Sphincteric**: ectopic ureterocele with an orifice distal to the bladder neck
- **Sphincterostenotic**: orifice is both stenostic and distal to the bladder neck
- **Cecoureterocele**: ectopic ureterocele that extends into the urethra, but the orifice is in the bladder

Presentation
Infants commonly present with symptoms of UTI. Association with duplicated ureters increases the risk of reflux and reflux nephropathy.

Ureteroceles can also cause obstruction and hydronephrosis, which may be identified on antenatal ultrasound (US) scan or present in children with an abdominal mass or pain.

A prolapsing ureterocele can present as a vaginal mass in girls.

Investigation
- **US** shows a thin-walled cyst in the bladder often associated with a duplex system.
- **Intravenous pyelogram (IVP)** may demonstrate deviation of upper-pole duplex kidney and delayed excretion of contrast signifying altered renal function. In single systems, contrast in the ureterocele gives the appearance of a cobra head.
- **Voiding cystourethrogram** can identify location, size, and associated reflux.
- **Cystoscopy** may reveal a defect near the trigone.
- **^{99m}Tc-DMSA** assesses renal segment function.

Treatment
Single-system ureterocele: Initial management is usually endoscopic incision of the ureterocele, which can be followed by surgical ureteric re-implantation to preserve renal function and prevent reflux.

Duplex-system ureterocele: Treatment options vary with the individual and include endoscopic incision, upper pole nephrectomy for a poorly functioning unit with ureterectomy (heminephroureterectomy), or, when there is useful renal function, ureteropyelostomy can be performed.

Ureteropelvic junction (UPJ) obstruction

Definition

UPJ obstruction is a blockage of the ureter at the junction with the renal pelvis resulting in a restriction of urine flow.

Boys are affected more than girls. The left side is affected more often than the right side. Obstruction is bilateral in up to 40% of patients.

Etiology

In children, most UPJ obstruction is congenital, due to either an intrinsic narrowing (secondary to aberrant development of ureteric/renal pelvis muscle, abnormal collagen, or ureteral polyps) or extrinsic causes (compression of the UPJ by aberrant vessels).

Coexisting vesicoureteric reflux (VUR) is found in 40% of patients.

Presentation

UPJ obstruction is the most common cause of hydronephrosis found on prenatal and early postnatal US (differential diagnoses include UVJ obstruction, VUR, renal abnormalities, and posterior urethral valves). Infants may also present with an abdominal mass, UTI, and hematuria.

Older children present with flank or abdominal pain (exacerbated by diuresis), UTI, nausea and vomiting, and hematuria following minor trauma.

Investigation

If prenatal US has shown a large or bilateral hydronephrosis, a follow-up renal tract ultrasound scan should be performed soon after birth. If there is a prenatal unilateral hydronephrosis (and the bladder is normal), the scan is deferred until days 3–7 (to allow normal physiological diuresis to occur, which may spontaneously improve or resolve hydronephrosis).

If upper tract obstruction persists, a voiding cystourethrogram (VCUG) is indicated (to rule out VUR and examine for posterior urethral valves), and a renogram can assess individual renal function and drainage (DTPA, MAG-3).

Treatment

Children may be observed with US and renogram if they remain stable and have good renal function and no other complications (such as persistent infection or stones).

If children are symptomatic or have a significant hydronephrosis with impaired renal function (<40%), pyeloplasty is recommended.

Hypospadias

Definition

Hypospadias is a congenital deformity in which the opening of the urethra (the meatus) occurs on the underside (ventral) part of the penis, anywhere from the glans to the perineum. It is often associated with a hooded foreskin and chordee (ventral curvature of the penile shaft).

It occurs in 1 in 250 live male births. There is an 8% incidence in offspring of an affected male, and a 14% risk in male siblings.

Classification

Hypospadias can be classified according to the anatomical location of the urethral meatus (Fig. 15.4).
- **Anterior** (or distal)—glandular, coronal, and subcoronal (~50%)
- **Middle**—distal penile, midshaft, and proximal penile (~30%)
- **Posterior** (or proximal)—penoscrotal, scrotal, and perineal (~20%)

Etiology

Hypospadias results from incomplete closure of urethral folds on the underside of the penis during embryological development. This is related to a defect in production or metabolism of fetal androgens, or the number and sensitivity of androgen receptors in the tissues.

Chordee is caused by abnormal urethral plate development, and the hooded foreskin is due to failed formation of the glandular urethra and fusion of the preputial folds (resulting in a lack of ventral foreskin but an excess of dorsal tissue).

Diagnosis

A full clinical examination will make the diagnosis. However, it is also important to seek out associated abnormalities that will need treatment (undescended testes, inguinal hernias, and hydroceles).

Patients with absent testes and severe hypospadias should undergo chromosomal and endocrine investigation to exclude intersex conditions.

Treatment

Surgery is indicated where deformity is severe, interferes with voiding, OR is predicted to interfere with sexual function. Surgery is now performed between 6 and 12 months of age. Local application of testosterone for 1 month preoperatively can help increase tissue size.

The aim of surgery is to correct penile curvature (orthoplasty), reconstruct a new urethra, and bring the new meatus to the tip of the glans using urethroplasy, glanuloplasty, and meatoplasty techniques.

Severe cases may require staged procedures. Common operations for anterior hypospadias include meatal advancement and glanuloplasty (MAGPI), meatal-based flaps (Mathieu procedure), and tubularization of the urethral plate.

Posterior defects require free grafts (buccal mucosa), on-lay grafts, and preputial transfer flaps.

Complications

These include bleeding, infection, urethral strictures, meatal stenosis, urethrocutaneous fistula, urethral diverticulum, and failed procedures requiring reoperation.

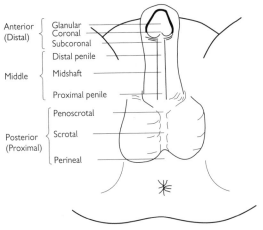

Figure 15.4 The anatomical classification of hypospadias according to the location of the urethral meatus. This figure was published in Walsh PC, et al. *Campbell's Urology*, 8th Edition, p. 2287. Copyright Elsevier 2002.

Normal sexual differentiation

Sexual differentiation and gonadal development is determined by the sex chromosomes (XY male, XX female). The gonads produce hormones that influence the subsequent differentiation of internal and external genitalia (Figs. 15.5 and 15.6).

Both sexes

Gonads develop from the genital ridges (formed by cells of the mesonephros and coelomic epithelium). At 5–6 weeks, primordial germ cells migrate from the yolk sac to populate the genital ridges. Primitive sex cords are formed, which support germ cell development.

From 4 weeks, the mesonephric (Wolffian) ducts are incorporated into the genital system, when renal function is taken over by the definitive kidney. At 6 weeks, coelomic epithelium creates the paramesonephric (Müllerian) ducts, which develop laterally and are fused to the urogenital sinus at their bases.

Males

The testis-determining gene (SRY) is located on the Y chromosome and stimulates medullary sex cords in the primitive testis to differentiate into Sertoli cells, which produce Müllerian inhibiting substance (MIS) at 7–8 weeks. This triggers regression of the paramesonephric ducts, testosterone secretion from Leydig cells of the testis, and the initial phase of testicular descent.

During weeks 8–12, mesonephric ducts differentiate into epididymis, vas deferens, seminal vesicles, and ejaculatory ducts. The prostate is formed from mesenchyme (capsule) and urethral endoderm.

After week 23, the testes rapidly descend from the abdomen (via the inguinal canal during weeks 24–28) and into the scrotal sac, guided by the gubernaculum. The scrotum is created by fusion of labioscrotal folds.

Testosterone and dihydrotestosterone (DHT) androgens are responsible for masculinization. DHT is made from testosterone by 5-α-reductase enzyme in the tissues.

Development of the external genitalia occurs from week 7. Urogenital folds develop around the opening of the urogenital sinus, and labioscrotal swellings form either side. The penile shaft and glans are formed by elongation of the genital tubercle and fusion of urogenital folds.

Incomplete production or activity of DHT in the male fetus will result in incompletely virilized male genitalia.

Females

The genital ridge forms secondary sex cords (primitive sex cords degenerate) that surround the germ cells to create ovarian follicles (week 15). These undergo meiotic division to become primary oocytes, which are later activated to complete gametogenesis at puberty.

Estrogen is produced from week 8 under the influence of the aromatase enzyme. In the absence of MIS, the mesonephric ducts regress, and the paramesonephric ducts become the fallopian tubes, uterus, and upper two-thirds of the vagina. The sinovaginal sinus develops at the junction of the paramesonephric ducts and the urogenital sinus. This forms the lower third of the vagina.

The genital tubercle forms the clitoris; the urogenital folds become the labia minora; and the labioscrotal swellings form the labia majora.

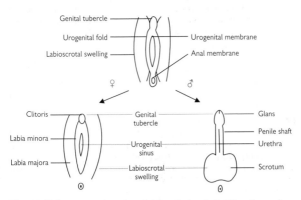

Figure 15.5 Differentiation of external genitalia (weeks 7–16).

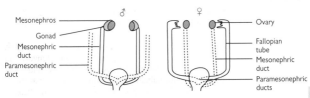

Figure 15.6 Differentiation of the genital tract.

Abnormal sexual differentiation

Disorders of sex development (DSD) are defined as congenital conditions in which the development of chromosomal, gonadal, or anatomical sex is atypical.

They are estimated to affect 1 in 4500 births, and have recently undergone changes in recommended nomenclature (Table 15.1).[1]

Sex chromosome DSD (disorders of gonadal differentiation)

These are subdivided into seminiferous tubule dysgenesis (Klinefelter syndrome XXY, 46XX males); Turner syndrome (45XO); true hermaphrodites (46XX or XY with both ovarian and testicular tissue); mixed gonadal dysgenesis (streak gonads and a spectrum of ambiguous genitalia); and pure gonadal dysgenesis (females with streak gonads).

46XY DSD (previously male pseudohermaphroditism)

Individuals have 46XY karyotype with differentiated testes. They have defects of testosterone production (3α-hydroxysteroid dehydrogenase, 17α-hydroxylase enzyme deficiencies) or androgen resistance (testicular feminization, 5α-reductase deficiency), resulting in varying degrees of feminization.

46XX DSD (previously female pseudohermaphroditism)

Individuals have 46XX karyotype with ovaries, a partially masculinized phenotype, and ambiguous genitalia. The most common type is **congenital adrenal hyperplasia** (CAH), due to 21-hydroxylase deficiency (in 95%; see Fig. 15.7). Formation of hydrocortisone is impaired, resulting in a compensatory increase in adrenocorticotrophin hormone (ACTH) and testosterone production.

Some forms have a salt-wasting aldosterone deficiency that can present in the first few weeks of life with adrenal crisis (severe vomiting and dehydration), requiring rehydration and steroid replacement therapy.

Evaluation

A detailed **history** may uncover a positive family history of intersex disorders. Maternal ingestion of drugs such as steroids or contraceptives during pregnancy should be ascertained.

General **examination** may show associated syndrome anomalies (Klinefelter and Turner syndromes) or failure to thrive and dehydration (salt-wasting CAH). Assess external genitalia for phallus size and location of urethral meatus. Careful palpation may confirm the presence of testes, excluding a diagnosis of female pseudohermaphroditism. Patients with bilateral undescended testes or unilateral undescended testis with hypospadias should be suspected of having an intersex disorder.

Pelvic US can help locate the gonads or, occasionally, laparotomy with gonadal biopsy is required for diagnosis.

1 Hughes IA, Houk C, Ahmed SF, et al. (2007). Consensus statement on management of intersex disorders. *Arch Dis Child* 554–563.

Table 15.1 Proposed revised nomenclature*

Previous terminology	Proposed new terminology (2007)
Intersex	Disorders of sex development (DSD)
Male pseudohermaphrodite	46,XY DSD
Female pseudohermaphrodite	46,XX DSD
True hermaphrodite	Ovotesticular DSD
Testicular feminization	Androgen insensitivity syndrome, complete (CAIS)
46XX male	46XX testicular DSD

* Hughes IA, Houk C, Ahmed SF, et al. (2007). Consensus statement on management of intersex disorders. *Arch Dis Child* 554–563.

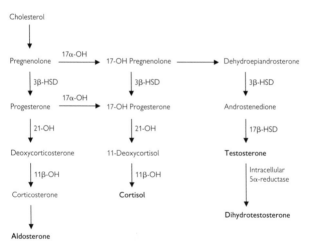

Key:
17-OH   17α-hydroxylase enzyme
21-OH*   21-hydroxylase
3β-HSD   3β-hydroxysteriod dehydrogenase
11β-OH   11β-hydroxylase

Figure 15.7 Metabolic pathways for adrenal steroid synthesis.

Chromosomal analysis confirms karyotype. Serum electrolytes, testosterone, and DHT analysis test for salt-wasting CAH. Serum 17-hydroxyprogesterone performed after day 3 can also diagnose 21-hydroxylase deficiency, and hCG stimulation test can diagnose androgen resistance and 5α-reductase deficiency.

Management

A multidisciplinary approach is required with full parental input. Gender assignment of ambiguous genitalia is guided by the functional potential of gonadal tissue, reproductive tracts, and genitalia, with the aim of optimizing psychosocial well-being and producing a stable gender identity.

Patients have a higher risk of gonadal malignancy, which requires surveillance and/or removal of gonadal tissues and hormone replacement.

Cystic kidney disease

Congenital cystic kidney disease can be classified into genetic and non-genetic types.

Genetic

Autosomal recessive polycystic kidney disease (ARPKD)

ARPKD is a disease of infancy and childhood, where renal collecting tubules and ducts become cystically dilated and numerous small cysts form in the renal cortex and medulla. Severe forms present early and have a poor prognosis.

Prenatal US demonstrates oligohydramnios (amniotic fluid <200 mL) and large, "bright" homogeneously hyperechogenic kidneys, which can cause obstructed labor and respiratory problems.

Neonates have large flank masses and limb and facial anomalies. All cases are associated with congenital hepatic fibrosis. Infants develop fatal uremia and respiratory failure; older children present with renal failure, hypertension, and portal hypertension. Most develop end-stage renal failure by adulthood, requiring hemodialysis and renal transplantation.

Autosomal dominant polycystic kidney disease (ADKD)

ADKDA Typically presents in adulthood, although older children can present with complications of hematuria, flank pain, flank mass, UTI, proteinuria, hypertension, and intracerebral bleeds (secondary to berry aneurysm rupture).

It is characterized by multiple expanding cysts of both kidneys that ultimately destroy the intervening parenchyma, and accounts for 10% of all chronic renal failure.

Familial juvenile nephronophthisis

This is an autosomal recessive disorder that develops in early childhood and accounts for up to 20% of pediatric renal failure. **Medullary cystic disease** is a similar (autosomal dominant) condition that develops in later childhood.

Histology shows interstitial nephritis associated with medullary and corticomedullary cysts. Disease progression causes a reduction in kidney size. Features include polyuria, polydipsia, anemia, growth retardation, and chronic renal failure.

Renal cysts are also a feature of autosomal dominant conditions, including **Von–Hippel–Lindau syndrome** (cerebellar hemangioblastomas, pheochromocytoma, renal cell carcinoma) and **tuberous sclerosis** (adenoma sebaceum, epilepsy, learning difficulties).

Nongenetic

Multicystic dysplastic kidney (MCDK)

MCDK is the most common cystic kidney disorder and second most common cause of abdominal mass in newborns (after UPJ obstruction). The cysts of a multicystic kidney are not due to dilatation of renal collecting ducts (as in polycystic disease); instead, the entire kidney is dysplastic, with immature dysplastic stroma and cysts of various sizes. The kidney does not have a renoform shape or a calyceal drainage system—the ureter is atretic.

Bilateral disease is incompatible with life. Unilateral disease is often associated with reflux (20–40%) or UPJ obstruction (10%) in the contralateral kidney. Affected kidneys may undergo renal aplasia, where they spontaneously shrink to a tiny remnant.

Ultrasound helps to distinguish this condition (noncommunicating cysts) from hydronephrosis. Renal scanning shows no function.

Most patients can be treated conservatively with close surveillance for the associated risks of hypertension and Wilms' tumor, which would be indications for surgery. It may involute spontaneously.

Multilocular cystic nephroma

This condition presents in young children, with unilateral flank mass. It is included in a spectrum of diseases that are closely associated with Wilms tumor, so the recommended treatment is partial or full nephrectomy.

There is bimodal distribution—male infants <2 and female adults >40 years of age.

Exstrophy

Bladder exstrophy results from defective development of the anterior bladder and lower abdominal walls, leaving the posterior bladder wall lying exposed on the abdomen.

Epidemiology

Incidence is 3.3 cases per 100,000 live births, with a male-to-female ratio >2:1. There is and increased risk in offspring of affected patients and with younger maternal age and increased parity.

Embryology

An embryological malformation results in the abnormal overdevelopment of the cloacal membrane, which prevents in-growth of lower abdominal tissues. The cloacal membrane normally perforates to form the urogenital and anal openings, but in exstrophy there is premature rupture, resulting in a triangular defect below the umbilicus.

    The timing of this rupture determines the type of defect (bladder exstrophy, cloacal exstrophy, OR epispadias).

Associated anomalies

- **Bone defects:** diastasis (widening) of the symphysis pubis due to outward rotation of the pelvic bones along the sacroiliac joints (Fig. 15.8)
- **Musculofascial defects:** umbilical hernias, inguinal hernias, abnormal pelvic floor
- **Genital defects:** *Males* have a short, broad epispadiac penis with lateral splaying of the corporal cavernosa, and short urethral plate. *Females* have a bifid clitoris, stenotic vaginal orifice, short vaginal canal, and vaginal prolase.
- **Urinary tract defects:** Most patients suffer vesicoureteric reflux (VUR) due to lateral displacement of the ureteric orifices.
- **GI defects:** anteriorly displaced anus, rectal prolapse; abnormal anal sphincter contributes to incontinence.

Investigation

Typical features seen on prenatal ultrasound scan include a lower abdominal wall mass, absent bladder filling, low-set umbilicus, small genitalia, and abnormal iliac crest widening. Diagnosis can help in planning of delivery in a center with facilities to perform early surgical correction.

Management

At birth, cover the bladder with plastic film and irrigate regularly with sterile saline. Trauma to the bladder mucosa can eventually result in squamous metaplasia, cystitis cystica, or adenocarcinoma and squamous cell carcinoma after chronic exposure.

Selected cases are suitable for one-stage repair, but most require a three-stage procedure:

• **Newborn:** pelvic osteotomy (cutting bone to correct deformity) with external fixation with closure of bladder, abdominal wall, and posterior urethra
• **6–12 months:** epispadias repair
• **4–5 years:** Bladder neck reconstruction (Young–Dees–Leadbetter procedure) and anti-reflux surgery (ureteric reimplantation) are performed when there is adequate bladder capacity and children can participate in voiding protocols. Where bladder capacity is too small, bladder augmentation or urinary diversion is required.

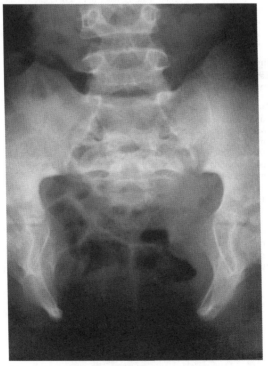

Figure 15.8 KUB from exstrophy patient shows characteristic wide separation of pubes.

Epispadias

In epispadias, the urethra opens onto the dorsal surface of the penis, any-where from the glans, penile shaft, or, most commonly, the penopubic region. An incomplete urethral sphincter mechanism results in a high risk of incontinence.

Epispadias is also associated with dorsal chordee (causing an upward curvature of the penis), with incomplete foreskin dorsally. Epispadias is part of the exstrophy–epispadias complex (which also includes bladder exstrophy and cloacal exstrophy) (see p. 560).

Associated anomalies

Diastasis of the symphysis pubis results in splaying of the corpora caver-nosa and shortening of the penile shaft. Females have a bifid clitoris and poorly developed labia and demonstrate a spectrum of urethral deformi-ties ranging from a patulous urethral orifice to a urethral cleft affecting the entire length of the urethra and sphincter.

There is a 40% risk of vesicoureteric reflux (VUR).

Incidence

Epispadias affects 1 in 117,000 males. It is rarely seen in females (male–female ratio is 5:1).

Management

This involves urethroplasty with functional and cosmetic reconstruction of the external genitalia (penile lengthening and correction of chordee) at 6–12 months.

The modified Cantwell–Ransley technique is commonly used in males. It describes mobilizing the urethra to the ventral aspect of the penis, with advancement of the urethral meatus onto the glans with a reverse MAGPI (meatal advancement-glanduloplasty). The corporal bodies are separated and rotated medially above the urethra and re-approximated.

From age 4–5 years, when children can be toilet trained, bladder neck reconstruction can be performed (Young–Dees–Leadbetter procedure). This achieves continence, and any bladder residuals may then be emptied by urethral catheterization.

If this surgery fails, insertion of artificial urinary sphincters or collagen injections of the sphincter may be tried.

Posterior urethral valves

Definition

Posterior urethral valves (PUV) are abnormal congenital mucosal folds in the prostatic (posterior) urethra causing lower urinary tract obstruction.

Classification

- **Type I** (90–95%): Membranes arise from the distal lateral aspect of the verumontanum,[1] which extend distally and anteriorly to fuse in the midline.
- **Type II:** Longitudinal folds extending from the verumontanum to bladder neck (of historical interest only)
- **Type III** (5%): A ring-like membrane found distal to the verumontanum

Incidence is 1 in >5000 males.

Etiology

Normal male urethra has small, paired lateral folds (plicae colliculi) found between the lateral, distal edge of verumontanum and lateral urethral wall. PUVs probably represent a congenital overgrowth of these folds from abnormal insertion of Wolffian ducts into the posterior urethra during fetal development.

Presentation

Prenatal US features

These include bilateral hydroureteronephrosis, dilated bladder with elongated ectatic posterior urethra, thick-walled bladder, oligohydramnios (reduced amniotic fluid), and renal dysplasia.

Early features are associated with poor prognosis.

Newborn and infants

These children have respiratory distress (secondary to pulmonary hypoplasia), palpable abdominal mass (hydronephrotic kidney or distended bladder), ascites, UTI, electrolyte abnormalities, and failure to thrive.

Older children

Milder cases may present later with recurrent UTI, poor urinary stream, incomplete bladder emptying, poor growth, and incontinence. There is a risk of renal failure, vesicoureteric reflux, and voiding dysfunction (overactive or underactive bladder), also described as valve bladder syndrome.

Associated features

POP-off valve syndrome is seen in 20%. It describes mechanisms by which high urinary tract pressure is dissipated to allow normal renal development. It includes leaking of urine from small bladder or renal pelvis ruptures (urinary ascites), reflux into a nonfunctioning kidney (vesicoureteral reflux with renal dysplasia [VURD]), and formation of bladder diverticuli.

Investigation

- **Ultrasound scan of kidneys and bladder**.
- **VCUG** shows distended and elongated posterior urethra (shield shaped; see Fig. 15.9); partially filled anterior urethra; bladder neck

hypertrophy; lucencies representing valve leaflets; thick-walled bladder (±diverticuli); incomplete bladder emptying; reflux (50%).
- **Isotope renal scan** (MAG-3, DMSA) assesses renal function.
- **Videourodynamics** allows diagnosis of associated voiding dysfunction.

Management

Commence prophylactic antibiotics immediately, check serum electrolytes, and drain the bladder with a pediatric feeding tube. If there is improvement, cystoscopy and transurethral ablation of valve (cuts at 5 and 7 o'clock with electrocautery) is recommended (complications include urethral strictures).

If upper tracts remain dilated with raised creatinine after bladder drainage, a temporary cutaneous vesicostomy is indicated (communicating stoma between the bladder dome and suprapubic abdominal wall, allowing free drainage of urine). An alternative is ureterostomy drainage. Valve ablation is performed at a later stage.

Prognosis

Prognosis is 35% of patients will have poor renal function; 20% develop end-stage renal failure.

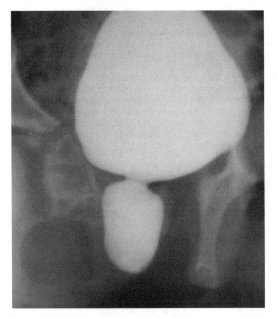

Figure 15.9 VCUG in infant with posterior urethral valves shows dilated elongated prostatic urethra and thickened bladder neck.

Non-neurogenic voiding dysfunction

Definition

This is an abnormal voiding pattern without an underlying organic cause (neurological disease, congenital malformation, or injury), which usually results in urinary incontinence (diurnal, nocturnal, or both). It is often associated with constipation and fecal retention.

Normal bladder control

- **Neonates:** Sacral spinal cord reflex triggers voiding when the bladder is full.
- **Infants:** Primitive reflexes are suppressed, bladder capacity increases, and voiding frequency is reduced.
- **2–4 years:** Development of conscious bladder sensation and voluntary control occurs.

Classification

Urinary incontinence can be divided into primary (never been dry) or secondary (re-emergence of incontinence after being dry for 6 months) types. Voiding dysfunction can be described as mild, moderate, or major.

- **Mild:** daytime urinary frequency syndrome; giggle incontinence; post-void dribbling (urine refluxes into the vagina, then dribbles into underwear on standing); nocturnal enuresis
- **Moderate:** lazy bladder syndrome (large capacity, poor contractility, infrequent voids); overactive bladder (detrusor overactivity associated with urgency and frequency). Children may demonstrate holding maneuvers (leg crossing, squatting, Vincent curtsey). There is increased risk of UTI, vesicoureteric reflux, and upper tract dilatation.
- **Major:** Hinman syndrome (non-neurogenic neurogenic bladder) involves dyscoordination between the bladder muscle and external urethral sphincter activity, resulting in a small, trabeculated bladder, VUR, UTI, hydronephrosis, and renal damage. It is caused by abnormal learned voiding patterns.

Evaluation

History

Enquire about UTIs; voiding habits (frequency, urgency, primary or secondary incontinence); family history; bowel problems; social history; and behavioral problems.

Examination

Conduct a full, noninvasive examination (palpable bladder or kidneys). Be vigilant for signs of sexual abuse in children with an atypical history (penile or vaginal discharge). Exclude an organic cause (hairy patch, lipoma, dimple on lower back may indicate lumbosacral spine abnormalities).

Investigations

Obtain urinalysis (infection, protein, glucose) and voiding diary and assess flow rate.

In selected cases, US of the renal tract (hydronephrosis, bladder size); VCUG (VUR, post-void residual), videourodynamics (over or underactive detrusor, sphincter dyssynergia), or MRI of the spine (if clinical suspicion of neurological cause) is indicated.

Management

This includes behavioral therapy (bladder retraining, timed voiding, change of voiding posture, psychological support); medication (antibiotics for infection, anticholinergics for bladder overactivity and urgency, laxatives or enemas for constipation); and intermittent catheterization to drain post-void residuals. Surgery is rarely indicated.

Prognosis

Fifteen percent of cases spontaneously resolve per year.

Nocturnal enuresis

Enuresis is normal but involuntary voiding that occurs at an inappropriate time or social setting, during the day, night, or both. *Nocturnal enuresis* describes any involuntary loss of urine during sleep.

Prevalence

Approximately 750,000 children over age 7 years will regularly wet the bed. The prevalence in adults is ~0.5%.

Prevalence		
Age (years)	Females	Males
5	10–15%	15–20%
7	7–15%	15–20%
9	5–10%	10–15%
16	1–2%	1–2%

Classification

- **Primary:** never been dry for more than a 6-month period
- **Secondary:** re-emergence of bed wetting after a period of being dry for at least 6 months

Etiology

- Familial
- Delay in functional bladder maturation
- Altered antidiuretic hormone (ADH) secretion; abnormal decrease in ADH levels at night causes increased urine production (nocturnal polyuria)
- Altered sleep/arousal mechanism
- Psychological factors
- UTI (1% of cases)

Evaluation

- **History:** frequency of episodes; daytime symptoms; new or recurrent; family history; UTIs; bowel problems; psychosocial history
- **Examination:** exclude organic causes (neurological disease)
- **Investigation:** urinalysis (infection, specific gravity is reduced in nocturnal polyuria, glucose, protein); voiding diary

Management

Behavioral

Provide reassurance; bladder training; motivational techniques to improve the child's self-esteem; conditioning therapy (an alarm is connected to the child's underwear, which is triggered with the first few drops of urine).

Pharmacological
- Imipramine—a tricyclic antidepressant with anticholinergic, antispasmodic properties.
- DDAVP or desmopressin (synthetic analogue of ADH) given intranasally or orally

Prognosis

Fifteen percent of patients have spontaneous resolution of symptoms per year.

Urological surgery and equipment

Preparation of the patient for urological surgery 572
Antibiotic prophylaxis in urological surgery 574
Complications of surgery in general: DVT and PE 576
Fluid balance and management of shock in the surgical
    patient 580
Patient safety in the operating room 582
Transurethral resection (TUR) syndrome 583
Catheters and drains in urological surgery 584
Guide wires 590
Irrigating fluids and techniques of bladder washout 592
JJ stents 594
Lasers in urological surgery 598
Diathermy 600
Sterilization of urological equipment 604
Telescopes and light sources in urological endoscopy 606
Consent: general principles 608
Cystoscopy 610
Transurethral resection of the prostate (TURP) 612
Transurethral resection of bladder tumor (TURBT) 614
Optical urethrotomy 616
Circumcision 618
Hydrocele and epididymal cyst removal 620
Nesbit procedure 622
Vasectomy and vasovasostomy 624
Orchiectomy 626
Urological incisions 628
JJ stent insertion 630
Nephrectomy and nephroureterectomy 632
Radical prostatectomy 634
Radical cystectomy 636
Ileal conduit 640
Percutaneous nephrolithotomy (PCNL) 642
Ureteroscopes and ureteroscopy 646
Pyeloplasty 650
Laparoscopic surgery 652
Endoscopic cystolitholapaxy and (open) cystolithotomy 654
Scrotal exploration for torsion and orchiopexy 656

Preparation of the patient for urological surgery

The degree of preparation is related to the complexity of the procedure. Certain aspects of examination (pulse rate, blood pressure) and certain tests (hemoglobin, electrolytes, and creatinine) are important not only to assess fitness for surgery but also as a baseline against which changes in the postoperative period may be measured.

- Assess cardiac status (angina, arrhythmias, previous myocardial infarction [MI], blood pressure, electrocardiogram [ECG], chest X-ray [CXR]). We assess respiratory function by pulmonary function tests (forced vital capacity [FVC], forced expiratory volume in 1 second [FEV_1]) for all major surgery and for any surgery where the patient has symptoms of respiratory problems or a history of chronic airways disease (e.g., asthma).
- Arrange an anesthetic review when there is, for example, cardiac or respiratory comorbidity.
- Culture urine, treat active (symptomatic) infection with an appropriate antibiotic starting a week before surgery, and give prophylactic antibiotics at the induction of anesthesia.
- Stop aspirin and nonsteroidal anti-inflammatory drugs (NSAIDs) 10 days prior to surgery.
- Obtain consent (see p. 608).
- Measure hemoglobin and serum creatinine and investigate and correct anemia, electrolyte disturbance, and abnormal renal function. If blood loss is anticipated, group and save a sample of serum or cross-match several units of blood, the precise number depending on the speed with which your blood bank can deliver blood if needed. Recommendations on blood products are as follows:

TURBT	Type and hold
TURP	Cross-match 2 units
Open prostatectomy	Cross-match 2 units
Simple nephrectomy	Cross-match 2 units
Radical nephrectomy	Cross-match 4 units
Cystectomy	Cross-match 4 units
Radical prostatectomy	Cross-match 2 units
PCNL	Cross-match 2 units

- The patient may choose to store his or her own blood prior to the procedure.

Bowel preparation

This is indicated if bowel is to be used (ileal conduit, bladder reconstruction). Use a mechanical prep (Fleets phosphasoda or polyethelen glycol 3350) and antimicrobial prep (neomycin and erythromycin base), starting at noon the day before surgery, with a clear fluid-only diet for the rest of the day.

Antibiotic prophylaxis in urological surgery

The precise antibiotic prophylaxis policy that you use will depend on your local microbiological flora. Your local microbiology department will provide regular advice and updates on which antibiotics should be used, both for prophylaxis and treatment. The policy shown below and in Table 16.1 is just a recommendation.

Culture urine before any procedure, and use specific prophylaxis (based on sensitivities) if culture positive.

We avoid ciprofloxacin in inpatients because it is secreted onto the skin and causes methicillin-resistant *Staphylococcus aureus* (MRSA) colonization. For most purposes, nitrofurantoin provides equivalent coverage without being secreted onto the skin.

We do use ciprofloxacin if there is known *Proteus* infection (all *Proteus* species are resistant to nitrofurantoin).

Patients with artificial heart valves

Patients with heart murmurs and those with prosthetic heart valves should be given 1 g IV amoxycillin with 80 mg gentamycin at induction of anesthesia, with an additional dose of oral amoxycillin, 500 mg 6 hours later (substituting vancomycin 1 g for those who are penicillin allergic).

Patients with joint replacements

The advice is conflicting.

AAOS/AUA advice

Joint advice of the American Academy of Orthopedic Surgeons (AAOS) and the American Urological Association (AUA) is that antibiotic prophylaxis is not indicated for urological patients with pins, plates, or screws, nor for most patients with total joint replacements.

It is recommended for all patients undergoing urological procedures, including TURP, *within 2 years of a prosthetic joint replacement*, for those who are immunocompromised (e.g., rheumatoid patients, those with systemic lupus erythematosus [SLE], drug-induced immunosuppression, including steroids), and for those with a history of previous joint infection, hemophilia, HIV infection, diabetes, or malignancy.

Antibiotic regime

Give a single dose of a quinolone, such as 500 mg of ciprofloxacin, 1–2 hours preoperatively + ampicillin 2 g IV + gentamicin 1.5 mg/kg 30–60 minutes preoperatively (substituting vancomycin 1 g IV for penicillin-allergic patients).

Table 16.1 Oxford urology procedure: specific antibiotic prophylaxis protocol for urological surgery

Procedure	Antibiotic prophylaxis
Catheter removal	Nitrofurantoin, 100 mg PO 30 min before catheter removal
Change of male long-term catheter	Gentamicin 1.5 mg/kg IM or IV 20 min before*
Flexible cystoscopy or GA cystoscopy	Nitrofurantoin 100 mg PO 30–60 min before procedure
Transrectal prostatic biopsy	Ciprofloxacin 500 mg PO 30 min pre-biopsy and for 48 hr post-biopsy (ciprofloxacin 500 mg bid)
ESWL	500 mg oral ciprofloxacin 30 min before treatment (nitrofurantoin does not cover *Proteus*, a common stone bacterium)
PCNL	Ampicillin 1 g + IV gentamicin at induction (1.5 mg/kg); before operation, and 2 doses postoperatively
Ureteroscopy	Gentamycin 1.5 mg/kg IV at induction
Urogynecological procedures (e.g., colposuspension)	Cefuroxime 1.5 g IV and metronidazole 500 mg IV at induction of anesthesia
TURPs and TURBTs — both for non-catheterized patients (i.e., elective TURP for LUTS) and patients with catheters (undergoing TURP for retention)	Ampicillin 1 g + IV gentamicin at induction (1.5 mg/kg); nitrofurantoin 100 mg PO 30 min before catheter removal
Radical prostatectomy	Ampicillin 1 g + IV gentamicin at induction (1.5 mg/kg); before operation
Cystectomy or other procedures involving the use of bowel (e.g., augmentation cystoplasty)	Ampicillin 1 g + IV gentamicin at induction (1.5 mg/kg); before operation
Artificial urinary sphincter insertion	Vancomycin 1 g 1.5 hr before leaving the ward (infuse over 100 min) + 1.5 mg IV cefuroxime + 3 mg/kg IV gentamicin at induction; continue IV cefuroxime, gentamicin, and vancomycin (1 g) for 48 hr

*Sepsis rate (necessitating admission to hospital) may be as high as 1% without antibiotic coverage.

Note: Cefuroxime has a short half-life. Whenever using cefuroxime, give a further dose 2 hours after the first dose. Further intraoperative top-up doses of vancomycin and gentamicin are not required as they have long half-lives.

Complications of surgery in general: DVT and PE

While venous thromboembolism (VTE) is uncommon after urological surgery, it is considered the most important nonsurgical complication of major urological procedures. Following TURP, 0.1–0.2% of patients experience a pulmonary embolus (PE)[1] and 1–5% of patients undergoing major urological surgery experience symptomatic VTE.[2]

The mortality of PE is on the order of 1%.[3]

Risk factors for DVT and PE

Increased risk for deep venous thromboembolism (DVT) and PE is with open (versus endoscopic) procedures, malignancy, and increasing age and depends on the duration of the procedure.

Categorization of VTE risk

American College of Chest Physicians (ACCP) Guidelines on prevention of venous thromboembolism[2] categorize the risk of VTE are as follows:

• *Low-risk patients*—those <40 years undergoing minor surgery (surgery lasting <30 minutes) and with no additional risk factors. No specific measures to prevent DVT are required in such patients other than early mobilization. Increasing age and duration of surgery increases risk of VTE.

• *High-risk patients*—include those undergoing non-major surgery (surgery lasting >30 minutes) who are age >60 years

Prevention of DVT and PE

See Box 16.1.

Diagnosis of DVT

Signs of DVT are nonspecific (i.e., cellulitis and DVT share common signs—low-grade fever, calf swelling and tenderness). If you suspect a DVT, arrange for a Doppler ultrasound. If the ultrasound probe can compress the popliteal and femoral veins, there is no DVT; if it can't, there is a DVT.

Diagnosis of PE

Small PEs may be asymptomatic.

Symptoms include breathlessness, pleuritic chest pain, and hemoptysis.

Signs include tachycardia, tachypnea, raised jugular venous pressure (JVP), hypotension, and pleural rubs pleural effusion.

---

1 Donat R, Mancey–Jones B (2002). Incidence of thromboembolism after transurethral resection of the prostate (TURP). *Scan J Urol Nephrol* 36:119–123.
2 Geerts WH, Heit JA, Clagett PG, et al. (2001). Prevention of venous thromboembolism. (American College of Chest Physicians [ACCP] Guidelines on prevention of venous thromboembolism) *Chest* 119:132S–175S.
3 Quinlan DJ, McQuillan A, Eikelboom JW (2004). Low molecular weight heparin compared with intravenous unfractionated heparin for treatment of pulmonary embolism. *Ann Intern Med* 140:175–183.

Tests
- *CXR* may be normal or show linear atelectasis, dilated pulmonary artery, and small pleural effusion.
- *ECG* may be normal or show tachycardia, right bundle branch block, and inverted T waves in V1–V4 (evidence of right ventricular strain). The classic SI, QIII, TIII pattern is rare.
- *Arterial blood gases* show low PO_2 and low PCO_2.
- *Imaging:* Computed tomography pulmonary angiogram (CTPA) has superior specificity and sensitivity compared with that of ventilation-perfusion (VQ) radioisotope scan.
- *Spiral CT:* A negative CTPA rules out a PE with similar accuracy to a normal isotope lung scan or a negative pulmonary angiogram.

Treatment of established DVT
- *Below-knee DVT:* above-knee thromboembolic stockings (AK-TEDs), if no peripheral arterial disease (enquire for claudication and check pulses) + unfractionated heparin (UFH) 5000 u SC 12 hourly
- *Above-knee DVT:* start a low molecular-weight heparin (LMWH) and warfarin, and stop heparin when INR is between 2 and 3. Continue treatment for 6 weeks for postsurgical patients; it should be lifelong if there is an underlying cause (e.g., malignancy).
- LMWH

Treatment of established PE
Fixed-dose, subcutaneous (SC) LMWH seems to be as effective as adjusted-dose, intravenous (IV) UFH for the treatment of PE found in conjunction with a symptomatic DVT.[3] Rates of hemorrhage are similar with both forms of heparin treatment.

Start warfarin at the same time and stop heparin when INR is 2–3. Continue warfarin for 3 months.

Box 16.1 Options for prevention of VTE

- Early mobilization.
- Above-knee thromboembolic stockings (AK-TEDs) (provide graduated, static compression of the calves, thereby reducing venous stasis). More effective than below-knee TEDS for DVT prevention.[1]
- Subcutaneous heparin (low-dose unfractionated heparin [LDUH] or low molecular weight heparin [LMWH]). In unfractionated preparations, heparin molecules are polymerized, with molecular weights from 5000 to 30,000 daltons. LMWH is depolymerized, with a molecular weight of 4000–5000 daltons.
- Intermittent pneumatic calf compression (IPC) boots, which are placed around the calves, are intermittently inflated and deflated, thereby increasing the flow of blood in calf veins.[2]
- For patients undergoing major urological surgery (radical prostatectomy, cystectomy, nephrectomy), AK-TEDS with IPC intra-operatively, followed by SC heparin (LDUH or LMWH) should be used. For TURP, many urologists use a combination of AK-TEDS and IPCs; relatively few use SC heparin.[3]

1 Howard A, et al. (2004). Randomized clinical trial of low molecular weight heparin with thigh-length or knee-length antiembolism stockings for patients undergoing surgery. *BJS* 91:842–847.
2 Soderdahl DW, Henderson SR, Hansberry KL (1997). A comparison of intermittent pneumatic compression of the calf and whole leg in preventing deep venous thrombosis in urological surgery. *J Urol* 157:1774–1776.
3 Golash A, Collins PW, Kynaston HG, Jenkins BJ (2002). Venous thromboembolic prophylaxis for transurethral prostatectomy: practice among British urologists. *J Roy Soc Med* 95:130–131.

Further reading

British Thoracic Society guidelines for management of suspected acute pulmonary embolism (2003) *Thorax* 58:1–14.

Kelly J, Rudd A, Lewis RR, Hunt BJ (2002). Plasma D-dimers in the diagnosis of venous thromboembolism. *Arch Intern Med* 162:747–756.

Kruip MJH, Slob MJ, Schijen JH, et al. (2002). Use of a clinical decision rule in combination with D-dimer concentration in diagnostic workup of patients with suspected pulmonary embolism. *Arch Intern Med* 162:1631–1635.

Fluid balance and management of shock in the surgical patient

Daily fluid requirement

This can be calculated according to patient weight:

- For the first 10 kg: 100 mL/kg per 24 hours (= 1000 mL)
- For the next 10 kg (i.e., 10–20 kg): 50 mL/kg per 24 hours (= 500 mL)
- For every kg above 20 kg: 20 mL/kg per 24 hours (= 1000 mL for a patient weighing 70 kg)

Thus, for every 24 hours, a 70 kg adult will require 1000 mL for their first 10 kg of weight, plus 500 mL for their next 10 kg of weight, and 1000 mL for their last 50 kg of weight = total 24-hour fluid requirement, 2500 mL.

Daily sodium requirement is ~100 mmol, and for potassium, ~70 mmol. Thus, a standard 24-hour fluid regimen is 2 L of 5% dextrose + 1 L of normal saline (equivalent to about 150 mmol Na^+), with 20 mmol K^+ for every liter of infused fluid.

Fluid losses from drains or nasogastric aspirate are similar in composition to plasma and should be replaced principally with normal saline.

Shock due to blood loss

Inadequate organ perfusion and tissue oxygenation occur. The causes are hypovolemia, cardiogenic, septic, anaphylactic, and neurogenic. The most common cause in the surgical patient is hypovolemia due to blood and other fluid loss. *Hemorrhage* is an acute loss of circulating blood volume. Hemorrhagic shock may be classified as follows:

- *Class I:* up to 750 mL of blood loss (15% of blood volume); normal pulse rate (PR), respiratory rate (RR), blood pressure (BP), urine output, and mental status
- *Class II:* 750–1500 mL (15–30% of blood volume); PR >100; decreased pulse pressure due to increased diastolic pressure; RR 20–30; urinary output 20–30 mL/hr
- *Class III:* 1500–2000 mL (30–40% of blood volume); PR >120; decreased BP and pulse pressure due to decreased systolic pressure; RR 30–40; urine output 5–15 mL/hr; confusion
- *Class IV:* >2000 mL (>40% of blood volume); PR >140; decreased pulse pressure and BP; RR >35; urine output <5 mL/hr; cold, clammy skin

Management

- Remember ABC (Airway, Breathing, Circulation): 100% oxygen to improve tissue oxygenation
- ECG, cardiac monitor, pulse oximetry
- Insert two short and wide IV cannulae in the antecubital fossa (e.g., 16G). A central venous line may be required.
- Infuse 1 L of warm Hartmann's solution or, if severe hemorrhage, then start a colloid instead. Aim for a urinary output of 0.5 mL/kg/hr and maintenance of blood pressure.

- Check complete blood count (CBC), coagulation screen, and cardiac enzymes.
- Cross-match 6 units of blood.
- Obtain arterial blood gases (ABG) to assess oxygenation and pH.

Obvious and excessive blood loss may be seen from drains, but drains can also block, so assume there is covert bleeding if there is a tachycardia (and low blood pressure).

If this regimen fails to stabilize pulse and blood pressure, return the patient to the operating room for exploratory surgery.

Further reading

American College of Surgeons Committee on Trauma (1999). *Advanced Trauma Life Support for Doctors—Student Course Manual*, 6th Edition.

Patient safety in the operating room

It is a fundamental part of safe surgical practice to cross-check that the following have been done prior to starting an operation or procedure. The process of cross-checking should be done with another member of staff (time out).

- Patient identification. Confirm that you are operating on the right patient by a process of active identification (i.e., ask the patient their name, date of birth, and their address to confirm that you are talking to the correct patient).
- Ensure you are doing the correct procedure and on the correct side by cross-checking with the notes and X-rays. For lateralized procedures (e.g., nephrectomy, PCNL), the correct side of the operation should be confirmed by cross-checking with the X-rays and with the X-ray report, as well as referring to the notes. Where it is possible for the sides of an IVP to be incorrectly labeled, this cannot happen with a CT scan, where the location of the liver (right side) and the spleen (left side) provide confirmation of what side is what. In addition, the patient should have the correct side mark on their body by the operating surgical team in the holding area.
- Check that appropriate antibiotic prophylaxis has been given.
- Check that DVT prophylaxis has been administered (e.g., heparin, AK-TEDS, intermittent pneumatic compression boots).
- Ensure that blood is available, if appropriate.
- The patient should be safely and securely positioned on the operating table—pressure points are padded, not touching metal (to avoid diathermy burns), body straps are securely in place.

Develop an approach to operating that involves members of your team. Listen to the opinions of staff members who are junior to you. They may sometimes be able to identify errors that are not obvious to you.

Cultivate the respect of the recovery room staff. They may express concern about a patient under their care—listen to their concerns, take them seriously, and, if all is well, reassure them.

It does no harm to your patients or to your reputation for you to develop the habit of visiting every patient in the recovery room in order to check that all is well. You may be able to identify a problem before it has developed into a crisis, and, at the very least, you will gain a reputation for being a caring surgeon.

Transurethral resection (TUR) syndrome

TUR syndrome arises from the infusion of a large volume of hypotonic irrigating solution into the circulation during endoscopic procedures (e.g., TURP, TURBT, PCNL). It occurs in 0.5% of TURPs.

Pathophysiology

Biochemical, hemodynamic, and neurological disturbances occur:

- Dilutional hyponatremia is the most important—and serious—factor leading to the symptoms and signs. The serum sodium usually has to fall to <125 mmol/L before the patient becomes unwell.
- Hypertension is due to fluid overload.
- Visual disturbances may be due to the fact that glycine is a neurotransmitter in the retina.

Diagnosis—symptoms, signs, and tests

These include confusion, nausea, vomiting, hypertension, bradycardia and visual disturbances, and seizures. If the patient is awake (spinal anesthesia), they may report visual disturbances (e.g., flashing lights).

Preventing development of TUR syndrome and definitive treatment

Use a continuous irrigating cystoscope (provides low-pressure irrigation), limit resection time, avoid aggressive resection near the capsule, and reduce the height of the irrigant solution.[1]

For prolonged procedures, where a greater degree of fluid absorption may occur, measure serum Na and give 20–40 mg of IV furosemide to start off-loading the excess fluid that has been absorbed. If the serum sodium comes back as being normal, you will have done little harm by giving the furosemide, but if it comes back at <125mmol/L, you will have started treatment already and thereby may have prevented the development of severe TUR syndrome.

Techniques for measuring fluid overload (not commonly done)

- Weighing machines can be added to the ordinary operating table.[2]
- Adding a little alcohol to the irrigating fluid and constantly monitoring the expired air with a breathalyser[3] allows an estimation of the volume of excess fluid that has been absorbed.

1 Madsen PO, Naber KG (1973). The importance of the pressure in the prostatic fossa and absorption of irrigating fluid during transurethral resection of the prostate. J Urol 109:446–452.

2 Coppinger SW, Lewis CA, Milroy EJG (1995). A method of measuring fluid balance during transurethral resection of the prostate. Br J Urol 76:66–72.

3 Hahn RG (1993). Ethanol monitoring of extravascular absorption of irrigating fluid. Br J Urol 72:766–769.

Catheters and drains in urological surgery

Catheters

Catheters are made from Latex or Silastic (for patients with Latex allergy or for long-term use—better tolerated by the urethral mucosa).

Types

- *Self-retaining* (also known as a Foley, balloon, or two-way catheter) (Fig. 16.1). An inflation channel can be used to inflate and deflate a balloon at the end of the catheter, which prevents the catheter from falling out.
- *Three-way catheter* (also known as an irrigating catheter). Has a third channel (in addition to the balloon inflation and drainage channels) that allows fluid to be run into the bladder at the same time as it is drained from the bladder (Fig. 16.2).

Size

The size of a catheter is denoted by its circumference in millimeters. This is known as the "French" or "Charriere" (hence Fr) gauge. Thus a 12 Fr catheter has a circumference of 12 mm.

Uses

- Relief of obstruction (e.g., BOO due to BPE causing urinary retention—use the smallest catheter that you can pass; usually a 12 Fr or 14 Fr is sufficient in an adult)
- Irrigation of the bladder for clot retention (use a 20 Fr or 22 Fr three-way catheter)
- Drainage of urine to allow the bladder to heal if it has been opened (trauma or deliberately, as part of a surgical operation)
- Prevention of ureteric reflux, maintenance of a low bladder pressure, where the ureter has been stented (post-pyeloplasty for UPJ obstruction)
- To empty the bladder before an operation on the abdomen or pelvis (deflating the bladder gets it out of harm's way)
- Monitoring of urine output postoperatively or in the critical patient
- For delivery of bladder instillations (e.g., intravesical chemotherapy or immunotherapy)
- To allow identification of the bladder neck during surgery (e.g., radical prostatectomy, operations on or around the bladder neck)

Drains

Drains are principally indicated for prevention of accumulation of urine, blood, lymph, or other fluids. They are particularly used after the urinary tract has been opened and closed by suture repair.

A suture line takes some days to become completely watertight, and during this time urine leaks from the closure site. A drain prevents accumulation of urine (a urinoma), the very presence of which can cause an ileus, and if it becomes infected, an abscess can develop.

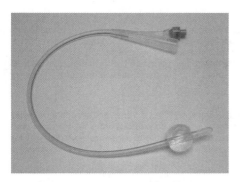

Figure 16.1 A Foley catheter with the balloon inflated.

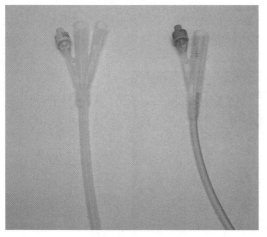

Figure 16.2 Two- and three-way catheters.

Tube drains

Tube drains (e.g., a Robinson drain) (Figs. 16.3 and 16.4) provide passive drainage (i.e., no applied pressure). They are used to drain suture lines at a site of repair or anastomosis of the urinary tract.

Avoid placing the drain tip on the suture line, as this may prevent healing of the repair. Suture it to adjacent tissues to prevent it from being dislodged.

Suction drains

Suction drains (e.g., Hemovac®) (Figs. 16.5 and 16.6) provide active drainage (i.e., air in the drainage bottle is evacuated, producing a negative pressure when connected to the drain tube to encourage evacuation of fluid). They are used for prevention of accumulation of blood (a hematoma) in superficial wounds.

Avoid using them in proximity to a suture line in the urinary tract—the suctioning effect may encourage continued flow of urine out of the hole, discouraging healing.

As a general principle, drains should be brought out through a separate stab wound, rather than through the main wound, since the latter may result in bacterial contamination of the main wound with subsequent risk of infection. Secure the drain with a silk suture to prevent it from inadvertently falling out.

To remove a urethral catheter that fails to deflate, see Box 16.2.

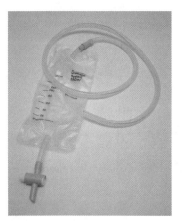

Figure 16.3 A Robinson (passive) drainage system.

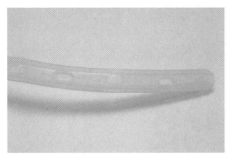

Figure 16.4 Note the eyeholes of the Robinson catheter.

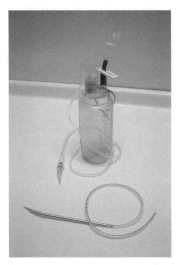

Figure 16.5 A Redivac suction drain showing the drain tubing attached to the needle used for insertion and the suction bottle.

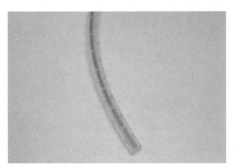

Figure 16.6 The eyeholes at the tip of the suction drain.

Box 16.2 Failure to deflate catheter balloon for removal of a urethral catheter

From time to time an inflated catheter balloon will not deflate when the time comes for removal of the catheter.

- Try inflating the balloon with air or water—this can dislodge an obstruction.
- Leave a 10 mL syringe firmly inserted in the balloon channel and come back an hour or so later.
- Try bursting the balloon by overinflation.
- Cut the end of the catheter off, proximal to the inflation valve—the valve may be stuck and the water may drain out of the balloon.
- In the female patient, introduce a needle alongside your finger into the vagina and burst the balloon by advancing the needle through the anterior vaginal and bladder wall.
- In male patients, balloon deflation with a needle can also be done under ultrasound guidance. Fill the bladder with saline using a bladder syringe so that the needle can be introduced percutaneously and directed toward the balloon of the catheter under ultrasound control.
- Pass a ureteroscope alongside the catheter and deflate the balloon with the rigid end of a guide wire or with a laser fiber (the end of which is sharp).

Guide wires

Guide wires are an essential tool for endourological procedures.

Uses

They are used as a track over which catheters or instruments can be passed into the ureter, collecting system of the kidney (retrograde or antegrade), or the bladder.

Types

Many different types of guide wire are available. They are classified according to their size, tip design, rigidity, and surface coating. These specific properties determine their use. All are radio-opaque so X-ray screening can be used to determine their position.

They come prepackaged in a coiled sheath to allow ease of handling and storage (Fig. 16.7).

Size

Size refers to diameter measured in inches (length is usually around 150 cm). The most common sizes are 0.035 inches and 0.038 inches. They are also available in 0.032 inches.

Tip design

The shape of the tip is either straight or angle (Fig. 16.8). A straight tip is usually adequate for most uses. Occasionally, an angle tip is useful for negotiating an impacted stone or for placing the guide wire in a specific position.

Similarly, a J-shaped tip can negotiate an impacted stone—the curved leading edge of this guide wire type can sometimes suddenly flick past the stone (in this situation, a straight guide wire can inadvertently perforate the ureter, thereby creating a false passage).

Surface coating

Most standard guide wires are coated with polytetrafluoroethylene (PTFE), which has a low coefficient of friction, thus allowing easy passage of the guide wire through the ureter and of instruments over them.

Some guide wires are coated with a polymer that when wet is very slippery (hydrophilic coating). In some cases, the entire length of the guide wire is so coated (e.g., Terumo Glidewire) and in others, just the tip (e.g., Sensor guide wire). The virtually friction-free surface of Glidewires makes them liable to slip out of the ureter, and they therefore make unreliable safety wires (they can be exchanged for a wire with greater friction via a ureteric catheter).

If allowed to become dry, these wires have a high coefficient of friction, which makes them difficult to manipulate.

Tip rigidity

The tip of all guide wires, over at least 3 cm, is soft and therefore flexible. This reduces—though does not completely remove—the risk of ureteric perforation.

Shaft rigidity

Stiff guide wires are easier to manipulate than floppy ones and help to straighten a tortuous ureter (e.g., Amplatz Ultrastiff is particularly useful for this). Very malleable wires such as the Terumo Glidewire can be very useful for passing an impacted stone (for the same reason as J-tip wires).

Some guide wires provide a combination of properties—a soft, floppy, hydrophilic-coated tip with the remainder of the guide wire being stiff (e.g., Sensor guide wire).

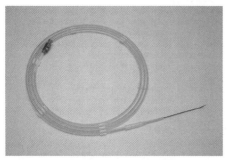

Figure 16.7 Guide wires come prepackaged in a sheath for ease of handling.

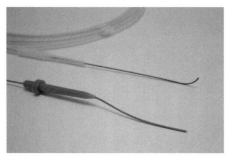

Figure 16.8 Examples of straight-tip and angle-tip guide wires.

Irrigating fluids and techniques of bladder washout

Glycine is used for endoscopic surgery requiring application of diathermy. Normal saline is used for the following:

- Irrigation of bladder following TURP, TURBT
- Irrigation during ureteroscopy, PCNL

Blocked catheter post -TURP and clot retention

To avoid catheter blockage following TURP, keep the catheter bag empty; ensure a sufficient supply of irrigant solution.

The bladder will be painfully distended. Irrigant flow will have stopped. A small clot may have blocked the catheter or a chip of prostate may have stuck in the eye of the catheter. Attach a bladder syringe to the end of the catheter and pull back (Fig. 16.9). This may suck out the clot or chip of prostate and flow may restart.

If it does not, draw some irrigant up into the syringe until it is about half-full and forcefully inject this fluid into the bladder. This may dislodge (and fragment) a clot that has stuck to the eye of the catheter.

If the problem persists, change the catheter. You may see the obstructing chip of prostate on the end of the catheter as it is withdrawn.

Blocked catheter post -TURBT

Use the same technique as for post-TURP catheter blockage, but avoid vigorous pressure on the syringe—the wall of the bladder will have been weakened at the site of tumor resection and it is possible to perforate the bladder, particularly in elderly women, who have thin bladder walls.

Blocked catheters following bladder augmentation or neobladder

The suture line of the augmented bladder is weak, and overvigorous bladder washouts can rupture the bladder.

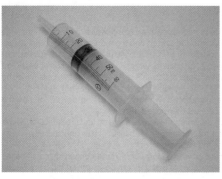

Figure 16.9 A bladder syringe—the tip is designed to fit onto a catheter.

JJ stents

These are hollow tubes, with a coil at each end, which are inserted through the bladder (usually), into the ureter, and from there into the renal pelvis. They are designed to bypass a ureteric obstruction (e.g., due to a stone) or drain the kidney (e.g., after renal surgery). They have a coil at each end (hence the alternative name of "double pigtail" stent—the coils have the configuration of a pig's tail—or the less accurate name of J stent).

JJ stents prevent migration downward (out of the ureter) or upward (into the ureter). They are therefore self-retaining.

They are made of polymers of variable strength and biodurability. Some stents have a hydrophilic coating that absorbs water and thereby makes them more slippery and easier to insert.

Stents are impregnated with barium- or bismuth-containing metallic salts to make them radio-opaque, so that they can be visualized radiographically to ensure correct positioning.

Types

Stents are classified by size and length. Common sizes are 6 Ch or 7 Ch (Fig. 16.10). Common lengths for adults are 22–28 cm. Multi-length stents are of variable length, allowing them to accommodate to ureters of different length.

Stent materials

These include polyurethane; silicone; C-flex; Silitek; Percuflex; and biodegradable material (the latter are experimental; they obviate the need for stent removal and eliminate the possibility of the "forgotten stent").

Indications and uses

- Relief of obstruction from ureteric stones, benign (i.e., ischemic) ureteric strictures, or malignant ureteric strictures. The stent will relieve the pain caused by obstruction and reverse renal impairment if present.
- Prevention of obstruction post-ureteroscopy
- Passive dilatation of ureter prior to ureteroscopy
- To ensure antegrade flow of urine following surgery (e.g., pyeloplasty) or injury to ureter
- Following endopyelotomy (endopyelotomy stents have a tapered end from 14 Fr. to 7 Fr., to keep the incised ureter open)

Symptoms and complications of stents

- Stent symptoms that are common include suprapubic pain, LUTS (frequency, urgency—stent irritates trigone), hematuria, and inability to work.
- Urinary tract infection. Development of bacteriuria after stenting is common. In a small proportion of patients sepsis can develop. In such cases, consider placement of a urethral catheter to lower the pressure in the collecting system and prevent reflux of infected urine.
- Incorrect placement: too high (distal end of stent in ureter; subsequent stent removal requires ureteroscopy; can be technically difficult;

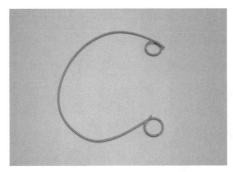

Figure 16.10 A JJ stent.

percutaneous removal may be required), or too low (proximal end not in renal pelvis; stent may not therefore relieve obstruction)
- Stent migration (up the ureter or down the ureter and into bladder)
- Stent blockage. Catheters and stents become coated with a biofilm when in contact with urine (a protein matrix secreted by bacteria-colonizing stent). Calcium, magnesium, and phosphate salts become deposited. Biofilm buildup can lead to stent blockage or stone formation on the stent (Fig. 16.11).
- The "forgotten stent is rare, but potentially very serious, as biofilm may become encrusted with stone, making removal technically very difficult. If the proximal end only is encrusted, PCNL may be required to remove the stone and then the stent. In some cases a combination of PCNL, ESWL, and ureteroscopy may be used. If the entire stent is encrusted, open removal via several incisions in the ureter may be necessary.

Commonly asked questions about stents

Does urine pass though the center of the stent?
No, it passes around the outside of the stent. Reflux of urine occurs through the center.

Should I place a JJ stent after ureteroscopy?
A stent should be placed if the following occur:
- There has been ureteric injury (e.g., perforation—indicated by extravasation of contrast)
- There are residual stones that might obstruct the ureter
- The patient has had a ureteric stricture that required dilatation

Routine stenting after ureteroscopy for distal ureteric calculi is unnecessary.[1] Many urologists will place a stent after ureteroscopy for proximal ureteric stones.

1 Srivastava A, et al. (2003). Routine stenting after ureteroscopy for distal ureteral calculi is unnecessary: results of a randomized controlled trial. *J Endourol* 17:871–874.

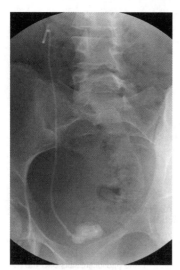

Figure 16.11 An encrusted stent.

Do stents cause obstruction?
In normal kidneys, stents cause a significant and substantial increase in intrarenal pressure that persists for up to 3 weeks.[1] (This can be prevented by placing a urethral catheter.)

Do stents aid stone passage?
Ureteric peristalsis requires coaptation of the wall of the ureter proximal to the bolus of urine to be transmitted down the length of the ureter. JJ stents paralyze ureteric peristalsis. In dogs, the amplitude of each peristaltic wave (measured by an intraluminal ureteric balloon) falls (from 50 to 15 mmHg) and the frequency of ureteric peristalsis falls (from 11 to 3 waves per minute).

Peristalsis takes several weeks to recover; 3 mm ball bearings placed within a nonstented dog ureter take 7 days to pass, compared with 24 days in a stented ureter.

Are stents able to relieve obstruction due to extrinsic compression of a ureter?
Stents are less effective at relieving obstruction due to extrinsic obstruction by, for example, tumor or retroperitoneal obstruction.[2] They are

1 Ramsay JW, et al. (1985). The effects of double J stenting on obstructed ureters. An experimental and clinical study. *Br J Urol* 57:630–634.
2 Docimo SG. (1989). High failure rate of indwelling ureteral stents in patients with extrinsic obstruction: experience at two institutions. *J Urol* 142:277–279.

much more effective for relieving obstruction by an intrinsic problem (e.g., a stone).

Placement of two stents may provide more effective drainage (figure-of-eight configuration may produce more space around the stents for drainage).

For acute, ureteric stone obstruction with a fever, should I place a JJ stent or a nephrostomy?

In theory, one might imagine that a nephrostomy is better than a JJ stent—it can be done under local anesthetic (JJ stent insertion may require a general anesthetic) and it lowers the pressure in the renal pelvis to 0 or a negative value. A JJ stent, by contrast, results in a persistently positive pressure, is less likely to be blocked by thick pus, and allows easier subsequent imaging (contrast can be injected down the ureter—a nephrostogram—to determine if the stone has passed).

In practice, both seem to be effective for relief of acute stone obstruction and associated infection.[3,4]

3 Pearle MS, et al. (1998). Optimal method of urgent decompression of the collecting system for obstruction and infection due to ureteral calculi. *J Urol* 160:1260–1264.
4 Ryan PC, et al. (1994). The effects of acute and chronic JJ stent placement on upper urinary tract motility and calculus transit. *Br J Urol* 74:434–439.

Lasers in urological surgery

Lasers involve light amplification by stimulated emission of radiation.

Photons are emitted when an atom is stimulated by an external energy source, and its electrons having been so excited revert to their steady state. In a laser the light is coherent (all the photons are in phase with one another), collimated (the photons travel parallel to each other), and of the same wavelength (monochromatic). The light energy is thus concentrated, allowing delivery of high energy at a desired target.

The holmium:YAG (yttrium aluminum garnet) laser is currently the principal urological laser. It has a wavelength of 2140 nm and is highly absorbed by water and thus by tissues, which are composed mainly of water. The majority of the holmium laser energy is absorbed superficially, resulting in a superficial cutting or ablation effect. The depth of the thermal effect is no greater than 1 mm.

The holmium:YAG laser produces a cavitation bubble that generates only a weak shock wave as it expands and collapses. Holmium laser lithotripsy occurs primarily through a photothermal mechanism that causes stone vaporization.

Lasers used in BPH treatments are summarized in Chapter 3 in the section entitled "Invasive Surgical Alternatives to TURP" (p. 86).

Uses

- Laser lithotripsy (ureteric stones, small intrarenal stones, bladder stones)
- Resection of the prostate (holmium laser prostatectomy)
- Division of urethral strictures
- Division of ureteric strictures, including PUJO
- Ablation of small bladder, ureteric, and intrarenal TCCs

Advantages

The holmium laser energy is delivered via a laser fiber (Fig. 16.12) that is thin enough to allow its use down a flexible instrument, without affecting the deflection of that instrument, and can therefore gain access to otherwise inaccessible parts of the kidney.

The zone of thermal injury adjacent to the tip of the laser fiber is limited to no more than 1 mm; the laser can safely be fired at a distance of 1 mm from the wall of the ureter.

A laser can be used for all stone types.

There is minimal stone migration effect because of minimal shock wave generation.

Disadvantages

- High cost
- Produces a dust cloud during stone fragmentation that temporarily obscures the view
- Can irreparably damage endoscopes if inadvertently fired near or within the scope
- Relatively slow stone fragmentation—the laser fiber must be "painted" over the surface of the stone to vaporize it.

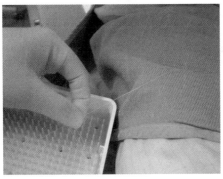

Figure 16.12 Holmium laser fiber.

Diathermy

Diathermy is the coagulation or cutting of tissues through heat.

Monopolar diathermy

When an electric current passes between two contacts on the body, there is an increase in temperature in the tissues through which the current flows. This increase in temperature depends on the volume of tissue through which the current passes, the resistance of the tissues, and the strength of the current. The stronger the current, the greater the rise in temperature.

If one contact is made large, the heat is dissipated over a wide area and the rise of temperature is insignificant. This is the earth or neutral electrode, and under this the rise in temperature is only 1 or 2°C. The working electrode or diathermy loop is thin, so that the current density is maximal and, therefore, so is the heating effect.

When a direct current is switched on or off, nerves are stimulated and muscles will twitch. If the switching on and off is rapid enough, there is the sustained contraction familiar to the physiology class as the tetanic contraction. If a high-frequency alternating current is used (300 kHz to 5 MHz), there is no time for the cell membranes of nerve or muscle to become depolarized, and nerves and muscles are not stimulated (they are stimulated at lower frequencies).

The effect of the diathermy current on the tissues depends on the heat generated under the diathermy loop. At relatively low temperatures, coagulation and distortion of small blood vessels occurs. If the current is increased to raise the temperature further, water within cells vaporizes and the cells explode. This explosive vaporization literally cuts the tissues apart.

Bipolar diathermy

Bipolar diathermy involves the passage of electrical current between two electrodes on the same handpiece. It is inherently safer than monopolar diathermy, since the current does not pass through the patient, and diathermy burns cannot therefore occur.

Potential problems with diathermy

The diathermy isn't working

• Do not increase the current.
• Check that the irrigating fluid is glycine (sodium chloride conducts electricity, causing the diathermy to short-circuit).
• Check that the diathermy plate is making good contact with the skin of the patient.
• Check that the lead is undamaged.
• Check that the resectoscope loop is securely fixed to the contact.

Modern diathermy machines have warning circuits that sound an alarm when there is imperfect contact between the earth plate and the patient.

Diathermy burns

If current returns to earth through a small contact rather than the broad area of the earth pad, then the tissues through which the current passes will be heated just like those under the cutting loop. If the pad is making good contact, the current will find it easier to run to earth through the pad and no harm will arise, even when there is accidental contact with some metal object.

The real danger arises when the diathermy pad is not making good contact with the patient. It may not be plugged in, or its wire may be broken. Under these circumstances the current must find its way to earth somehow, and any contact may then become the site of a dangerous rise in temperature.

Pacemakers and diathermy

See Box 16.3 for diathermy problems and their prevention.

Box 16.3 Pacemakers and diathermy: problems and their prevention

- *Pacemaker inhibition.* The high frequency of diathermy current may simulate the electrical activity of myocardial contraction so the pacemaker can be inhibited. If the patient is pacemaker dependent, the heart may stop.
- *Phantom reprogramming.* The diathermy current may also simulate the radiofrequency impulse by which the pacemaker can be reprogrammed to different settings. The pacemaker may then start to function in an entirely different mode.
- The *internal mechanism* of the pacemaker may be *damaged* by the diathermy current if this is applied close to the pacemaker.
- *Ventricular fibrillation.* If the diathermy current is channeled along the pacemaker lead, ventricular fibrillation may be induced.
- *Myocardial damage.* Another potential effect of channeling of the diathermy current along the pacemaker lead is burning of the myocardium at the tip of the pacemaker lead. This can subsequently result in ineffective pacing.

It was formerly recommended that a magnet be placed over the pacemaker to overcome pacemaker inhibition and to make the pacemaker function at a fixed rate. This can, however, result in phantom reprogramming. For demand pacemakers, it is better to program the pacemaker to a fixed rate (as opposed to demand pacing) for the duration of the operation. Consult the patient's cardiologist for advice.

Other precautions

- The patient plate should be sited such that the current path does not go right through the pacemaker. Ensure that the indifferent plate is correctly applied, as an improper connection can cause grounding of the diathermy current through the ECG monitoring leads, and this can affect pacemaker function. The indifferent plate should be placed as close as possible to the prostate (e.g., over the thigh or buttock).
- The diathermy machine should be placed well away from the pacemaker and should certainly not be used within 15 cm of it.
- The heartbeat should be continually monitored, and a defibrillator and external pacemaker should be at hand.
- Try to use short bursts of diathermy at the lowest effective output.
- Give antibiotic prophylaxis (as for patients with artificial heart valves).
- Because the pacemaker-driven heart will not respond to fluid overload in the normal way, the resection should be as quick as possible, and fluid overload should be avoided.

Sterilization of urological equipment

Techniques for sterilization

Autoclaving

Modern cystoscopes and resectoscopes, including components such as light leads, are autoclavable. Standard autoclave regimens heat the instruments to 121°C for 15 minutes or 134°C for 3 minutes.

Chemical sterilization

This involves soaking instruments in an aqueous solution of chlorine dioxide (Cidex), an aldehyde-free chemical (there has been a move away from formaldehyde because of health and environmental concerns). Chlorine dioxide solutions kill bacteria, viruses (including HIV and hepatitis B and C), spores, and mycobacteria.

Cameras cannot be autoclaved. Use a camera sleeve or sterilize the camera between cases.

Sterilization and prion diseases

Variant Creutzfeldt Jakob disease (vCJD) is a neurodegenerative disease caused by a prion protein (PrP). Other examples of neurodegenerative prion diseases include classic CJD, kuru, sheep scrapie, and bovine spongiform encephalopathy (BSE). Variant CJD and BSE are caused by the same prion strain and represent a classic example of cross-species transmission of a prion disease.

There has been much recent concern about the potential for transmission of vCJD between patients via contaminated surgical instruments. Classic CJD may be transmitted by neurosurgical and other types of surgical instruments because normal hospital sterilization procedures do not completely inactivate prions.[1] It is not possible at present to quantify the risks of transmission of prion diseases by surgical instruments. To date, iatrogenic CJD remains rare, with 267 cases having been reported worldwide, up to the year 2000.[2]

The risk of transmission of CJD may be higher with procedures performed on organs containing lymphoreticular tissue, such as tonsillectomy and adenoidectomy, because vCJD targets these tissues and is found in high concentrations there. For this reason there was a move toward the use of disposable, once-only-use instruments for procedures such as tonsillectomy. However, these instruments have been associated with a higher postoperative hemorrhage rate.[3]

Prions are particularly resistant to conventional chemical (ethylene oxide, formaldehyde, and chlorine dioxide) and standard autoclave regimens, and dried blood or tissue remaining on an instrument could harbor prions that will not then be killed by the sterilization process. Once

---

1 Collinge J (1999). Variant Creutzfeldt-Jakob disease. *Lancet* 354:317–323.
2 Collins SJ, Lawson VA, Masters CL (2004). Transmissible spongiform encephalopathies. *Lancet* 363:51–61.
3 Nix P (2003). Prions and disposable surgical instruments. *Int J Clin Pract* 57:678–680.

proteinaceous material such as blood or tissue has dried on an instrument, it is very difficult to subsequently be sure that the instrument has been sterilized.[4] Sterilization should include the following:

- *Presterilization cleaning:* Initial low-temperature washing (<35°C) with detergents and an ultrasonic cleaning system removes and prevents coagulation of prion proteins—sonic cleaners essentially shake attached material from the instrument.
- Hot wash
- Air drying
- *Thermal sterilization:* Longer autoclave cycles at 134–137°C for at least 18 minutes (or 6 successive cycles with holding times of 3 minutes) or 1 hour at conventional autoclave temperatures may result in a substantial reduction in the level of contamination with prions.

The latest models of presterilization cleaning devices—automated thermal washer disinfectors—perform all of these cleaning tasks within one unit.
  Enzymatic proteolytic inactivation methods are under development.

4 The Advisory Committee on Dangerous Pathogens and Spongiform Encephalopathy (1998). Transmissible spongiform encephalopathy agents: safe working and the prevention of infection. London: HM Stationery Office.

Telescopes and light sources in urological endoscopy

There are three types of modern urological telescopes—rigid, semi-rigid, and flexible. These endoscopes may be used for inspection of the urethra and bladder (cystoscourethroscopes, usually simply called cystoscopes), the ureter and collecting system of the kidney (ureteroscopes and ureterorenoscopes) and, via a percutaneous access track, the kidney (nephroscopes).

The light sources and image transmission systems are based on the innovative work of Professor Harold Hopkins, University of Reading.

The Hopkins rod-lens system

The great advance in telescope design was the development of the rod-lens telescope, which replaced the conventional system of glass lens with rods of glass, separated by thin air spaces that essentially were air lenses (Fig. 16.13). By changing the majority of the light transmission medium from air to glass, the quantity of light that could be transmitted was doubled. The rods of glass were also easier to handle during manufacture, and therefore their optical quality was greater.

The angle of view of the telescope can be varied by placing a prism behind the objective lens. 0°, 12°, 30° and 70° scopes are available.

Lighting

Modern endoscopes (urological and those used to image the gastrointestinal tract) use fiber-optic light bundles to transmit light to the organ being inspected. Each glass fiber is coated with glass of a different refractive index so that light entering at one end is totally internally reflected and emerges at the other end (Fig. 16.14).

These fiber-optic bundles can also be used for image (as well as light) transmission, as long as the arrangement of the fibers at either end of the instrument is the same (coordinated fiber bundles are not required for simple light transmission). The fiber bundles are tightly bound together only at their end (for coordinated image transmission). In the middle, the bundles are not bound—this makes the instrument flexible (e.g., flexible cystoscope and flexible ureteroscope).

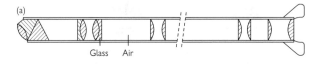

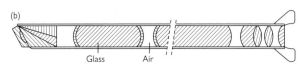

Figure 16.13 (a) Diagram of conventional cystoscope. The glass lenses are held in place by metal spacers and separated by air spaces. (b) Rod-lens telescope with "lenses" of air, separated by "spaces" of glass, with no need for metal spacers. Reprinted with permission from Blandy J, Fowler C (1996) *Urology*. Wiley-Blackwell, pp. 3–5.

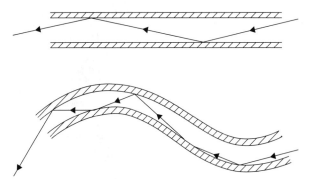

Figure 16.14 Total internal reflection permits light to travel along a flexible glass fiber. Reprinted with permission from Blandy J, Fowler C (1996) *Urology*. Wiley-Blackwell, pp. 3–5.

Consent: general principles

Consent is required before you examine, treat, or care for a competent adult (a person age 16 or older).

Think of obtaining consent as a *process* rather than as an *event*. In order to give consent, a patient must understand the nature, purpose, and likely effects (outcomes, risks) of the treatment. From the information they receive, the patient must be able to weigh the risks against the benefits and so arrive at an informed choice. They must not be coerced into making a decision (e.g., by the doctor in a hurry). Giving the patient time to reach a decision is a good way of avoiding any accusation that they were pressured into a decision.

To reiterate—think of consent as a *process* rather than as an *event*.

Giving information

How much information should you give? What options and risks should you mention? A doctor is not guilty of negligence if he or she acted in accordance with a practice accepted by a responsible body of medical people skilled in that particular art. (That body of medical people must be a competent and reasonable body and the opinion expressed must have a logical basis—the *Bolitho* modification of the *Bolam* defense.)

You have a duty to discuss the range of treatment options available (the alternatives), regardless of their cost, in a form the patient can understand, as well as the side effects and risks that are relevant to the *individual patient's* circumstances.

A *risk* is defined as a material one (one that matters, one that is important) if a reasonable person in the patient's circumstances, if warned of that risk, would attach significance to it (e.g., loss of the tip of a little finger may be of little long-term consequence to many people, but for the concert pianist it could be a disaster). Thus, the amount and type of information you give is different in every case.

Remember, it can be argued that the consent was not valid because the amount of information you gave was not enough or was in a form the patient could not understand.

Recording

Remember to record the consent discussion in the notes. If you do not record what you said, you might as well not bother saying it. If a patient later claims that they were not told of a particular risk or outcome, it will be difficult to refute this if your notes do not record what you said.

Writing "risks explained" is inadequate. When cases do come to court, this is usually several years after the events in question. You will have forgotten precisely what you said to the patient and it will not take much effort of a lawyer to suggest that you might not have said everything that you thought you said. If you give a written information sheet, record that you have done so and put a copy of the version you gave in the notes.

The consent form

The consent form is designed to record the patient's decision and, to some extent, the discussions that took place during the consent process (although the space available for recording the discussion, even on the consent form, is limited). It is not proof that the patient was properly informed—that valid consent was obtained.

Avoid, if possible, technical abbreviations such as TURBT. A patient could reasonably claim not to have understood what this was.

Try to avoid standing over the patient, waiting for them to sign the form. It is good practice to leave the form with the patient and to return after a few minutes—they will feel less pressured and can ask further questions if they wish.

Children

Children less than 16 years of age may give consent as long as they fully understand what is involved in the proposed examination or treatment (a parent cannot override the competent child's consent to treatment).

However, a child cannot *refuse* consent to treatment (i.e., a parent can override a child's refusal to consent—the parent can consent on the child's behalf if the child refuses consent, though such situations are rare).

Cystoscopy

Cycstoscopy is a basic skill of the urologist. It allows direct visual inspection of the urethra and bladder.

Indications
- Hematuria
- Irritative LUTS (marked frequency and urgency) where intravesical pathology is suspected (e.g., carcinoma in situ, bladder stone)
- For bladder biopsy
- Follow-up surveillance of patients with previously diagnosed and treated bladder cancer
- Retrograde insertion of ureteric stents and removal
- Cystoscopic removal of stones

Technique

Flexible cystoscopy
A flexible cystosope is easily passed down the urethra and into the bladder following instillation of lubricant gel (with or without local anesthetic). This is principally diagnostic, but small biopsies can be taken with a flexible biopsy forceps, small tumors can be fulgurated (with a diathermy probe) or vaporized (with a laser fiber), and JJ stents can be inserted and removed using this type of cystoscope.

Rigid cystoscopy
This is a rigid, metal instrument that can be passed under local anesthetic in women (short urethra), but usually requires general anesthetic. It is preferred over flexible cystoscopy when deeper biopsies will be required or as an antecedent to TURBT or cystolitholapaxy when it is anticipated that other pathology will be found (tumor, stone).

The flexible cystoscope uses fiber optics for illumination and image transmission. It can be deflected through 270°.

Common postoperative complications and their management
Mild burning discomfort and hematuria are common after both flexible and rigid cystoscopy. These usually resolve within hours.

Procedure specific consent form—recommended discussion of adverse events

Serious or frequently occurring complications of flexible cystoscopy
Warn the patient that if the cystoscopy is being done because of hematuria, it is possible that a bladder cancer may be found, which may require further treatment. You should specifically seek consent for biopsy (removal of tissue if an abnormality is found).

Common
- Mild burning or bleeding on passing urine for a short period after operation
- Biopsy of an abnormal area in the bladder may be required.

Occasional
- Infection of bladder requiring antibiotics

Rare
- Temporary insertion of a catheter
- Delayed bleeding requiring removal of clots or further surgery
- Injury to urethra causing delayed scar formation (a stricture)

Serious or frequently occurring complications of rigid cystoscopy
- As for flexible cystoscopy
- Use of heat (diathermy) may be required to cauterize biopsy sites.
- Very rarely, perforation of the bladder can occur, requiring temporary insertion of a catheter or open surgical repair.

Transurethral resection of the prostate (TURP)

Indications
- Bothersome LUTS that fail to respond to changes in lifestyle or medical therapy
- Recurrent acute urinary retention
- Renal impairment due to bladder outlet obstruction (high-pressure *chronic* urinary retention)
- Recurrent hematuria due to benign prostatic enlargement
- Bladder stones due to prostatic obstruction

Postoperative care
A three-way catheter is left in situ after the operation, through which irrigation fluid (normal saline) is run to dilute the blood so that a clot will not form to block the catheter. The rate of inflow of the saline is adjusted to keep the outflow a pale pink rosé color and, as a rule, the rate of inflow can be cut down after about 20 minutes. The irrigation is continued for ~12–24 hours.

The catheter is removed the day after (second postoperative day) if the urine has cleared to a normal color (trial without catheter [TWOC] or trial of void [TOV]).

Common postoperative complications and their management

Blocked catheter post-TURP
This is common. The catheter may become blocked with clot or a prostatic chip that was inadvertently left in the bladder at the end of the operation.
- Apply a bladder syringe to the end of the catheter to try to dislodge the obstruction.
- If this fails, withdraw some irrigant into the syringe and flush the catheter.
- If this fails, change the catheter. The obstructing chip of prostate may be found stuck in one of the eyeholes of the catheter.
- Pass a new catheter, on an introducer.

If the bladder has been allowed to become so full of clot that a simple bladder washout is unable to evacuate it all, return the patient to the operating room for clot evacuation.

Hemorrhage
Minor bleeding after TURP is common and will stop spontaneously. A simple system to allow communication between staff is to describe the color of the urine draining through the catheter as the same as a rosé wine (minor hematuria), a dark red wine (moderate hematuria), or frank blood (bright red bleeding, suggesting serious hemorrhage).

The rosé urine requires no action. Dark red urine should be managed by increasing the flow of irrigant and by applying gentle traction to the catheter (with the balloon inflated to 40–50 mL), thereby pulling it onto the bladder neck or into the prostatic fossa to tamponade bleeding for 20 minutes or so. This will usually result in the urine clearing.

An attempt at controlling heavier bleeding by these techniques may be tried, but at the same time you should make preparations to return the patient to the operating room because it is unlikely that bleeding of this degree will stop. The bleeding vessel(s), if seen, is controlled with diathermy.

If bleeding persists, open surgical control is required—the prostatic capsule is opened, the bleeding vessels sutured, and the prostatic bed packed. Postoperative bleeding requiring a return to the operating room occurs in ~0.5% of cases.[1]

Procedure-specific consent form—recommended discussion of adverse events

Serious or frequently occurring complications of TURP

- Temporary mild burning on passing urine, urinary frequency, hematuria
- Retrograde ejaculation in 75% of patients
- Failure of symptom resolution
- Permanent inability to achieve an erection adequate for sexual activity
- UTI requiring antibiotic therapy
- 10% of patients require re-do surgery for recurrent prostatic obstruction
- Failure to pass urine after the postoperative catheter has been removed
- In ~10% of patients, prostate cancer is found on subsequent pathological examination of the resected tissue.
- Urethral stricture formation requiring subsequent treatment
- Incontinence (loss of urinary control)—may be temporary or permanent
- Absorption of irrigating fluid causing confusion and heart failure (TUR syndrome)
- Very rarely, perforation of the bladder requiring a temporary urinary catheter or open surgical repair

Alternative therapy

This includes observation, drugs, a catheter, stent, or open operation.

1 Ryan PC, et al. (1994). The effects of acute and chronic JJ stent placement on upper urinary tract motility and calculus transit. *Br J Urol* 74:434–439.

Transurethral resection of bladder tumor (TURBT)

Indications
- Local control of non-muscle-invasive bladder cancer (i.e., stops bleeding tumors)
- Staging of bladder cancer—to determine whether the cancer is non-muscle invasive or muscle invasive, so that subsequent treatment and appropriate follow-up can be arranged

Postoperative care
A two- or three-way catheter is left in situ after the operation, depending on the size of the tumor and, therefore, on the likelihood that bleeding requiring irrigation will be required. As for TURP, normal saline is run through the catheter to dilute the blood so that a clot will not form to block the catheter. It is particularly important to avoid catheter blockage post-TURBT, since this could lead to distension of the bladder already weakened by resection of a tumor.

The period of irrigation is usually shorter than that required after TURP, and for small tumors the catheter may be removed the day after the TURBT. For larger tumors, remove it 2 days later.

Common operative and postoperative complications and their management

Bladder perforation during TURBT
Small perforations into the perivesical tissues (extraperitoneal) are not uncommon when resecting small tumors of the bladder. So long as you have secured good hemostasis and all the irrigating fluid is being recovered, no additional steps are required, except that perhaps one should leave the catheter in for 4 rather than 2 days.

Intraperitoneal perforations (through the wall of the bladder, through the peritoneum, and into the peritoneal cavity) are uncommon, but far more serious.

Is it an extraperitoneal or intraperitoneal perforation? Establishing this can be difficult. Both can cause marked distension of the lower abdomen—an intraperitoneal perforation by allowing escape of irrigating solution directly into the abdominal cavity, and an extraperitoneal perforation by expanding the retroperitoneal space, with fluid then diffusing directly into the peritoneal cavity.

The fact that a suspected intraperitoneal perforation was actually extraperitoneal becomes apparent only at laparotomy when no hole can be found in the peritoneum overlying the bladder (the peritoneum over the bladder is *not* breached in an extraperitoneal perforation).

When there is no abdominal distension, the volume of extravasated fluid is likely to be low and, if the perforation is small, it is reasonable to manage the case conservatively. Achieve hemostasis and pass a catheter.

Make frequent postoperative assessments of the patient's vital signs and abdomen (worsening abdominal pain, distension, and tenderness suggest the need for laparotomy).

Where there is marked abdominal distension, regardless of whether the perforation is extraperitoneal or intraperitoneal, explore the abdomen, principally to drain the large amount of fluid (which can compromise respiration in an elderly patient) by splinting the diaphragm, but also to check that loops of bowel adjacent to the site of perforation have not been injured at the same time.

Failing to make the diagnosis of an intraperitoneal perforation, particularly if bowel has been injured, is a worse situation than performing a laparotomy for a suspected intraperitoneal perforation but then finding that the perforation was "only" extraperitoneal.

Open bladder repair

Use a Pfannenstiel incision or lower midline abdominal incision, open the bladder, evacuate the clot, control bleeding, and repair the hole. Open the peritoneum and inspect the small and large bowel for perforations. Leave a urethral catheter and a drain in place.

Blocked catheter post-TURBT

The catheter may become blocked with clot. Use the same technique for unblocking it as for TURP, but avoid vigorous washouts of the bladder because of the risk of bladder perforation.

Hemorrhage

Minor bleeding after TURBT is common and will stop spontaneously. The only technique for controlling it is to ensure adequate flow of irrigant is maintained (to dilute the blood and thereby prevent clots from forming). If bleeding persists, return the patient to the OR for endoscopic control.

TUR syndrome

This is uncommon after TURBT, unless the tumor is large and the resection therefore long.

Procedure-specific consent form—recommended discussion of adverse events

Serious or frequently occurring complications of TURBT

Common complications
- Mild burning on passing urine
- Additional treatment (intravesical chemotherapy or immunotherapy) may be required to reduce the risk of future tumor recurrence.
- UTI
- No guarantee of bladder cancer cure
- Tumor recurrence is common.

Rare complications
- Delayed bleeding requiring removal of clots or further surgery
- Damage to drainage tubes from kidney (ureters) requiring additional therapy
- Development of a urethral stricture
- Bladder perforation requiring a temporary urinary catheter or open surgical repair

Alternative treatment includes open removal of bladder, chemotherapy, and radiation.

Optical urethrotomy

Indications
• Short (<1 cm) bulbar urethral strictures (longer and recurrent strictures are now best treated by open urethroplasty incorporating excision and/or grafts—usually buccal mucosa—or penile skin flaps)

Anesthesia
Use regional or general anesthetic.

Postoperative care
• Leave a catheter for 3–5 days (longer catheterization does not reduce long-term restricturing).

Common postoperative complications and their management
• Septicemia
• Restricturing is the most common long-term problem occurring after optical urethrotomy.

Procedure-specific consent form—recommended discussion of adverse events

Common
• Mild burning on passing urine for short periods of time after operation
• Temporary insertion of a catheter
• Need for self-catheterization to keep the narrowing from closing down again

Occasional
• Infection of bladder, requiring antibiotics
• Permission for telescopic removal if stone is found, biopsy of bladder abnormality
• Recurrence of stricture necessitating further procedures or repeat incision

Rare
• Decrease in quality of erections, requiring treatment

Alternative therapy includes observation, urethral dilatation, and open (nontelescopic) repair of stricture.

Circumcision

Indications
- Phimosis
- Recurrent paraphimosis
- Penile cancer confined to the foreskin
- Lesions on the foreskin of uncertain histological nature

Anesthesia
Local or general anesthetic can be used.

Postoperative care
A nonadhesive dressing may be applied to the end of the penis, but this is difficult to keep on for more than an hour or two and is unnecessary. Warn the patient that the penis may be bruised and swollen after the operation, but that this resolves spontaneously over a week or two.

Common postoperative complications and their management
You might think that circumcision is about as simple an operation as you can get, but it can cause both the patient (or, in the case of little boys, their parents) and you considerable concern if the cosmetic result is not what was expected, or if complications occur about which the patient was not warned.

As with any procedure, it should be performed with care and with the potential complications always in mind so that steps can be taken to avoid these. If complications do occur, manage them appropriately.

Hemorrhage
Most frequently this occurs from the frenular artery on the ventral surface of the penis. If local pressure does not stop the bleeding (and if it is from the frenular artery, it usually won't), return the patient to the operating room and, either under ring-block local anesthesia or general anesthetic, suture ligature the bleeding vessel.

Be careful not to place the suture through the urethra!

Necrosis of the skin of the shaft of the penis
In most cases of suspected skin necrosis, there is none. Not infrequently, a crust of coagulated blood develops around the circumference of the penis after circumcision. As blood oxidizes it turns black and this appearance can be mistaken for necrosis of the end of the penis. Reassurance of the patient (and the referring doctor!) is all that is needed.

If necrosis has occurred because, for example, adrenaline was used in the local anesthetic, wait for the necrotic tissue to demarcate before assessing the extent of the problem. The penis has a superb blood supply and has remarkable healing characteristics.

Separation of the skin of the coronal sulcus from the shaft skin
If limited to a small area this will heal spontaneously. If a larger circumference of the wound has dehisced, resuture in the operating room.

Wound infection is rare.

Urethrocutaneous fistula is due to hemostatic sutures (placed to control bleeding from the frenular) passing through the urethra, the wound later breaking down.

Urethral damage is due to a stitch placed through the urethra as the frenular artery is suture ligatured.

Excessive removal of skin

Re-epithelialization can occur if the defect between the glans and shaft skin is not too great. If the defect is too great, the end result will be a buried penis—the glans retracts toward the skin at the base of the penis.

Procedure-specific consent form—recommended discussion of adverse events

Serious or frequently occurring complications of circumcision

- Bleeding of the wound occasionally needing a further procedure
- Infection of incision requiring further treatment
- Permanent altered sensation of the penis
- Persistence of absorbable stitches after 3–4 weeks, requiring removal
- Scar tenderness, rarely long-term
- You may not be completely cosmetically satisfied
- Occasional need for removal of excessive skin at a later date
- Permission for biopsy of abnormal area of glans if malignancy a concern

Alternative therapy includes drugs to relieve inflammation or leaving the penis uncircumcised.

Hydrocele and epididymal cyst removal

Hydrocele repair (removal)

Indications include primary (idiopathic) hydrocele repair; this is not indicated for secondary hydrocele repair.

Anesthesia: local or general

Techniques
- Lord's plication technique—for small to medium-sized hydroceles (minimal interference with surrounding scrotal tissues, which minimizes risk of postoperative hematoma)
- Jaboulay procedure—for large hydroceles. Excision of hydrocele sac

Hydrocele aspiration
Strict attention to asepsis is vital, since introduction of infection into a closed space could lead to abscess formation. Avoid superficial blood vessels (if you hit them, a large hematoma can result).

Postoperative care involves nothing specific.

Postoperative complications and their management
- Scrotal swelling, which resolves spontaneously
- Hematoma formation. If it is large, surgical drainage is best performed, as spontaneous resolution may take many weeks. It can be difficult to identify the bleeding vessel. Leave a small drain to prevent reaccumulation of the hematoma.
- Hydrocele recurrence

Epididymal cyst removal (spermatocelectomy)
- Avoid in young men who wish to maintain fertility, since epididymal obstruction can occur.
- An alternative to surgical removal is aspiration, though recurrence is usual.

Procedure-specific consent form—recommended discussion of adverse events

Hydrocele removal
Occasional
- Recurrence of fluid collection can occur.
- Collection of blood around the testes which resolves slowly or requires surgical removal
- Possible infection of incision or testis requiring further treatment

Alternative therapy
- Observation
- Removal of fluid with a needle

Epididymal cyst removal

Occasional

- Recurrence of fluid collection can occur
- Collection of blood around the testes which resolves slowly or requires surgical removal
- Possible infection of incision or testis requiring further treatment.

Rare

- Scarring can damage the epididymis, causing infertility

Alternative therapy includes observation; removal of fluid with a needle.

Nesbit procedure

This is a penile straightening procedure for correcting penile curvature. Wait for at least 6 months after the patient has experienced no more pain, and wait for the penile curvature to stabilize (there is no point in repairing the curvature if it is still progressing).

Indications

This procedure can used in Peyronie's disease for men with deformity who still obtain rigid erections.

Anesthesia

Local or general anesthetic can be used.

Postoperative care

The patient should avoid intercourse for 2 months. Edema can be managed with cold compresses.

Procedure-specific consent form—recommended discussion of adverse events

Serious or frequently occurring complications

Common

- Some mild shortening of the penis
- Possible dissatisfaction with the cosmetic or functional result
- Temporary swelling and bruising of the penis and scrotum

Occasional

- Circumcision is sometimes required as part of the procedure.
- There is no guarantee of total correction of the bend.
- Bleeding or infection may require further treatment.

Rare

- Impotence or difficulty maintaining an erection
- Nerve injury with temporary or permanent numbness of penis

Alternative treatment includes observation, drugs, and other surgical procedures plication and graft procedures.

Vasectomy and vasovasostomy

Vasectomy

This is the removal of a section of the vas deferens from each side with the aim of achieving infertility.

Indications: a method of birth control

Anesthesia: local or general

Postoperative care and common postoperative complications and their management

Postoperative hematoma can occur. If large, evacuation may be required. Infection can occur, but is usually superficial.

Two semen samples are required, usually at 10 and 12 weeks post-vasectomy, before unprotected intercourse can take place. Viable sperm can remain distal to the site of vasectomy (in the distal vas deferens or seminal vesicles) for some weeks after vasectomy, and even longer.

Occasionally, a persistently positive semen analysis is an indication that the vas was not correctly identified at the time of surgery and has not been ligated (or, very rarely, that there were two vas deferens on one side). The potential for fertility remains in those with positive semen analysis, and re-exploration is indicated. Warn the patient that the vas deferens can later recanalize, thereby restoring fertility.

Sperm granuloma is a hard, pea-sized lump in the region of the cut ends of the vas, forming as a result of an inflammatory response to sperm leaking out of the proximal cut end of the vas. It can be a cause of persistent pain, in which case it may have to be excised or evacuated and the vas cauterized or re-ligated.

Vasovasostomy

This is vasectomy reversal.

Anesthesia

This tends to be done under general or spinal anesthesia, as it takes far longer than a vasectomy.

Postoperative care and common postoperative complications and their management

They are much the same as for vasectomy. The patient should avoid sexual intercourse for 2 weeks or so.

Vasectomy: procedure-specific consent form— recommended discussion of adverse events

Serious or frequently occurring complications

Common

- Irreversible
- Small amount of scrotal bruising
- Two semen samples are required before unprotected intercourse, both of which must show no spermatozoa.

Occasional
- Bleeding requiring further surgery or bruising

Rare
- Inflammation or infection of testis or epididymis, requiring antibiotics
- Rejoining of vas ends resulting in fertility and pregnancy (1 in 2000)
- Chronic testicular pain (5%) or sperm granuloma

Alternative treatment is other forms of contraception (male or female).

Vasovasostomy: procedure-specific consent form—recommended discussion of adverse events

Serious or frequently occurring complications

Common
- Small amount of scrotal bruising
- No guarantee that sperm will return to semen
- Sperm may return but pregnancy is not always achieved
- If storing sperm, check that appropriate forms have been filled out

Occasional
- Bleeding requiring further surgery

Rare
- Inflammation or infection of testes or epididymis, requiring antibiotics
- Chronic testicular pain (5%) or sperm granuloma

Alternative therapy includes IVF, sperm aspiration, and ICSI.

Orchiectomy

Indications

There are two types—radical orchiectomy and simple orchiectomy.

Radical (inguinal) orchiectomy

This is done for excision of testicular cancer. This approach is used for three reasons:

- To allow ligation of the testicular lymphatics as high as possible as they pass in the spermatic cord and through the internal inguinal ring, thereby removing any cancer cells that might have started to metastasize along the cord.
- To allow cross-clamping of the cord prior to manipulation of the testis which, theoretically at least, could promote dissemination of cancer cells along the lymphatics (In reality, this probably doesn't occur.)
- To prevent the potential for dissemination of tumor cells into the lymphatics that drain the scrotal skin that could occur if a scrotal approach is used. These lymphatics drain to inguinal nodes. Thus, direct spread of tumor to scrotal skin and violation of another lymphatic field (the groin nodes) is avoided. Historically, this was important because the only adjuvant therapy for metastatic disease was radiotherapy. The morbidity of groin and scrotal irradiation was not inconsiderable (severe skin reactions to radiotherapy, irradiation of femoral artery and nerve).

Obtain serum markers before surgery (α-fetoprotein, β-hCG, and lactic acid dehydrogenase [LDH]) and get a CXR. A full staging CT scan can wait until after surgery. If the contralateral testis has been removed or is small, offer sperm storage—there is usually time to do this.

Warn the patient that, very occasionally, what appears clinically and on ultrasound to be a malignant testis tumor turns out to be a benign tumor on subsequent histological examination.

Simple orchiectomy

This is done for hormonal control of advanced prostate cancer, via a scrotal incision, with ligation and division of the cord and complete removal of the testis and epididymis.

Alternatively, a subcapsular orchiectomy may be done, where the tunica of the testis is incised and the seminiferous tubules contained within are excised. There is the potential with this approach to leave a small number of Leydig cells that can continue to produce testosterone.

Anesthesia

Local, regional, and general anesthesia can be used. Few men will require or opt for local anesthetic.

Postoperative care and common postoperative complications and their management

For both simple and radical orchiectomy

Scrotal hematoma can occur. Drain it if it is large or enlarging or if there are signs of infection (fever, discharge of pus from the wound).

For radical orchiectomy

Damage to the ileoinguinal nerve can lead to an area of loss of sensation overlying the scrotum.

Orchiectomy ± testicular implant: procedure-specific consent form—recommended discussion of adverse events

Serious or frequently occurring complications

Occasional

- Cancer, if found, may not be cured by orchiectomy alone.
- There may be a need for additional surgery, radiotherapy, or chemotherapy.
- Loss of future fertility
- Biopsy of contralateral testis may be required if an abnormality is found (small testis or history of maldescent).

Rare

- On pathological examination cancer may not be found, or the pathological diagnosis may be uncertain.
- Infection of incision may occur, requiring further treatment and possibly removal of the implant if this has been inserted.
- Pain requiring removal of implant
- Cosmetic expectation not always met
- Implant may lie higher in the scrotum than the normal testis did
- A palpable stitch may be felt at one end of the implant.
- Long-term risks of silicone implants are not known.

Urological incisions

Midline, transperitoneal

Indications

These include access to the peritoneal cavity and pelvis for radical nephrectomy, cystectomy, reconstructive procedures, etc.

Technique

Divide skin, subcutaneous fat. Divide fascia in midline. Find the midline between the rectus muscles. Dissect the muscles free from the underlying peritoneum. Place two clips on either side of the midline, and pinch between the two to ensure no bowel has been trapped. Elevate the clips, and divide between them with a knife. Extend the incision in the peritoneum up and down, ensuring no bowel is in the way.

Closure

Use a nonabsorbable (e.g., nylon) or very slowly absorbable (e.g., PDS) suture.

Specific complications

These include dehiscence (classically around day 10 postoperative and preceded by pink serous discharge, then sudden herniation of a bowel through incision).

Lower midline, extraperitoneal

Indications

Access to pelvis (e.g., radical prostatectomy, colposuspension) is needed.

Technique

Divide skin, subcutaneous fat. Divide fascia in midline. Find the midline between the rectus muscles and dissect the muscles free from the underlying peritoneum. If you make a hole in it, repair the defect with vicryl. Divide the fascia posterior to the rectus muscles in the midline, thus exposing the extravesical space.

Closure is as for midline, transperitoneal incisions.

Pfannenstiel

Indications

Access to pelvis (e.g., colposuspension, open prostatectomy, open cysto-lithotomy) is needed.

Technique

Divide the skin 2 cm above the pubis and the tissues down to the rectus sheath, which is cut in an arc, avoiding the inguinal canal. Apply clips to the top flap (and afterward, the bottom flap) and use a combination of scissors and your fingers to separate the rectus muscle from the sheath.

For maximum exposure you must elevate the anterior rectus sheath from the recti, cranially to just below the umbilicus and caudally to the pubis. Take care to diathermy a perforating branch of the inferior epigastric artery on each side.

Apply two Babcock forceps to the inferior belly of the rectus on either side of the midline. Elevate and cut in the midline, the lower part of the fascia (transversalis fascia) between the recti. Separate the recti in the midline (do not divide them).

Closure

Tack the divided transversalis fascia together and then close the transversely divided rectus sheath with vicryl.

Supra-12th rib incision

Indications

Access to kidneys, renal pelvis, or upper ureter is needed.

Technique

Make the incision over the tip of the 12th rib through skin and subcutaneous fascia. Palpate the tip of the 12th rib. Make a 3 cm cut with diathermy, through the muscle (latissimus dorsi) overlying the tip of the 12th rib so you come down onto the tip of the 12th rib, and then cut anterior to the tip of the 12th rib, down through external and internal oblique, transversus abdominis, to Gerota's fascia and the perirenal fat. Sweep anteriorly with a finger to push the peritoneum and intraperitoneal organs out of harm's way.

Cut the muscles overlying the rib, cutting centrally along the length of the rib, in so doing avoiding the pleura. Cut with scissors along the top edge of the rib to free the intercostal muscle from the rib—watch out for the pleura! Insert a Gillies forceps between the pleura and overlying intercostal muscle and divide the muscle fibers, protecting the pleura.

Dissect fibers of the diaphragm away from the inner surface of the 12th rib—as you do so, the pleura will rise upward with the detached diaphragmatic fibers, out of harm's way. At the posterior end of the incision feel for the sharp edge of the costovertebral ligament.

Insert heavy scissors, with the blades just open, on the top of the rib (to avoid the XIth intercostal nerve) and divide the costovertebral ligament. You should now be on top of Gerota's fascia.

Specific complications

These include damage to the pleura. If you make a hole in the pleura, repair it at the end of the operation. Pass a small-bore catheter (e.g., Jacques) through the hole, close all the muscle layers, inflate the lung, and then, before closing the skin, remove the catheter.

Complications common to all incisions

These include hernia, wound infection, and chronic wound pain.

JJ stent insertion

Preparation

This can be done under sedation or general anesthetic.

With sedation

Use oral ciprofloxacin 250 mg; lidocaine gel for urethral anesthesia and lubrication; sedoanalgesia (diazepam 2.5–10 mg IV, meperidine 50–100 mg IV). Monitor pulse and oxygen saturation with a pulse oximeter.

Technique

A flexible cystoscope is passed into the bladder and rotated through 180°. This allows greater deviation of the end of the cystoscope and makes identification of the ureteric orifice easier.

A 0.9 mm hydrophilic guide wire (Terumo Corporation, Japan) is passed into the ureter under direct vision. The guide wire is manipulated into the renal pelvis using C-arm digital fluoroscopy.

The cystoscope is placed close to the ureteric orifice and its position, relative to bony landmarks in the pelvis, is recorded by frame grabbing a fluoroscopic image.

The flexible cystoscope is then removed and a 4 Fr ureteric catheter is passed over the guide wire, into the renal pelvis. A small quantity of non-ionic contrast medium is injected into the renal collecting system, to outline its position and to dilate it.

The Terumo guide wire is replaced with an ultra-stiff guide wire (Cook Spencer) and the 4 Fr ureteric catheter is removed. We use a variety of stent sizes depending on the patient's size (6–8 Fr, 20–26 cm) (Boston Scientific).

The stent is advanced to the renal pelvis under fluoroscopic control, checking that the lower end of the stent is not inadvertently pushed up the ureter by checking the position of the ureteric orifice on the previously frame-grabbed image.

The guide wire is then removed.

Further reading

Hellawell GO, Cowan NC, Holt SJ, Mutch SJ (2002). A radiation perspective for treating loin pain in pregnancy by double-pigtail stents. *Br J Urol Int* 90:801–808.

McFarlane J, Cowan N, Holt S, Cowan M (2001). Outpatient ureteric procedures: a new method for retrograde ureteropyelography and ureteric stent placement. *Br J Urol Int* 87:172–176.

Nephrectomy and nephroureterectomy

Indications
- Renal cell cancer
- Nonfunctioning kidney containing a staghorn calculus
- Persistent hemorrhage following renal trauma

Anesthesia
General anesthesia is used.

Postoperative care
Nephrectomy
Cardiovascular status and urine output should be carefully monitored in the immediate postoperative period. Hemorrhage from the renal pedicle or, for left-sided nephrectomy, the spleen, is rare, but will present with an increasing tachycardia, cool peripheries, falling urine output, and eventually a drop in blood pressure.

A drain is usually not left in place, but if it is, there may be excessive drainage of blood from the drain. However, do not be lulled into a false sense of security by the absence of drainage—this does not mean that hemorrhage is not occurring, as the drain may be blocked but hemorrhage may be ongoing.

For nephrectomy via a posterolateral (rib-based) incision, watch for pneumothorax. Arrange for a CXR on return from the recovery room. Arrange routine chest physiotherapy to reduce the risk of chest infection. Regular chest examination is important, looking specifically for pneumothorax and pleural effusion.

Mobilize the patient as quickly as possible, to reduce the risk of DVT and PE.

Nephroureterectomy
Where the ureter has been excised from the bladder, a urethral catheter is left in place at the end of the procedure, to allow the hole in the bladder to heal. This is usually removed 10–14 days after surgery.

Common postoperative complications and their management
- Hemorrhage—see above.
- Wound infection is rare. If superficial, treat with antibiotics. If an underlying collection of pus is suspected, open the wound to allow free drainage, and pack the wound daily.
- Pancreatic injury is rare, but would be indicated by excessive drainage of fluid from the drain, if present, which will have a high amylase level. If no drain is present, an abdominal collection will develop, which may be manifested by a prolonged ileus.

Procedure-specific consent form—recommended discussion of adverse events

Serious or frequently occurring complications of nephrectomy or nephroureterectomy

Simple nephrectomy

Common
- Temporary insertion of a bladder catheter
- Occasional insertion of a wound drain

Occasional
- Bleeding requiring further surgery or transfusion
- Entry into lung requiring temporary insertion of a drainage tube

Rare
- Involvement or injury to nearby structures—blood vessels, spleen, lung, liver, pancreas, bowel, requiring further extensive surgery
- Infection, pain, or hernia of incision, requiring further treatment
- Anesthetic or cardiovascular problems, possibly requiring intensive care admission (including chest infection, pulmonary embolus, stroke, deep vein thrombosis, heart attack)

Alternative therapy includes observation, laparoscopic approach.

Radical nephrectomy

Complications are as above plus the following:
- *Occasional:* need for further therapy for cancer
- *Rare:* may be an abnormality other than cancer on microscopic analysis

Alternative therapy includes observation, embolization, immunotherapy, and laparoscopic approach.

Nephroureterectomy

Complications are the same as those listed above.

Radical prostatectomy

Indications
This is performed for localized prostate cancer.

Anesthesia
General or regional anesthesia is required.

Postoperative care
Mobilize the patient as quickly as possible and continue subcutaneous heparin and use of AK-TEDS until discharge to reduce the risk of DVT and PE. Remove the drains when drainage is minimal.

If there is persistent leak of fluid from the drains, send a sample for urea and creatinine, and if it is urine, get a cystogram to determine the size of the leak at the vesicourethral junction.

Urethral catheters are left in situ after radical prostatectomy for a variable time depending on the surgeon who performs the operation. Some surgeons leave a catheter for 3 weeks and others for just 1 week.

Common postoperative complications and their management
Hemorrhage

This is managed in the usual way (transfusion; return to surgery when bleeding persists or when there is cardiovascular compromise).

Ureteric obstruction

This usually results from edema of the bladder, obstructing the ureteric orifices. Retrograde ureteric catheterization is rarely possible (this would require urethral catheter removal and it is difficult to see the ureteric orifices because of the edema).

Arrange for placement of percutaneous nephrostomies.

Lymphocele

Drain by radiologically assisted drain placement. If the lymphocele recurs after drain removal, create a window from the lymph collection into the peritoneal cavity so the lymph drains into the peritoneum from which it is absorbed.

Displaced catheter post radical prostatectomy

If the catheter falls out a week after surgery, the patient may well void successfully, and in this situation no further action need be taken. If, however, the catheter inadvertently falls out the day after surgery, gently attempt to replace it with a 12 Fr. catheter that has been well lubricated.

If this fails, pass a flexible cystoscope, under local anesthetic, into the bulbar urethra and attempt to pass a guide wire into the bladder, over which a catheter can then safely be passed. If this is not possible, another option is to hope that the patient voids spontaneously and does not leak urine at the site of the anastomosis.

An ascending urethrogram may provide reassurance that there is no leak of contrast and that the anastomosis is watertight. If there is a leak or the patient is unable to void, a suprapubic catheter can be placed (percutaneously or under general anesthetic via an open cystostomy).

Fecal fistula
This is due to rectal injury, either recognized and repaired at the time of surgery and later breaking down, or not immediately recognized. Formal closure is often required.

Contracture at the vesicourethral anastomosis
Gentle dilatation may be tried. If the stricture recurs, instruct the patient in ISC, in an attempt to keep the stricture open. If this fails, a bladder neck incision may be tried.

Procedure-specific consent form—recommended discussion of adverse events

Serious or frequently occurring complications of radical prostatectomy
Common
- Temporary insertion of a bladder catheter and wound drain
- High chance of impotence due to unavoidable nerve damage
- No semen is produced during orgasm, causing infertility

Occasional
- Blood loss requiring transfusion or repeat surgery
- Urinary incontinence—temporary or permanent, requiring pads or further surgery
- Discovery that cancer cells are already outside the prostate, needing observation or further treatment at a later date if required, including radiotherapy or hormonal therapy

Rare
- Anesthetic or cardiovascular problems possibly requiring intensive care admission (including chest infection, pulmonary embolus, stroke, deep vein thrombosis, heart attack)
- Pain, infection, or hernia in area of incision
- Rectal injury, very rarely needing temporary colostomy

Alternative therapy includes watchful waiting, radiotherapy, brachytherapy, hormonal therapy, and perineal or laparoscopic removal.

Radical cystectomy

Indications
- Muscle-invasive bladder cancer
- Adenocarcinoma of bladder (radioresistant)
- Squamous carcinoma of bladder (relatively radioresistant)
- Non-muscle-invasive TCC bladder that has failed to respond to intravesical chemotherapy or immunotherapy
- Recurrent TCC bladder post-radiotherapy

Combined with urethrectomy if
- There are multiple bladder tumors
- There is involvement of the bladder neck or prostatic urethra

Anesthesia
General anesthesia is used.

Postoperative care and common post-operative complications and their management
Monitor cardiovascular status, urine output, and respiratory status carefully in the first 48 hours. Routine chest physiotherapy is started early in the postoperative period to reduce the chance of chest infection. Mobilize the patient as early as possible to minimize the risk of DVT and PE.

Drains are removed when they stop draining. Some surgeons prefer to leave them for a week or so, so that late leaks (urine, intestinal contents) will drain via the drain track and not cause peritonitis.

Try to remove the nasogastric tube, if used, as soon as possible to assist respiration and reduce the risks of chest infection. The patient usually starts to resume their diet within a week or so. If the ileus is prolonged, start parenteral nutrition.

Hemorrhage
Persistent bleeding that fails to respond to transfusion should be managed by re-exploration.

Wound dehiscence requires resuturing under general anesthetic.

Ileus is common. It usually resolves spontaneously within a few days.

Small bowel obstruction
This occurs from herniation of small bowel through the mesenteric defect created at the junction between the two bowel ends. Continue nasogastric aspiration. The obstruction will usually resolve spontaneously.

Reoperation is occasionally required when the obstruction persists or when there are signs of bowel ischemia.

Leakage from the intestinal anastomosis
This can lead to the following:
- *Peritonitis*—requiring reoperation and repair or refashioning of the anastomosis
- *An enterocutaneous fistula*—bowel contents leak from the intestine and through a fistulous track onto the skin. A low-volume leak (<500

mL/24 hr) will usually heal spontaneously. Normal (enteral) nutrition may be maintained until the fistula closes (which usually occurs within a matter of days or a few weeks). If the leak is high volume, spontaneous closure is less likely and reoperation to close the fistula may be required.

Pelvic abscess

Formal surgical (open) exploration of the pelvis is indicated with drainage of the abscess and careful inspection to see if the underlying cause is a rectal injury, in which case a defunctioning colostomy should be performed.

Partial cystectomy

Indications

This is done to remove primary, solitary bladder tumors at a site that allows 2 cm of normal tissue around it in a bladder that will have adequate capacity and compliance after operation.

There should be the following:
- No prior history of bladder cancer
- No carcinoma in situ
- A solitary muscle-invasive tumor located well away from the ureteral orifices which includes 2 cm of normal surrounding bladder

High-grade tumors should not be excluded if these criteria are met. The lesions most commonly amenable to partial cystectomy are G2 or G3 TCCs or adenocarcinomas located on the posterior wall or dome.

Contraindications

These include associated carcinoma in situ, deeply invasive tumors, and tumors at the bladder base (i.e., near the ureteric orifices).

Procedure-specific consent form—recommended discussion of adverse events

Serious or frequently occurring complications of radical cystectomy

See also consent for ileal conduit if this is the planned form of urinary diversion.

Common
- Temporary insertion of a nasal tube, drain, and stent
- High chance of impotence (lack of erections) due to unavoidable nerve damage
- No semen is produced during orgasm (dry orgasm), causing infertility.
- Blood loss requiring transfusion or repeat surgery
- In women, pain or difficulty with sexual intercourse from narrowing or shortening of vagina and need for removal of uterus and ovaries (causing premature menopause in those not at menopause)

Occasional
- Cancer may not be cured with surgery alone.
- Need to remove penile urinary pipe as part of procedure

Rare
- Infection or hernia of incision, requiring further treatment

- Anesthetic or cardiovascular problems possibly requiring intensive care admission (including chest infection, pulmonary embolus, stroke, deep vein thrombosis, heart attack)
- Decreased renal function with time

Very rarely
- Rectal injury, very rarely needing temporary colostomy
- Diarrhea due to shortened bowel, vitamin deficiency requiring treatment
- Bowel and urine leak, requiring reoperation
- Scarring of bowel or ureters, requiring operation in the future
- Scarring, narrowing, or hernia formation around stomal opening, requiring revision

Alternative treatment includes radiotherapy, neobladder formation rather than ileal conduit urinary diversion.

Formation of neobladder with bowel
Common
- Need to perform intermittent self-catheterization if bladder fails to empty.

Ileal conduit

Indications
- For urinary diversion following radical cystectomy
- Intractable incontinence for which anti-incontinence surgery has failed or is not appropriate

Postoperative care and common postoperative complications and their management
Oliguria or anuria: Try a fluid challenge.

Wound infection: Treat with antibiotics and wound care. Open the superficial layers of the wound to release pus.

Wound dehiscence is rare. It requires resuturing in the operating room, under general anesthetic.

Ileus is common. It usually resolves spontaneously within a few days.

Small bowel obstruction
This occurs from herniation of small bowel through the mesenteric defect created at the junction between the two bowel ends. Continue nasogastric aspiration. The obstruction will usually resolve spontaneously.

Reoperation is occasionally required when the obstruction persists or there are signs of bowel ischemia.

Leakage from the intestinal anastomosis
This can lead to the following:
- *Peritonitis*—requiring reoperation and repair or refashioning of the anastomosis
- *An enterocutaneous fistula*—bowel contents leak from the intestine and through a fistulous track onto the skin. A low-volume leak (<500 mL/24 hr) will usually heal spontaneously. Normal (enteral) nutrition may be maintained until the fistula closes (which usually occurs within a matter of days or a few weeks). If high volume, spontaneous closure is less likely, and reoperation to close the fistula may be required.

Leakage from the ureteroileal junction
Leakage may be suspected because of a persistently high output of fluid from the drain. Test this for urea. Urine will have a higher urea and creatinine concentration than serum. If the fluid is lymph, the urea and creatinine concentration will be the same as that of serum.

Arrange for a loopogram. This will confirm the leak. Place a soft, small catheter (12 Fr) into the conduit to encourage antegrade flow of urine and assist healing of the ureteroileal anastomosis. If the leakage continues, arrange for bilateral nephrostomies to divert the flow of urine away from the area and encourage wound healing.

Occasionally, a ureteroileal leak will present as a urinoma (this causes a persistent ileus). Radiologically assisted drain insertion can result in a dramatic resolution of the ileus, with subsequent healing of the ureteroileal leak.

Hyperchloremic acidosis
This may be associated with obstruction of the stoma at its distal end or from infrequent emptying of the stoma back (leading to back-pressure on the conduit). Catheterize the stoma relieves the obstruction. In the long term, the conduit may have to be surgically shortened.

Acute pyelonephritis is due to the presence of reflux combined with bacteriuria.

Stomal stenosis
The distal (cutaneous) end of the stoma may become narrowed, usually as a result of ischemia to the distal part of the conduit. Revision surgery is required if this stenosis causes obstruction leading to recurrent UTIs or back-pressure on the kidneys.

Parastomal hernia formation
Hernias occur around the site through which the conduit passes, through the fascia of the anterior abdominal wall. Many hernias can be left alone. The indications for repairing a hernia are as follows:
• Bowel obstruction
• Pain
• Difficulty with applying the stoma bag (distortion of the skin around the stoma by the hernia can lead to frequent bag detachment).

Repair the hernia defect by placing mesh over the hernia site, via an incision sited as far as possible from the stoma itself, to reduce the risk of wound infection.

Procedure-specific consent form—recommended discussion of adverse events

Serious or frequently occurring complications of ileal conduit formation
Common
• Temporary drain, stents, or nasal tube
• Urinary infections, occasionally requiring antibiotics

Occasional
• Diarrhea due to shortened bowel
• Blood loss requiring transfusion or repeat surgery
• Infection or hernia of incision requiring further treatment

Rare
• Bowel and urine leakage from anastomosis requiring reoperation
• Scarring to bowel or ureters requiring operation in future
• Scarring, narrowing, or hernia formation around urine opening requiring revision
• Decreased renal function with time

Alternative treatment includes catheters, continent diversion of urine.

Percutaneous nephrolithotomy (PCNL)

Indications
- Stones >3 cm in diameter
- Stones that have failed ESWL and/or an attempt at flexible ureteroscopy and laser treatment
- Staghorn calculi

Preoperative preparation
- CT scan to assist planning the track position and to identify a retrorenal colon[1]
- Stop aspirin 10 days prior to surgery
- Culture urine (so appropriate antibiotic prophylaxis can be given)
- Cross-match 2 units of blood
- Start IV antibiotics the afternoon before surgery to reduce the chance of septicemia (many stones treated by PCNL are infection stones). If urine is culture negative, use 1.0 g IV ampicillin and IV gentamicin (1.5 mg/kg). Routine antibiotic prophylaxis also reduces the incidence of postoperative UTI.[2]

Postoperative management
Once the stone has been removed, a nephrostomy tube is left in situ for several days (Fig. 16.15). This drains urine in the postoperative period and tamponades bleeding from the track.

Complications of PCNL and their management
Bleeding
Some bleeding is inevitable, but an amount severe enough to threaten life is uncommon. In most cases it is venous in origin and stops following placement of a nephrostomy tube (which compresses bleeding veins in the track).

If bleeding persists, clamp tube for 10 minutes. If bleeding continues despite this, order urgent angiography, looking for an arteriovenous fistula or pseudoaneurysm, both of which require selective renal artery embolization (required in 1% of PCNLs[3]) or open exposure of kidney to control bleeding by suture ligation, partial nephrectomy, or nephrectomy.

Septicemia
This occurs in 1–2% of cases. Incidence is reduced by prophylactic antibiotics. Track damage; it is essentially minimal. Cortical loss from track is estimated to be <0.2% of total renal cortex in animal studies.[4]

---

1 Hopper KD, Sherman JL, Williams MD, et al. (1987). The variable anteroposterior position of the retroperitoneal colon to the kidneys. *Invest Radiol* 22:298–302.
2 Inglis JA, Tolly DA (1988). Antibiotic prophylaxis at the time of percutaneous stone surgery. *J Endourol* 2:59–62.
3 Martin X (2000). Severe bleeding after nephrolithotomy: results of hyperselective embolisation. *Eur Urol* 37:136–139.

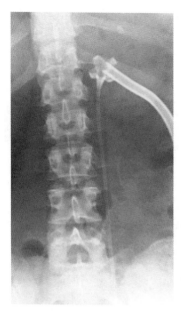

Figure 16.15 A Malecot catheter, which has wide drainage eyeholes and an extension at the distal end which passes down the ureter to prevent fragments of stone from passing down the ureter.

Colonic perforation

The colon is usually lateral or anterolateral to the kidney and is therefore not usually at risk of injury unless a very lateral approach is made. The colon is retrorenal in 2% of individuals (more commonly in thin females with little retroperitoneal fat[1]).

The perforation usually occurs in an extraperitoneal part of the colon and is managed by JJ stent placement and withdrawal of the nephrostomy tube into the lumen of the colon to encourage drainage of bowel contents away from that of the urine, thereby encouraging healing without development of a fistula between the bowel and kidney.

A radiological contrast study a week or so later confirms that the colon has healed and that there is no leak of contrast from the bowel into the renal collecting system.

Damage to the liver or spleen is very rare in the absence of splenomegaly or hepatomegaly.

---

4 Clayman J (1987). Percutaneous nephrostomy: assessment of renal damage associated with semi-rigid (24F) and balloon (36F) dilation. *J Urol* 138:203–206.

Damage to the lung and pleura leading to pneumomothorax or pleural effusion can occur with supra-12th rib puncture.

Nephrocutaneous fistula

When the nephrostomy tube is removed from the kidney, a few days after surgery, the 1 cm incision usually closes within 2 days or so.

Occasionally, urine continues to drain percutaneously for a few days and a small stoma bag must be worn. In most of these cases the urine leak will stop spontaneously, but if it fails to do so after a week or so, place a JJ stent to encourage antegrade drainage of urine.

Outcomes

For small stones, the stone-free rate after PCNL is on the order of 90–95%. For staghorn stones, the stone-free rate of PCNL, when combined with postoperative ESWL for residual stone fragments, is on the order of 80–85%.

Procedure-specific consent form—recommended discussion of adverse events

Serious or frequently occurring complications of PCNL

Common

- Temporary insertion of a bladder catheter and ureteric stent or kidney tube needing later removal
- Transient hematuria
- Transient temperature

Occasional

- More than one puncture site may be required
- No guarantee of removal of all stones and need for further operations
- Recurrence of stones

Rare

- Severe kidney bleeding requiring transfusion, embolization, or, at last resort, surgical removal of kidney
- Damage to lung, bowel, spleen, or liver requiring surgical intervention
- Kidney damage or infection needing further treatment
- Overabsorption of irrigating fluids into the blood system, causing strain on heart function

Alternative treatment includes external shock wave treatments, open surgical removal of stones, observation.

Ureteroscopes and ureteroscopy

Instruments

Two types of ureteroscope are in common use—the semi-rigid uretero-scope and the flexible ureteroscope.

Semi-rigid ureteroscopes

These instruments have high-density fiber-optic bundles for light (noncoherently arranged) and image transmission (coherently arranged to maintain image quality). For equivalent light and image transmission using glass rod lenses, thicker lenses are required than with fiber-optic bundles.

Consequently, semi-rigid ureteroscopes can be made smaller, while maintaining the size of the instrument channel. In addition, the instrument can be bent by several degrees without the image being distorted.

The working tip of most current models is on the order of 7 to 8 Fr., with the proximal end of the scope being on the order of 11 to 12 Fr. There is usually at least one working channel of at least 3.4 Fr.

Flexible ureteroscopes

The fiber-optic bundles in flexible ureteroscopes are the same as those in semi-rigid scopes, only of smaller diameter. Thus, image quality and light transmission are not as good as with semi-rigid scopes, but are usually adequate.

The working tip of most current models is on the order of 7 to 8 Fr., with the proximal end of the scope being on the order of 9 to 10 Fr. There is usually at least one working channel of at least 3.6 Fr.

The great advantage of the flexible ureteroscope over the semi-rigid variety is the ability to perform controlled deflection of the end of the scope (active deflection). Behind the actively deflecting tip of the scope is a segment of the scope that is more flexible than the rest of the shaft. This section is able to undergo passive deflection—when the tip is fully actively deflected, by advancing the scope further, this flexible segment allows even more deflection.

Flexible ureteroscopes have recently been developed that have two actively deflecting segments.

Flexible ureteroscopes are intrinsically more intricate and are therefore less durable than semi-rigid scopes.

Ureteroscopic irrigation systems

Normal saline is used (high-pressure irrigation with glycine or water would lead to fluid absorption from pyelolymphatic or venous backflow). Irrigation by gravity pressurization alone (the fluid bag suspended above the patient without any applied pressure) will produce flow that is inadequate for visualization because the long, fine-bore irrigation channels of modern ureteroscopes are inherently high resistance.

Several methods are available—hand-inflated pressure bags, foot pumps, and hand-operated syringe pumps. Whatever system is chosen, use the minimal flow required to allow a safe view so as to avoid flushing the stone out of the ureter and into the kidney; you may not be able to retrieve it from there.

Ureteric dilatation

Some surgeons use this, others don't. Those who don't, argue that dilatation is unnecessary in the era of modern, small-caliber ureteroscopes. Those who do, cite a higher chance of being able to pass the ureteroscope all the way up to the kidney. Ureteric dilatation may be helpful when multiple passes of the ureteroscope up and down the ureter are going to be required for stone removal (alternatively, use a ureteric access sheath).

Some surgeons prefer to place two guide wires into the ureter, one to pass the ureteroscope over ("railroading") and the other to act as a safety wire, so that access to the kidney is always possible if difficulties are encountered. The second guide wire is most easily placed via a dual-lumen catheter that has a second channel, through which the second guide wire can be easily passed into the ureter, without requiring repeat cystoscopy. This dual lumen catheter has the added function of gently dilating the ureteric orifice to about 10 Fr. There is probably no long-term harm done to the ureter as a consequence of dilatation.[1]

Ureteric access sheaths, which have outer diameters from 10 to 14 Fr, may facilitate access to the ureter and are particularly useful if it is anticipated that the ureteroscope will have to be passed up and down the ureter on multiple occasions (to retrieve fragments of stone). In addition, they facilitate the outflow of irrigant fluid from the pelvis or the kidney, thereby maintaining the field of view and decreasing intrarenal pressures.

Patient position

The patient is positioned as flat as possible on the operating table to "iron out" the natural curves of the ureter. A cystoscopy is performed with either a flexible or rigid instrument. A retrograde ureterogram can be done to outline pelvicalyceal anatomy.

A guide wire is then passed into the renal pelvis. We use a Sensor guide wire (Microvasive, Boston Scientific), which has a 3 cm long floppy, hydrophilic tip that can usually easily be negotiated up the ureter. The remaining length of the wire is rigid and covered in smooth PTFE.

Both properties aid passage of the ureteroscope.

Technique of flexible ureteroscopy and laser treatment for intrarenal stones

Flexible ureteroscopy and laser treatment can be performed with topical urethral local anesthesia and sedation. However, trying to fragment a moving stone with the laser can be difficult and, ideally, ureteroscopy is most easily done under general anesthesia with endotracheal intubation (rather than a laryngeal mask) to allow short periods of suspension of respiration and so stop movement of the kidney and its contained stone.

Empty the bladder to prevent coiling of the scope in the bladder. Pass the scope over a guide wire. This requires two people—the surgeon holds the shaft of the scope and the assistant applies tension to the guide wire to fix the latter in position without pulling it down. This allows the scope to progress easily up the ureter.

1 Emberton M, et al. (1995). The National Prostatectomy Audit: the clinical management of patients during hospital admission. *Br J Urol* 75:301–316.

The assistant also ensures that acute angulation of the scope where the handle meets the shaft does not occur. The flexible ureteroscope should slide easily up the ureter and into the renal pelvis.

With modern active secondary deflection ureteroscopes, access to most, if not all, parts of the renal collecting system is possible.

Laser lithotripsy

The main drawback of laser lithotripsy is the dust cloud effect that occurs as the stone is fragmented. This temporarily obscures the view and must be washed away before the laser can safely be reapplied.

To stent or not to stent after ureteroscopy

JJ stent insertion does not increase stone-free rates and is therefore not required in routine cases. A stent should be placed if

- There has been ureteric injury (e.g., perforation—indicated by extravasation of contrast)
- There are residual stones that might obstruct the ureter
- The patient has had a ureteric stricture that required dilatation
- There are solitary kidneys

Routine stenting after ureteroscopy for distal ureteric calculi is unnecessary.[2] Many urologists will place a stent after ureteroscopy for proximal ureteric stones.

Complications of ureteroscopy

These include septicemia; ureteric perforation requiring either a JJ stent or, very occasionally, a nephrostomy tube where JJ stent placement is not possible; and ureteric stricture (<1%).

Procedure-specific consent form—recommended discussion of adverse events

Serious or frequently occurring complications of ureteroscopy for treatment of ureteric stones

Common

- Mild burning or bleeding on passing urine for a short period after the operation
- Temporary insertion of a bladder catheter may be required.
- Insertion of a stent may be required with a further procedure to remove it.
- Urinary infections occasionally requiring antibiotics

Occasional

- Inability to get stone or movement of stone back into kidney when it is not retrievable
- Kidney damage or infection requiring further treatment
- Failure to pass scope if ureter is narrow
- Recurrence of stones

2 Srivastava A, et al. (2003). Routine stenting after ureteroscopy for distal ureteral calculi is unnecessary: results of a randomized controlled trial. *J Endourol* 17:871.

Rare
• Damage to ureter with need for open operation or placement of a
  nephrostomy tube into the kidney

Alternative treatment includes open surgery, shock wave therapy, or observation to allow spontaneous passage.

Further reading

Harmon WJ, et al. (1997). Ureteroscopy: current practice and long-term complications. *J Urol* 157:28–32.

Pyeloplasty

Indications
This is used for UPJ obstruction.

Anesthesia
General anesthesia is used.

Postoperative care
A JJ stent, bladder catheter, and a drain are left in situ. The bladder catheter serves to prevent reflux of urine up the ureter, which can lead to increased leakage of urine from the anastomosis site (reflux occurs because of the presence of the JJ stent).

The drain is removed when the drain output is minimal. The stent is left in position for 6 weeks.

Common postoperative complications and their management

Hemorrhage

This usually arises from the nephrostomy track (if a nephrostomy tube has been left in place—some surgeons leave a JJ stent and a perinephric drain, with no nephrostomy). Clamp the nephrostomy tube, in an attempt to tamponade the bleeding.

If the bleeding continues, consider angiography and embolization of the bleeding vessel if seen, or exploration.

Urinary leak

This can occur within the first day or so. If a urethral catheter has not been left in place, catheterize the patient to minimize bladder pressure and therefore the chance of reflux, which might be responsible for the leak. If the drainage persists for more than a few days, shorten the drain—if it is in contact with the suture line of the anastomosis it can keep the anastomosis open, rather than letting it heal.

If the leak continues, identify the site of the leak by either a nephrostogram (if a nephrostomy has been left in situ) or a cystogram (if a JJ stent is in place—contrast may reflux up the ureter and identify the site of leakage) or an IVP. Some form of additional drainage may help dry up the leak (a JJ stent if only a nephrostomy has been left in situ, or a nephrostomy if one is not already in place).

Obstruction at UPJ

This is uncommon, and if it occurs it is usually detected once all the tubes have been removed and a follow-up renogram has been done. If the patient had symptomatic UPJO but remains asymptomatic, then no further treatment may be necessary. If they develop recurrent flank pain, reoperation may be necessary.

Acute pyelonephritis

Manage with antibiotics.

Procedure-specific consent form—recommended discussion of adverse events

Serious or frequently occurring complications of pyeloplasty

Common
- Temporary insertion of a bladder catheter and wound drain
- Further procedure to remove ureteric stent, usually a local anesthetic

Occasional
- Bleeding requiring further surgery or transfusion

Rare
- Recurrent kidney or bladder infections
- Recurrence can occur, needing further surgery

Very rarely
- Entry into lung cavity requiring insertion of temporary drainage tube
- Anesthetic or cardiovascular problems possibly requiring intensive care admission (including chest infection, pulmonary embolism, stroke, deep vein thrombosis, heart attack)
- Need to remove kidney at a later time because of damage caused by recurrent obstruction
- Infection, pain, or hernia of incision requiring further treatment

Alternative therapy
This includes observation, telescopic incision, dilation of area of narrowing, temporary placement of plastic tube through narrowing, and laparoscopic repair.

Laparoscopic surgery

Virtually every urological procedure can be done laparoscopically. It is particularly suited to surgery in the retroperitoneum (nephrectomy for benign and malignant disease and for kidney donation at transplantation, pyeloplasty for UPJO), but is also suited to pelvic surgery (lymph node biopsy, radical prostatectomy).

Reconstructive surgery requiring laparoscopic suturing and using bowel is technically very challenging, but is possible. Laparoscopic surgery offers the following advantages over open surgery:

- Reduced postoperative pain
- Smaller scars
- Less disturbance of bowel function (less postoperative ileus)
- Reduced recovery time and reduced hospital stay

Contraindications to laparoscopic surgery

- Severe COPD (avoid use of CO_2 for insufflation)
- Uncorrectable coagulopathy
- Intestinal obstruction
- Abdominal wall infection
- Massive hemoperitoneum
- Generalized peritonitis
- Suspected malignant ascites

Laparoscopic surgery is difficult or potentially hazardous in the morbidly obese (inadequate instrument length, decrease range of movement of instruments, higher pneumoperitoneum pressure required to lift the heavier anterior abdominal wall, excess intra-abdominal fat limiting the view); those with extensive previous abdominal or pelvic surgery (adhesions); those with previous peritonitis leading to adhesion formation; in those with organomegaly; in the presence of ascites; in pregnancy; in patients with a diaphragmatic hernia; and in those with aneurysms.

Potential complications unique to laparoscopic surgery

These include gas embolism (potentially fatal), hypercarbia (acidosis affecting cardiac function—e.g., arrhythmias), post-operative abdominal crepitus (subcutaneous emphysema), pneumothorax, pneomomediastinum, pneumopericardium, barotraumas.

Bowel, vessel (aorta, common iliac vessels, IVC, anterior abdominal wall injury), and other viscus injury are not unique to laparoscopic surgery, but are a particular concern during port access. Perforation of small or large bowel is the most common trocar injury. Rarely, the bladder is perforated.

Failure to progress with a laparoscopic approach or vessel injury with uncontrollable hemorrhage requires conversion to an open approach. Postoperatively, bowel may become entrapped in the trocar sites, or there may be bleeding from the sheath site.

An acute hydrocele can develop from irrigation fluid accumulating in the scrotum. It resorbs spontaneously. Scrotal and abdominal wall bruising commonly occurs.

Procedure specific consent forms

For all laparoscopic procedures

Common

- Temporary shoulder tip pain
- Temporary abdominal bloating
- Temporary insertion of a bladder catheter and wound drain

Occasional

- Infection, pain, or hernia of incision requiring further treatment

Rare

- Bleeding requiring conversion to open surgery or transfusion
- Entry into lung cavity requiring insertion of a temporary drainage tube

Very rarely

- Recognized (and unrecognized) injury to organs or blood vessels requiring conversion to open surgery or deferred open surgery
- Anesthetic or cardiovascular problems possibly requiring intensive care admission (including chest infection, pulmonary embolus, stroke, deep vein thrombosis, heart attack)

Laparoscopic pyeloplasty

Common

- Further procedure to remove ureteric stent, usually under local anesthesia

Occasional

- Recurrence can occur needing further surgery
- Short-term success rates are similar to those with open surgery, but long-term results are unknown.

Very rarely

- Need to remove kidney at a later time because of damage caused by recurrent obstruction

Alternative therapy includes observation, telescopic incision, dilation of area of narrowing, temporary placement of a plastic tube through narrowing, and conventional open surgical approach.

Laparoscopic simple nephrectomy

Occasional

- Short-term success rates are similar to those with open surgery, but long-term results are unknown.

Alternative therapy includes observation and conventional open surgical approach.

Laparoscopic radical nephrectomy

- *Occasional:* Short-term success rates are similar to those with open surgery, but long-term results are unknown.
- *Rare:* A histological abnormality other than cancer may be found

Alternative therapy includes observation, embolization, chemotherapy, immunotherapy, and conventional open surgical approach.

Endoscopic cystolitholapaxy and (open) cystolithotomy

Indications
- **Endoscopic cystolitholapaxy** is generally indicated for stones <6 cm in diameter. Electrohydraulic lithotripsy (EHL) is usually used.
- **Open cystolithotomy:** for stones >6 cm in diameter; patients with urethral obstruction that precludes endoscopic access to bladder

Anesthesia
Regional or general anesthesia is used.

Postoperative care
A catheter is left in the bladder for a day or so, since hematuria is common, particularly after fragmentation of large stones. Irrigation may be required if the hematuria is heavy.

Common postoperative complications and their management
- **Hematuria** requiring bladder washout or return to surgery is rare.
- **Septicemia** is uncommon.

Bladder perforation
This is uncommon, but it can occur with the use of stone punches, which grab the stone between powerful cutting jaws. Grasping the bladder wall in the jaws of the stone forceps or punch is easily done, and can cause perforation.

Procedure-specific consent form—recommended discussion of adverse events
Serious or frequently occurring complications of endoscopic cystolitholapxy
Common
- Mild burning or bleeding on passing urine for short periods after operation
- Temporary insertion of a catheter

Occasional
- Infection of bladder requiring antibiotics
- Permission for removal/biopsy of bladder abnormality if found
- Recurrence of stones or residual stone fragments

Rare
- Delayed bleeding requiring removal of clots or further surgery
- Injury to urethra causing delayed scar formation

Very rarely
- Perforation of bladder requiring a temporary urinary catheter or return to theatre for open surgical repair

Alternative therapy includes open surgery, observation.

Scrotal exploration for torsion and orchiopexy

Indications

Scrotal exploration is used for suspected testicular torsion.

Technique

A midline incision is used, since this allows access to both sides so that they may both be fixed within the scrotum. Untwist the testis and place in a warm, saline-soaked swab for 10 minutes.

If it remains black, remove it, having ligated the spermatic cord with a transfixion stitch of absorbable material. If it pinks up, fix it. If uncertain about its viability, make a small cut with the tip of a scalpel. If the testis bleeds actively, it should be salvaged (close the small wound with an absorbable suture). If not, it is dead and should be removed. Whatever you do, fix the other side, since the predisposing "bell clapper" deformity tends to be bilateral.

Fixation technique

Some surgeons fix the testis within the scrotum with suture material, inserted at 3 points (3-point fixation). Some use absorbable sutures and others, nonabsorbable sutures. Those who use the latter argue that absorbable sutures may disappear, exposing the patient to the risk of retorsion.[1]

Those who use absorbable sutures argue that the fibrous reaction around the absorbable sutures prevents retorsion and argue that the patient may be able to feel nonabsorbable sutures, which can be uncomfortable. The sutures should pass through the tunica albuginea of the testis, and then through the parietal layer of the tunica vaginalis lining the inner surface of the scrotum.

Others say the testis should be fixed within a dartos pouch,[2] arguing that suture fixation breaches the blood–testis barrier, exposing both testes to the risk of sympathetic orchiopathia (an autoimmune reaction caused by development of antibodies against the testis).

For dartos pouch fixation, open the tunica vaginalis, bring the testis out and untwist it. Develop a dartos pouch in the scrotum by holding the skin with forceps and dissecting with scissors between the skin and the underlying dartos muscle. Enlarge this space by inserting your two index fingers and pulling them apart. Place the testis in this pouch.

Use a few absorbable sutures to attach the cord near the testis to the inside of the dartos pouch to prevent retorsion of the testes. The dartos may then be closed over the testis and the skin can be closed in a separate layer.

Postoperative care and potential complications and their management

As with all procedures involving scrotal exploration, a scrotal hematoma may result that may have to be surgically drained.

Procedure-specific consent form—recommended discussion of adverse events

Serious or frequently occurring complications of scrotal exploration

Common

- The testis may have to be removed if nonviable.

Occasional

- You may be able to feel the stitch used to fix the testis.
- Blood collection around the testes, which slowly resolves or requires surgical removal
- Possible infection of incision or testis requiring further treatment

Rare

- Loss of testicular size or atrophy in future if testis is saved
- No guarantee of fertility

Alternative therapy includes observation for risks of loss of testis and autoimmune reaction.

Chapter 17

Basic science of relevance to urological practice

Physiology of bladder and urethra 660
Renal anatomy: renal blood flow and renal function 661
Renal physiology: regulation of water balance 664
Renal physiology: regulation of sodium and potassium
    excretion 665
Renal physiology: acid–base balance 666

Physiology of bladder and urethra

Bladder

The bladder consists of an endothelial lining (urothelium) on a connective tissue base (lamina propria), surrounded by smooth muscle (the *detrusor*), with an outer connective tissue, *adventitia*.

The urothelium consists of a multilayered transitional epithelium. It has numerous tight junctions that render it impermeable to water and solutes. The detrusor muscle is a homogeneous mass of smooth muscle bundles.

The bladder base is known as the *trigone*—a triangular area with the two ureteric orifices and the internal urinary meatus forming the corners. Intravesical pressure during filling is low. The main excitatory input to the bladder is via parasympathetic innervation (S2–4; cholinergic postganglionic fibers that when activated cause contraction; see p. 500).

Urethra

The bladder neck is normally closed during filling. It is composed of a circular smooth muscle (sympathetic innervation). High pressure is generated at the midpoint of the urethra in women, and at the level of the membranous urethra in men, where the urethral wall is composed of a longitudinal and circular smooth muscle coat, surrounded by striated muscle (*external sphincter*).

The striated part of the sphincter receives motor innervation from the somatic pudendal nerve (S3,4) and has voluntary control (ACh, or acetylcholinesterase mediates contraction).

The smooth muscle component of the sphincter has myogenic tone and receives excitatory and inhibitory innervation from the autonomic nervous system. Contraction is enhanced by sympathetic input (noradrenaline) and ACh. Inhibitory innervation is nitrergic (nitric oxide).

Micturition

Voiding is mediated by the pontine micturition center in the brain. During urine storage, bladder neck and sphincter smooth muscle are constricted, and ganglia in the bladder wall are inhibited by sympathetic input, while somatic innervation causes contraction of the striated sphincter muscle. As the bladder fills, sensory nerves respond to stretch and send information about bladder filling to the CNS.

At a socially acceptable time, the voiding reflex is activated. Stimulation of detrusor smooth muscle by parasympathetic anticholinergic nerves causes the bladder to contract. Simultaneous activation of nitrergic nerves reduces the intraurethral pressure, inhibition of somatic input relaxes the striated sphincter muscle, and sympathetic inhibition causes coordinated bladder neck and sphincter smooth muscle relaxation, resulting in bladder emptying.

Renal anatomy: renal blood flow and renal function

The kidneys and ureters lie within the retroperitoneum (literally behind the peritoneal cavity). The hila of the kidneys lie on the transpyloric plane (vertebral level—L1).

Each kidney is composed of a cortex, surrounding the medulla, which forms projections—papillae, which drain into cup-shaped epithelial-lined pouches called *calyces* (the calyx draining each papilla is known as a minor calyx, and several minor calyces coalesce to form a major calyx, several of which drain into the central renal pelvis).

The renal artery, which arises from the aorta at vertebral level L1/2, branches to form interlobar arteries, which in turn form arcuate arteries, and then cortical radial arteries from which the afferent arterioles are derived. Venous drainage occurs into the renal vein.

There are two capillary networks in each kidney—a glomerular capillary network (lying within Bowman's capsule) that drains into a peritubular capillary network, surrounding the tubules (proximal tubule, loop of Henle, distal tubule, and collecting ducts).

The anterior relations of the right kidney are, from top to bottom, the suprarenal gland, the liver, and the hepatic flexure of the colon. Medially, anterior to the right renal pelvis is the second part of the duodenum.

The anterior relations of the left kidney are, from top to bottom, the suprarenal gland, the stomach, the spleen, and the splenic flexure of the colon. Medially lies the tail of the pancreas.

The posterior relations of both kidneys are, superiorly, the diaphragm and lower ribs and, inferiorly (from lateral to medial), transversus abdominis, quadratus lumborum, and psoas major.

Renal blood flow (RBF)

The kidneys represent <0.5% of body weight, but they receive 25% of cardiac output (~1300 mL/min through both kidneys; 650 mL/min per kidney). Combined blood flow in the two renal veins is about 1299 mL/min, and the difference in flow rates represents the urine production rate (i.e., ~1 mL/min).

Autoregulation of RBF

RBF is defined as the pressure difference between the renal artery and renal vein divided by the renal vascular resistance. The glomerular arterioles are the major determinants of vascular resistance.

RBF remains essentially constant over a range of perfusion pressures (~80–180 mmHg) (i.e., RBF is *autoregulated*).

Autoregulation requires no innervation and probably occurs via the following:

- A myogenic mechanism (increased pressure in the afferent arterioles causes them to contract, thereby preventing a change in RBF)
- Tubuloglomerular feedback—the flow rate of tubular fluid is sensed at the macula densa of the juxtaglomerular apparatus (JGA), and in some way this controls flow through the glomerulus to which the JGA is opposed.

Other factors that influence RBF

- Sympathetic nerves innervate the glomerular arterioles. A reduction in circulating volume (such as blood loss) can stimulate sympathetic nerves, causing the release of NA (which acts on ₁-adrenoceptors on the afferent arteriole) to cause vasoconstriction. This results in reduced RBF and GFR (glomerular filtration rate).
- Angiotensin II constricts efferent arterioles and afferent arterioles and reduces RBF.
- Antidiuretic hormone (ADH), ATP, and endothelin all cause vasoconstriction and reduce RBF and GFR.
- Nitric oxide causes vasorelaxation and increases RBF.
- Atrial natriuretic peptide (ANP) causes afferent arteriole dilatation and increases RBF and GFR.

Renal function

Each kidney has 1 million functional units, or nephrons (Fig. 17.1), the functional unit of the kidney consisting of a glomerular capillary network, surrounded by podocytes (epithelial cells) of Bowman's capsule, which drains into a tubular system (proximal convoluted tubule, loop of Henle, distal convoluted tubule, collecting tube, and collecting duct) (Fig. 17.1).

Blood is delivered to the glomerular capillaries by an afferent arteriole and drained by an efferent arteriole. An ultrafiltrate of plasma is formed within the lumen of Bowman's capsule, driven by Starling forces across the glomerular capillaries. Reabsorption of salt and water occurs in the proximal tubule, loop of Henle, distal tubule, and collecting ducts.

Clearance is the volume of *plasma* that is completely cleared of solute by the kidney per minute.

Glomerular filtration rate (GFR) is the clearance for any substance that is freely filtered and is neither reabsorbed, secreted, nor metabolized by the kidney.

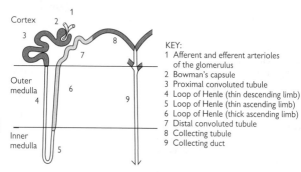

KEY:
1 Afferent and efferent arterioles of the glomerulus
2 Bowman's capsule
3 Proximal convoluted tubule
4 Loop of Henle (thin descending limb)
5 Loop of Henle (thin ascending limb)
6 Loop of Henle (thick ascending limb)
7 Distal convoluted tubule
8 Collecting tubule
9 Collecting duct

Figure 17.1 The nephron.

For a substance that is freely filtered at the glomerulus, is neither secreted nor reabsorbed by the renal tubules, and is not metabolized (catabolized), clearance is equivalent to GFR. When a substance is both filtered at the glomerulus and secreted by the renal tubules, its clearance will be greater than GFR. When a substance is filtered at the glomerulus, but reabsorbed by the renal tubules, its clearance will be less than GFR.

GFR is directly related to RBF.

Experimentally, GFR can be accurately measured by measuring the clearance of inulin (a substance that is freely filtered by the glomerulus and is neither secreted nor reabsorbed by the kidneys). Thus, the volume of plasma from which in 1 minute the kidneys remove all inulin is equivalent to GFR. Normally about one-fifth (120 mL/min) of the plasma that flows through the glomerular capillaries (600 mL/min) is filtered.

Clinically, GFR is estimated using serum and urine creatinine, and is ~80–125 mL/min in an adult male and 75–115 mL/min in an adult female.

Clearance of a substance from the plasma can be expressed mathematically as

Clearance = $U \times V / P$

where U is the concentration of a given substance in urine, P is its concentration in plasma, and V is the urine flow.

Clinically, a serum and 24-hour urine can be obtained to measure creatine clearance by the formula:

$$\text{Clearance} = \frac{(\text{Urine creatinine} \times \text{total urine volume})}{(\text{plasma creatinine} \times \text{time})}$$

where time = 1440 minutes for a 24-hour urine collection

Alternatively, the eGFR (estimated GFR) is based on serum creatinine combined with other factors such as age, sex, and race is used more commonly than the 24-hour urine collection. Various on-line calculators are available for this eGFR calculation, such as http://www.nkdep.nih.gov/professionals/gfr_calculators/idms_con.htm.

The Modification of Diet in Renal Disease (MDRD) eGFR equation does not require weight as results are normalized to 1.73^2 body surface area (BSA), an accepted "average" adult BSA.[1] The National Kidney Disease Education Program, sponsored by the NIH, recommends reporting estimated GFR values greater than or equal to 60 mL/min/1.73 m^2 simply as "≥60 mL/min/1.73 m^2," not an exact number.

$$\text{eGFR (mL/min/1.73 } m^2) = 186 \times (S_{cr})^{-1.154} \times (\text{Age})^{-0.203}$$
$$\times (0.742 \text{ if female}) \times (1.212 \text{ if African American}) \text{ (conventional units)}$$

1 Levey AS, Bosch JP, Lewis JB, et al. (1999). A more accurate method to estimate glomerular filtration rate from serum creatinine: a new prediction equation. Modification of Diet in Renal Disease Study Group. *Ann Intern Med* 130(6):461–470.

Renal physiology: regulation of water balance

Total body water (TBW) is 42 L. It is contained in two major compartments—the intracellular fluid (ICF or the water inside cells) which accounts for 28 L and the extracellular fluid (ECF or water outside cells) representing 14 L.

ECF is further divided into interstitial fluid (ISF, 11 L), transcellular fluid (1 L), and plasma (3 L). Hydrostatic and osmotic pressures influence movement between the compartments. Water is taken in from fluids, food, and oxidation of food.

Water is lost from urine, feces, and insensible losses. Intake and losses usually balance (~2 L/day) and TBW remains relatively constant.

Antidiuretic hormone (ADH or vasopressin)

ADH is secreted from the posterior pituitary in response to stimuli from changes in plasma osmolarity (detected by osmoreceptors in the hypothalamus) or changes in blood pressure or volume (detected by baroreceptors in the left atrium, aortic arch, and carotid sinus). These changes also stimulate the thirst center in the brain.

The action of ADH on the kidney
• Increases collecting duct permeability to water and urea
• Increases loop of Henle and collecting duct reabsorption of NaCl
• Increases vasoconstriction

Conditions of water excess

Water excess occurs when body fluids become hypotonic and ADH release and thirst are suppressed. In the absence of ADH, the collecting duct is impermeable to water and a large volume of hypotonic urine is produced, thus restoring normal plasma osmolarity.

Conditions of water deficit

When body fluids are hypertonic, ADH secretion and thirst are stimulated. The collecting duct becomes permeable, water is reabsorbed into the lumen, and a small volume of hypertonic urine is excreted.

The ability to concentrate or dilute urine depends on the countercurrent multiplication system in the loop of Henle. Essentially, a medullary concentration gradient is generated (partly by the active transport of NaCl), which provides the osmotic driving force for the reabsorption of water from the lumen of the collecting duct when ADH is present.

Children have a circadian rhythm in ADH secretion—high at night and low during the day. Adults essentially have a constant ADH secretion over a 24-hour period, with slight increases occurring around mealtimes. At these times, increased ADH secretion probably acts to prevent sudden increases in plasma osmolality that would otherwise occur due to ingestion of solutes in a meal.

Renal physiology: regulation of sodium and potassium excretion

Sodium regulation

NaCl is the main determinant of ECF osmolality and volume. Osmolality = osmoles per kg water (osmol/kg). Osmolarity = osmoles per liter of solution (osmol/L.

Low-pressure receptors in the pulmonary vasculature and cardiac atria, and high-pressure baroreceptors in the aortic arch and carotid sinus recognize changes in the circulating volume. Decreased blood volume triggers increased sympathetic nerve activity and stimulates ADH secretion, which results in reduced NaCl excretion.

Conversely, when blood volumes are increased, sympathetic activity and ADH secretion are suppressed, and NaCl excretion is enhanced (natriuresis).

A variety of natriuretic peptides have been isolated that cause a natriuresis. Under physiological conditions, renal natriuretic peptide (urodilatin) is the most important of these. Atrial natriuretic hormone (ANP) may influence sodium output under conditions of heart failure.

Renin–angiotensin–aldosterone system

Renin is an enzyme made and stored in the juxtaglomerular cells found in the walls of the afferent arteriole. Factors increasing renin secretion are as follows:

- Reduced perfusion of the afferent arteriole
- Sympathetic nerve activity
- Reduced Na^+ delivery to the macula densa

Renin acts on angiotensin to create angiotensin I. This is converted to angiotensin II in the lungs by angiotensin-converting enzyme (ACE). Angiotensin II performs several functions, which result in the retention of salt and water:

- Stimulates aldosterone secretion (resulting in NaCl reabsorption)
- Vasoconstriction of arterioles
- Stimulates ADH secretion and thirst
- Enhances NaCl reabsorption by the proximal tubule

Potassium regulation

K^+ is critical for many cell functions. A large concentration gradient across cell membranes is maintained by the Na^+-K^+-ATPase pump. Insulin and adrenaline also promotes cellular uptake of K^+.

The kidney excretes up to 95% of K^+ ingested in the diet. The distal tubule and collecting duct are able to both reabsorb and secrete K^+. Factors promoting K^+ secretion include the following:

- Increased dietary K^+ (driven by the electrochemical gradient)
- Aldosterone
- Increased rate of flow of tubular fluid (i.e., diuretics)
- Metabolic alkalosis (acidosis exerts the opposite effect)

Renal physiology: acid–base balance

The normal pH of extracellular fluid (ECF) is 7.4 ([H^+] = 40 nmol/L). Several mechanisms are in place to eliminate acid produced by the body and maintain body pH within a narrow range.

Buffering systems limiting [H^+] fluctuation in the blood

Buffer bases that take up H^+ ions in the body include the following:[1]

Bicarbonate buffer system $H^+ + HCO_3^- \leftrightarrow H_2CO_3 \leftrightarrow H_2O + CO_2$

Phosphate system $H^+ + HPO_4^{-2} \leftrightarrow H_2PO_4^-$

Protein buffers $H^+ + Protein^- \leftrightarrow HProtein$

The Henderson–Hasselbalch equation describes the relationship between pH and the concentration of conjugate acid and base:

From this equation, it can be seen that alterations in bicarbonate [HCO_3^-] or CO_2 will affect pH. Metabolic acid–base disturbances relate to a change in bicarbonate, and respiratory acid–base disorders relate to alterations in CO_2.

Bicarbonate reabsorption along the nephron

Bicarbonate is the main buffer of ECF and is regulated by both the kidneys and lungs; 85% is reabsorbed in the proximal convoluted tubule (Fig. 17.2).

Carbonic acid is first produced from CO_2 and water (accelerated by carbonic anhydrase). The carbonic acid dissociates, and an active ion pump (Na^+/H^+ antiporter) extrudes intracellular H^+ into the tubule lumen in exchange for Na^+. Secretion of H^+ ions favors a shift of the carbonic acid–bicarbonate equilibrium toward carbonic acid, which is rapidly converted into carbon dioxide and water.

CO_2 diffuses into the tubular cells down its diffusion gradient and is reformed into carbonic acid by intracellular carbonic anhydrase. The bicarbonate formed by this reaction is exchanged for chloride and passes into the circulation. Essentially, with each H^+ ion that enters the kidney, a bicarbonate ion enters the blood, which bolsters the buffering capacity of the ECF.

The remaining bicarbonate is absorbed in the distal convoluted tubule, where cells actively secrete H^+ into the lumen via an ATP-dependent pump. The distal tubule is the main site that pumps H^+ into the urine to ensure the complete removal of bicarbonate. Once the bicarbonate has gone, phosphate ions and ammonia buffer any remaining H^+ ions.

---

1 H_2O = water; CO_2 = carbon dioxide; HCO_3^- = bicarbonate; H_2CO_3 = carbonic acid; H^+ = hydrogen ions; $H_2PO_4^{2-}$ = dihydrogen phosphate; H_3PO_4 = phosphoric acid.

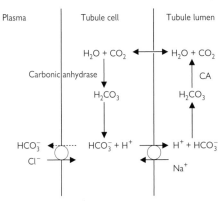

Figure 17.2 Diagram showing bicarbonate reabsorption in the proximal convoluted tubule.

Urological eponyms

Alcock's canal: canal for the internal pudendal vessels and nerve in the ischiorectal fossa.

Benjamin Alcock (1801–?). Professor of Anatomy, Physiology, and Pathology (1837) at the Apothecaries Hall in Dublin.

Anderson–Hynes pyeloplasty: dismembered pyeloplasty for UPJO.
James Anderson and Wilfred Hynes. Surgeons, Sheffield United Hospitals.

BCG (Bacille Calmette–Guerin): attenuated TB bacillus used for immunotherapy of carcinoma in situ of bladder.

Leon Charles Albert Calmette (1863–1933). A pupil of Pasteur in Paris, later becoming first director of the Pasteur Institute.

Camille Guerin (1872–1961). A veterinary surgeon at the Calmette Institute in Lille, who, along with Calmette, developed BCG vaccine.

Bonney test: elevation of bladder neck during vaginal examination reduces leakage of urine during coughing (used to diagnose stress incontinence).

William Bonney (1872–1953). Studied at Barts and The Middlesex Hospitals. On the staff of the Royal Masonic Hospital and The Chelsea Hospital for Women. He was a highly skilled surgeon with an international reputation.

Bowman's capsule: epithelial-lined cup surrounding the glomerulus in the kidney.

Sir William Paget Bowman (1816–1892). Surgeon to Birmingham General Hospital. Elected FRS in 1841. FRCS 1844. Won the Royal Medal of the Royal Society for his description of the Malpihgian body of the kidney. Proposed the theory of urine production by filtration of plasma. Described as the father of histology. 1846 became surgeon to Moorfields Eye Hospital. He was an early proponent of the opthalmoscope and the first in England to treat glaucoma by iridectomy (1862).

Camper fascia: superficial layer of superficial fascia (fat) of abdomen and inguinal region.

Pieter Camper (1722–1789). Physician and anatomist in Leyden, The Netherlands.

Charrière system: system of measurement for sizing catheters and stents.

Joseph Charrière (1803–1876). Surgical instrument maker in Paris.

Clutton sounds: metal probes for dilating the urethra (originally used for "sounding" for bladder stones).

Henry Clutton (1850–1909). Surgeon to St. Thomas's Hospital, London.

Colles fascia: superficial fascia of the perineum.

Abraham Colles (1773–1843). Professor of Anatomy and Surgery in Dublin.

Denonvilliers fascia: rectovesical fascia.

Charles Denonvilliers (1808–1872). Professor of Anatomy, Paris and later Professor of Surgery.

Dormia basket: basket for extracting stones from the ureter.
   Enrico Dormia. Assistant Professor of Surgery, Milan.

(Pouch of) Douglas: rectouterine pouch (in females), rectovesical pouch (in males).
   James Douglas (1675–1742). Anatomist; physician to the Queen.

Foley catheter: balloon catheter, designed to be self-retaining.

Foley pyeloplasty
   Frederic Foley (1891–1966). Urologist, St Paul, Minnesota.

Fournier gangrene: fulminating gangrene of external genitalia and lower abdominal wall.
   Jean Fournier (1832–1914). Professor of Dermatology, Hôpital St Louis, Paris. Also recognized the association between syphilis and tabes dorsalis.

Gerota's fascia: the renal fascia.
   Dumitru Gerota (1867–1939). Professor of Surgery, University of Budapest.

(Loop of) Henle: U-shaped segment of the nephron between the proximal and distal convoluted tubules.
   Friedrich Henle (1809–1885). Professor of Anatomy, Zurich and Göttingen.

von Hippel–Lindau syndrome: syndrome of multiple renal cancers
   Eugen von Hippel (1867–1939). Opthalmologist in Berlin.
   Arvid Lindau (1892–1958). Swedish pathologist.

Hunner's ulcer: ulcer in bladder in interstitial cystitis.
   Guy Hunner (1868–1957). Professor of Gynaecology, Johns Hopkins.

Jaboulay procedure: operation for hydrocele repair (excision of hydrocele sac).
   Mathieu Jaboulay (1860–1913). Professor of Surgery, Lyon.

Klinefelter syndrome: male hypogonadism with XXY chromosome complement.
   Harry Klinefelter (1912–1990). Associate Professor of Medicine, Johns Hopkins.

Kocherization of the duodenum: Mobilization of the second part of the duodenum. Used to expose the inferior vena cava and right renal vein during radical nephrectomy.
   Emil Kocher (1841–1917). Professor of Surgery, Berne University. A founder of modern surgery. He won the Nobel Prize in 1909 for work on the physiology, pathology, and surgery of the thyroid gland.

Lahey forceps: curved forceps used during surgery.
   Frank Lahey (1880–1953). Head of Surgery, The Lahey Clinic, Boston.

Langenbeck retractor: commonly used retractor during surgery.
   Bernard von Langenbeck (1810–1887). Professor of Surgery, Kiel and Berlin. A great teacher and surgeon.

Leydig cells: interstitial cells of the testis.
Franz von Leydig (1821–1908). Professor of Histology, Würtzburg, Tübingen, Bonn.

Malécot catheter: large-bore catheter, used for drainage of kidney following PCNL.
Achille Malécot (1852–?). Surgeon in Paris.

Millin's prostatectomy: retropubic open prostatectomy.
Terence Millin (1903–1980). Irish Surgeon, trained in Dublin. Surgeon at the Middlesex and Guy's Hospitals and, later, the Westminster Hospital. He became President of the British Association of Urological Surgeons and then President of the Royal College of Surgeons of Ireland.

Peyronie's disease: fibrosis of shaft of penis causing a bend of the penis during erection.
Francois Peyronie (1678–1747). Surgeon to Louis XV in Paris.

Pfannenstiel incision: suprapubic incision used for surgery to the bladder and uterus.
Hermann Pfannenstiel (1862–1909). Gynecologist from Breslau.

(Space of) Retzius: prevesical space.
Andreas Retzius (1796–1860). Professor of Anatomy and Physiology at the Karolinska Institute, Stockholm.

Santorini plexus: plexus of veins on the ventral surface of the prostate
Giandomenico Santorini (1681–1738). Professor of Anatomy and Medicine in Venice. Wrote a great work on anatomy, Observationes anatomicae, published in Venice in 1724.

Scarpa fascia: deep layer of the superficial fascia of the abdominal wall.
Antonio Scarpa (1747–1832). Professor of Anatomy in Modena and Pavia.

Sertoli cells: supportive cells of testicular epithelium.
Entrico Sertoli (1842–1910). Professor of Experimental Physiology, Milan.

Trendelenburg position: head-down operating position.
Friedrich Trendelenburg (1844–1924). Langenbeck's assistant in Berlin, and was then Professor of Surgery at Rostock, Bonn, and then Leipzig.

Weigert's law: inverse position of ectopic ureter (the ureter of the upper moiety of a duplex system) drains distally into the bladder (or below, into the urethra), whereas the lower pole ureter drains into a proximal position in the bladder.
Carl Weigert (1845–1904). German pathologist.

Wilms tumor: nephroblastoma of kidney.
Max Wilms (1867–1918). Surgical assistant to Trendelenburg in Leipzig and subsequently Professor of Surgery in Leipzig. Later, Professor of Surgery in Basle and Heidelberg.

Young's prostatectomy: perineal prostatectomy.
Hugh Hampton Young (1870–1945). Professor of Urology, John Hopkins School of Medicine.

Index

A

Abdominal aortic aneurysm
(AAA), 43
Abdominal distension, 25
Abdominal examination in
urological disease, 24–5
abdominal distension, 25
enlarged bladder, 25
enlarged kidney, 24
enlarged liver, 24
enlarged spleen, 24
umbilicus, 25
causes of, 25
Acid–base balance, 667–7
Acquired renal cystic
disease (ARCD)
associated disorders, 338
definition, 338
epidemiology, 338
etiology, 338
investigation, 338
pathology, 338
presentation, 338
treatment, 339
Active surveillance, 232
Acute inflammatory
demyelinating
polyneuropathy, 525–6
Adenocarcinoma, 212,
251, 268
Adenoma, 188–9
Adrenaline, 618
Adrenal steroid synthesis,
metabolic pathways
for, 555
α-Adrenergic blockers,
511
α-Adrenoceptor (AR), 76
AdVance, 129
Albendazole, 178, 179
ALFIN study, 80–1
Alfuzosin, 76, 390–1
Allopurinol, 384
5α-reductase (AR), 64
5α-reductase inhibitors,
78–9, 80–1
and α-blocker, 80–1
efficacy, 78
for hematuria due to BPH,
78–9
and risk of urinary
retention, 78
side effects, 78

α-blocker
and 5α-reductase
inhibitor, 80–1
classification, 76
efficacy, 76
indications for treatment,
76
side effects, 76–7
therapy, 76
α-fetoprotein (AFP), 299
Alprostadil (MUSE;
Caverject), 490
American Urological
Association (AUA), 5–6,
84, 84–5
Amoxicillin, 520–1, 534, 574
Ampicillin, 148–9, 160–1,
534
Androgen deprivation,
mechanisms of, 234–6
Androgen-independent/
castration-resistant
disease, 240–1
Androgen-independent
phase, 240
Androgen replacement
therapy, 490
Angiogenic factors, 188–9
Angiomyolipoma (AML),
276–7
pathology, 277
presentation, 277
investigations, 277
treatment, 277
Angiomyolipoma, 188–9
Anterior urethra, 106
Anterior urethral injuries,
452
complete rupture, 452
diagnosis and subsequent
management,
confirming, 452
history and examination,
452
partial rupture, 452
penetrating anterior
urethral injuries, 452
Antiandrogens, 236
Antibiotic prophylaxis
low-dose, 143–4
post-intercourse, 144
self-start therapy, 145
in urological surgery, 574
Anticholinergics, 82, 122

Antidiuretic hormone
(ADH), 665
deficiency, 14–15
Antiestrogens, 480
Antimicrobial drug therapy,
146
Artificial urinary sphincter
(AUS), 120–1
complications and long-
term outcomes, 121
indications and patient
selection, 120
patient evaluation, 120
results, 120
Assisted conception, 481
Assisted reproductive
techniques (ART), 481
Asymptomatic inflammatory
prostatitis, 169
Atypical small acinar
proliferation (ASAP),
193
Augmentation
enterocystoplasty, 124
Auto-augmentation, 124
Autoclaving, 604
Autonomic dysreflexia
(AD), management
of, 523
Autosomal dominant
polycystic kidney disease
(ADPKD), 558
associated disorders, 340
definition, 340
differential diagnosis, 340
epidemiology, 340
etiology, 340
investigation, 341
pathology, 340
presentation, 340
treatment, 341
Autosomal recessive
polycystic kidney disease
(ARPKD), 558
Azoospermia, 476–8
Aztreonam, 148–9

B

Bacille Calmette–Guérin
(BCG), 258–9
Back pain, 68
Baclofen, 122
Bacterial prostatitis, 168–9

Bacterial resistance to drug therapy, 146
Bacteriuria, 134–5
Balanitis, 182
Balanitis xerotica obliterans (BXO), 107, 310–3
Balanoposthitis, 182
Ball et al. study, 74–5
Basic science of relevance to urological practice, 659–67
bladder, physiology of, 660
micturition, physiology of, 660
renal anatomy, 661–3
renal blood flow (RBF), 661–2
renal function, 662–3
renal physiology
acid–base balance, 668–9
sodium and potassium excretion, regulation of, 665
water balance, regulation of, 664
urethra, physiology of, 660
Bed-wetting, 21, 68
Behavioral exercises, 126
Benign prostatic hyperplasia (BPH), 10–3, 39, 198–9
androgens' role in, 64
and bladder outlet obstruction (BOO), 66
and lower urinary tract symptoms (LUTS), 70–1, 72–3
medical management
5α-reductase inhibitors, 78–9
α-blockers, 76–7
alternative drug therapy, 82
combination therapy, 80–1
minimally invasive management of, 84–5
and prostate growth regulation, 64
Benign prostatic obstruction (BPO), 68
clinical practice guidelines, 68
prostatism vs. LUTS vs. LUTS/BPH, 68
urinary symptoms, 68
Benign renal masses, 276–7
angiomyolipoma (AML), 276–7
oncocytoma, 276
β subunit (B-hCG), 299
Bevacizumab, 293
Bicalutamide, 232, 236

Bicarbonate reabsorption along nephron, 668, 669
Bilateral obstruction of a ureter (BUO), 414
Bilateral orchiectomy, 234
side effects, 236
Bilateral ureteric obstruction, 463
immediate treatment, 463
Biofeedback, 126
Birt-Hogg-Dubé (BHD) syndrome, 279
Bladder. See also Neuropathic bladder
abnormalities, 112
afferent innervation of, 500–1
augmentation, 512–13
behavior in patient with neurological disease, 506–7
characteristics and causes of, 25
diagnosis, 444
extraperitoneal perforation, 444
imaging studies, 444–6
injuries, 444–6
associated with pelvic fractures, 440–2
intraperitoneal perforation, 444
motor innervation of, 500
parasympathetic, 500
sympathetic, 500, 502
physiology of, 660
situations, 444
treatment, 447
Bladder cancer, 14. See also Muscle-invasive bladder cancer
diagnosis and staging, 254–5
staging investigations, 255
transurethral resection of bladder tumor (TURBT), 254
epidemiology and etiology, 246
pathology and staging, 248–51
adenocarcinoma, 251
histological grading, 248
squamous cell carcinoma (SCC), 250
staging, 248
tumor spread, 248
urothelial carcinoma, 248–50
presentation, 252
signs, 252
symptoms, 252

risk factors, 246
urinary diversion after cystectomy, 266–8
continent diversion, 266–8
ileal conduit, 266
ureterosigmoidostomy, 266
Bladder management techniques, for neuropathic patient, 510–3
bladder augmentation, 512–13
deafferentation, 513
external sphincterotomy, 511
indwelling catheters, 511
intermittent self-catheterization (ISC), 511
medical therapy, 511
sacral neuromodulation, 512
urinary diversion, 513
Bladder neck stenosis, 222–3
Bladder outlet obstruction (BOO), 10–3, 66, 242
acute urinary retention definition, pathophysiology, and causes, 90–1
initial and definitive management, 94
benign prostatic hyperplasia (BPH)66
α-blockers, 76–7
5α-reductase inhibitors, 78–9
alternative drug therapy, 82
combination therapy, 80–1
and lower urinary tract symptoms (LUTS), 70–1, 72–3
minimally invasive management of, 84–5
and prostate growth regulation, 64
uncomplicated, 74–5
benign prostatic obstruction (BPO), 68
high-pressure chronic retention (HPCR), 102
lower urinary tract symptoms (LUTS), 70–1, 72–3
nocturia and nocturnal polyuria, management of, 100–1

pathophysiological consequences of, 66
and retention in women, 104–5
suprapubic catheterization, 98–9
transurethral resection of the prostate (TURP)
invasive surgical alternatives to, 86–7
and open prostatectomy, 88–9
surgical alternatives to, 84–5
urethral catheterization, 96–7
urethral stricture disease, 106–7
Bladder outlet obstruction and retention in women, 104–5
voiding studies in women, 104
treatment of, 104
Fowler syndrome, 104–5
Bladder pressure, 60–1
Bladder stones, 400
Bladder syringe, 593
Bleeding
during PCNL, 642
in testicular injuries, 454
Blocked catheters, 552–3
Blood, in urine, 36
Blunt injures, 420
Blunt trauma, testicular ultrasound in, 454
Boari flap, 437
Bonney test, 114
Bosniak classification, of CT appearance of simple and complex cysts, 333
Bothersome symptoms, 72
Botulinum toxin A (BTX-A) injection therapy, 124–5
Bowen disease, 310–3
Bowenoid papulosis, 310
Brachytherapy (BT), 228–9
BT plus EBRT, outcomes of, 229
and RP and EBRT, 229
complications, 228
contraindications to, 228
indications for
with EBRT, 228
as monotherapy, 228
outcomes of, 228–9
rising PSA post-BT, 229
Brainstem lesions, bladder dysfunction in, 525
Bristol flow rate nomogram, 55
Buck fascia, 453
Buffering systems, 666

Bulbocavernosus reflex (BCR), 29, 488
Burch colposuspension, 117
Buschke–Löwenstein tumor, 310–3
Butterfly bruising in anterior urethral rupture, 453

C

Calcium oxalate, 362
Calcium oxalate stone formation, prevention of, 398–9
Calcium phosphate, 363
Calyceal diverticulum, 334
Canal of Nück, 31
Carbonic acid, 668
Carcinoma in situ (CIS), 188–9, 248–50
Carcinomas, 188–9
Castration resistant disease, 233
Castration-resistant prostate cancer (CRPC), 241
Casts, 37
Catheters, 584, 585, , 588
Catheters and sheaths and neuropathic patient, 516–17
condom catheter sheaths, 517
intermittent catheterization (IC), 516
long-term catheterization, 516–17
Cauda equina compression, 464
Cavernosography, 488–9
Cefaclor, 534
Cefalexin, 534
Cefotaxime, 158–9, 534
Ceftriaxone, 148–9, 158–9
Cefuroxime, 164, 534
Cephalexin, 144
Cephalosporins, 158–9, 534
Cerebrovascular accidents (CVAs), bladder dysfunction after, 525
Cervix, MRI of, 93
Chemical sterilization, 604
Chemotherapy, 319
adjuvant intravesical, 258–9
Chlorine dioxide (Cidex), 604
Chromophobe RCC, 278–9
Chronic flank pain, 18
nonurological causes, 19
urological causes, 18
Chronic pelvic pain syndrome (CPPS), 169

Chronic pyelonephritis, 154
Ciprofloxacin, 148–9, 169, 520, 520–1, 574
Ciprofloxin, 148–9
Circumcision, 618–19
Cisplatin, 265
Clamshell ileocystoplasty, 124
Clearance of substance, 663–4
Clear cell renal cell carcinoma, 278
Clindamycin, 160–1
Clonal expansion, 188–9
Clot/tumor colic, 17
CO_2, 668
Colonic perforation during PCNL, 643
Color Doppler ultrasonography, 162, 488–9
CombAT study, 80–1
Completely patent urachus, 25
Computed tomography (CT), 6, 50
CT cystography, 444–6
CT urography (CTU), 254–5, 403
contrast-enhanced, 6
uses, 50
Condom catheter sheaths, 517
Condyloma acuminatum, 310
Congential adrenal hyperplasia (CAH), 554–6
Contact laser prostatectomy, 86
Continent diversion, 266–8
Corticosteroids, 480
Creatinine, serum, 102
Cryotherapy, 230
Cutaneous horn, 310–3
Cyst, complex, 333
Cyst, simple
differential diagnosis, 332
etiology, 332
investigation
CT, 333
renal ultrasound, 332–3
presentation, 332
prevalence, 332–3
treatment, 333
Cystic renal disease, 558–9.
See also Acquired renal cystic disease (ARCD); Autosomal dominant (adult) polycystic kidney disease (ADPKD); Calyceal diverticulum; Medullary sponge kidney (MSK); Simple cyst

Cystine, 364
Cystine stones, 384–5
Cystography, 48
Cystometrogram, 21
Cystometry, 60–1
Cystoscopy, 5–6, 610–1
  flexible, 610
  rigid, 610
Cytology, urine collections
  for, 38
Cytotoxic chemotherapy,
  240–1

D

Daily fluid requirement, 580
Dantec flowmeter, 55
Darifenicin, 122
Deafferentation, 513
Deep venous
  thromboembolism
  (DVT), 576–8
  diagnosis, 576
  risk factors for, 576
  treatment, 576
Degree of hematuria,
  422, 423
Desmopressin (DDAVP),
  100–1, 122, 569
Detrusor-external sphincter
  dyssynergia (DESD),
  506–7
Detrusor hyperreflexia
  (DH), 506–7
Detrusor leak point
  pressure (DLPP), 115
Detrusor myectomy, 124
Detrusor overactivity (DO),
  506–7
Detrusor sphincter
  dyssynergia (DSD), 66,
  104, 506–7, 511
Devitalized segments of
  kidney, 426
Dexamethasone, 182, 293
Diabetes insipidus (DI),
  14–15
Diagnostic radiological
  imaging, 388
Diathermy, 602
Diathermy, 601–3
  bipolar, 600
  monopolar, 600
  and pacemakers, 602
  potential problems with,
  600–1
Dietary oxalate, 399
Dietary risk factors for
  stone disease, 357
Diethylcarbamazine, 179
Diffuse bone pain, 243
Digital rectal examination
  (DRE), 28–9, 196

abnormal, 197
  features to elicit in, 29
  and PSA, 70
Dihydrotestosterone
  (DHT), 64, 78–9, 190,
  233, 552
Dimercaptosuccinic acid
  (DMSA) scanning, 53
Dimethylsulfoxide (DMSO),
  174
Dipstick hematuria, 2
Dipstick testing, 36–7
Disorders of sex
  development (DSD),
  554–6
Disseminated intravascular
  coagulation (DIC), 243
Dissolution therapy, 384–5
Distal urethral sphincter
  mechanism, 501
Diuretics, 100
Docetaxel, 265
Doxazosin, 76, 169, 511
D-penicillamine, 384–5
Drains, 584–6
Ductal dysplasia. See
  Prostatic intraepithelial
  neoplasia (PIN)
Dutasteride, 78–9, 80–1

E

Early prostate cancer
  antigen-2 (EPCA-), 00
Early versus delayed
  hormone therapy, 238
Ectopic ureter, 546
Eection and ejaculation
  impotence
  evaluation of, 488–9
  treatment, 490–1
  Peyronie's disease, 494–5
  physiology, 484–5
  priapism, 496–8
  retrograde ejaculation, 492
eGFR (estimated GFR),
  663–4
Electrohydraulic lithotripsy
  (EHL), 374
Electromyographic (EMG)
  activity, 104–5
Embryonal cell, 33
Emphysematous
  pyelonephritis, 152, 153
Endoscopic cystolitholapaxy
  (and (open)
  cystolithotomy), 654
  anesthesia, 654
  common postoperative
  complications and
  management, 654
  indications, 654
  postoperative care, 654

procedure-specific
  consent form, 654
Enterococcus, 542
Enucleation, 86–7
Enuresis, 568–9
Ephedrine sulfate, 492
Epididymal cyst 33
  removal of, 620
Epididymitis, 22, 162–3, 33
  chronic epididimitis, 163
  differential diagnosis, 162
  treatment, 162–3
Epididymo-orchitis, 22
Erectile dysfunction
  (ED), 222–3. See also
  Impotence
ERSPC (European
  Randomized Study of
  Screening for Prostate
  Cancer) trial, 194
Escherichia coli (*E. coli*), 542
Estrogen replacement
  therapy, 143
Estrogens, 190
Ethambutol, 258–9
European Association of
  Urology (EUA) guideline,
  84–5
Everolimus, 293
Exstrophy, 560–1
External beam radiotherapy
  (EBRT), 226–7
External sphincterotomy,
  511
Extracorporeal lithotripsy
  (ESWL), 372–3, 396–7
Extracorporeal shock wave
  lithotripsy (ESWL), 334
Extraperitoneal perforation,
  444, 447

F

False negative urine
  dipstick, 2
False positive urine
  dipstick, 2
Familial juvenile
  nephronophthisis, 558
Femoral aneurysm, 31
Femoral hernia, 30
Finasteride, 78–9, 78,
  80–1, 82
Fine needle aspiration,
  274–5
Five centers' study, 74–5
Flank pain, acute, 16
  non-stone, urological
  causes, 17
  nonurological causes,
  17–18
Flank pain, 16–19
  acute flank pain, 16

non-stone, urological causes, 17
nonurological causes, 17–18
chronic flank pain, 18
nonurological causes, 19
urological causes, 18
urological and nonurological flank pain, 18
Flavoxate, 82
Flexible ureteroscopes, 378–9, 646
technique, 646
Flomax, 390–1
Fluid restriction, 100
Fluorescent in situ hybridization (FISH), 254–5
Fluoroquinolones, 144, 145, 148–9, 158–9
Focal bone pain, 243
4-glass test, 167
Fournier gangrene, 160–1
diagnosis, 160
presentation, 160
treatment, 160–1
Fowler syndrome, 91, 104–5
Free-to-total (F:T) ratio, 200
Frontal lobe lesions, bladder dysfunction in, 525
Fructose, 472–4

G

Gabapentin, 163
Gamete intrafallopian transfer (GIFT), 481
Gemcitabine, 265
Genital filariasis, 179
Genital symptoms, 22–3
priapism, 23
scrotal pain, 22
testicular tumors, acute presentations of, 22–3
Genital tract, differentiation of, 553
Gentamicin, 158–9, 160–1, 164, 168, 520–1, 574
Germ cell tumors (GCT), 188–9, 300
Gleason score, 212, 213
Glomerular filtration rate (GFR), 663–4
Glycine, 592
Gonococcal urethritis (GU), 140–1
Granulomatous prostatitis, 170
Greenlight Laser Prostatectomy, 87
Groin, lumps in. See Lumps in groin

Gross hematuria, 422, 426
Guide wires, 590–1
Gunshot injuries, 420

H

Helical CT, 50
Hematospermia, 8–9
causes, 8
examination, 8
investigation, 8
treatment, 8–9
Hematuria, 36
Hematuria, macroscopic, 68
Hematuria I, 2
definition, 2
microscopic/dipstick hematuria, 2
Hematuria II, 4–7
common causes, 4
and cystoscopy, 5–6
diagnostic cystoscopy, 5
further investigation, 6–7
medical (nephrological), 4
surgical (urological), 4
upper tract imaging study, 6
urological investigation, 5
Heme test, urine dipsticks test for, 2
Hemoglobin, 36
Hemorrhage
after circumcision, 618
during pyeloplasty, 650
after TURP, 612–13
after TURBT, 615
Hemorrhagic shock, 580
Hemospermia. See Hematospermia
Hemostasis, 88–9
Heparin, 577–8
Hereditary papillary RCC (HPRCC), 279
Hernia, 30
High-dose radiation (HDR), 228–9
High-flow priapism, 23
High-grade prostatic intraepithelial neoplasia (HGPIN), 190, 193
High-intensity focused ultrasound (HIFU), 85, 227, 230–1
High-pressure chronic retention (HPCR), 102
acute treatment, 102
definitive treatment, 102
High-pressure sphincter, 508, 518
High-riding prostate, 442
HIV in urological surgery, 180–1
diagnosis, 180

needle stick injury, 181
pathogenesis, 180
urological sequelae, 180–1
Holmium laser, 598–600, 598, 599
Holmium laser enucleation of the prostate (HoLEP), 86–7
Holmium laser prostatectomy, 86–7
Holmium laser resection of the prostate (HoLRP), 86–7
Holmium-only laser ablation of the prostate (HoLAP), 86–7
Hopkins rod-lens system, 606
Hormone assay, in male infertility, 472, 473, 476–7
Hormone therapy, 232
additional therapies, 238–9
androgen deprivation, mechanisms of, 234–6
androgen-independent/castration-resistant disease, 240–1
castration-resistant prostate cancer, 241
cytotoxic chemotherapy, 240–1
early versus delayed hormone therapy, 238
hormone dependence of prostate cancer, 233
intermittent hormone therapy, 238
monitoring treatment, 238
prognostic factors, 233
second-line hormone therapy, 240
Horseshoe kidney, 348, 349
HPC-1 gene, 9
Human chorionic gonadotrophin, 299
Hunner's ulcer, 173
Hydatid disease, 178
Hydrocele, 31, 32, 620
Hydronephrosis, 41, 406–8
bilateral, 408
causes, 409
diagnostic approach, 406–8
management of, 522
of pregnancy, 402, 536
ultrasound, 406
unilateral, 407
Hyoscyamine, 511
Hypercalcemia, 362
Hypercalciuria, 356, 362
Hyperchloremic acidosis, 641

Hypernephroma. *See* Renal cell carcinoma (RCC)
Hyperoxaluria, 362
Hypertension and renal injury, 429
Hyperuricosuria, 362
Hypocitraturia, 362
Hypofractionation, 226–7
Hypospadias, 550–1
Hypothalamic–pituitary–testicular axis, 466, 467

I

Iatrogenic renal injury, 429
IL-2 (Aldesleukin), 9
Ileal conduit, 266, 640–1
  complications, 266
  indications, 640
  postoperative care and common post-operative complications and management, 640–1
  procedure-specific consent form, 641
Ileal loopogram, 48
Imipramine, 122, 492, 569
Impotence
  causes, 489
  evaluation, of, 488–9
  treatment, 490–1
Incontinence, C4
  causes and pathophysiology, 112–13
  classification, 110–1
    mixed urinary incontinence, 110–1
    nocturnal enuresis, 110–1
    overflow incontinence, 110–1
    post-micturition dribble, 110–1
    stress urinary incontinence (SUI), 110–1
    urge urinary incontinence (UUI), 110–1
  definition, 110
  in elderly patient, 132
    management, 132
    prevalence, 132
    transient causes (DIAPPERS), 132
  evaluation, 114–15
  investigation, 114–15
    bladder diaries, 114
    blood tests, X-ray imaging, cystoscopy, 114
  screening tests, 115
  sphincter electromyography (EMG), 115
  urodynamic investigations, 115
  mixed incontinence, 126
  in neuropathic patient, 518–19
    causes, 518
    empirical treatment, 518–19
    investigations, 518
  overactive bladder (OAB)
    conventional treatment, 122
    options for failed conventional therapy, 124–5
  physical examination, 114
  post-prostatectomy incontinence, 128–9
  prevalence, 110
  sphincter weakness incontinence, treatment of
    artificial urinary sphincter, 120–1
    injection therapy, 116
    pubovaginal slings, 118
    retropubic suspension, 117
  vesicovaginal fistula (VVF), 130–1
Indinavir, 358–9
Indwelling catheters, 511
Infections and inflammatory conditions
acute pyelonephritis, 148–9, 153
  chronic pyelonephritis, 154
  emphysematous pyelonephritis, 152, 153
  epididymitis and orchitis, 162–3
  Fournier gangrene, 160–1
  granulomatous prostatitis, 170
  HIV in urological surgery, 180–1
  interstitial cystitis, 172–4
  lower urinary tract infection, 140–1
  parasitic infections, 178–9
  of penis, 182–3
  perinephric abscess, 153, 164
  prostatic abscess, 170
  prostatitis
    epidemiology and classification, 166–7
  presentation, evaluation, and treatment, 168–9
  pyonephrosis, 153
  pyonephrosis and perinephric abscess, 150
  recurrent urinary tract infection, 142–5
  septicemia and urosepsis, 156–9
  tuberculosis, 176–7
  urinary tract infection, 134–7
    antimicrobial drug therapy, 146
    bacterial resistance to drug therapy, 146
    bacterial virulence, factors increasing, 138–9
    complicated, 138
    definitive treatment, 146–7
    host defenses, 139
    route of infection, 138
    uncomplicated, 138
    xanthogranulomatous pyelonephritis, 152–3
Infertility
  azoospermia, 476–8
  definition, 470
  etiology and evaluation, 470–1
  lab investigation, 472–6
  male reproductive physiology, 466–8
    hypothalamic–pituitary–testicular axis, 466
    mature sperm, 466–8
    spermatogenesis, 466
    testosterone, 466
  oligospermia, 476
  treatment options, 480–1
    assisted conception, 481
    assisted reproductive techniques (ART), 481
    medical treatment, 480
    surgical treatment, 480–1
  varicocele, 478–80
Inguinal hernia, 30, 32
Inguinal lymphadenectomy, 320
Injection therapy, for urinary incontinence, 116
Insulin-like growth factor type 1 (IGF-), 39
Interferon A-2b, 9
Intermittent catheterization (IC), 516
Intermittent hormone therapy, 238

Intermittent self-catheterization (ISC), 511
Internal (optical) urethrotomy, 107
International Germ Cell Cancer Collaborative Group (IGCCCG), 303
International Prostate Symptom Score (IPSS), 11, 10–3, 68, 70, 74–5
Interstitial cystitis, 172–4
  associated disorders, 172
  epidemiology, 172
  evaluation, 172–4
  pathogenesis, 172
  treatment, 172
Interstitial laser prostatectomy (ILP), 86
Intracavernosal therapy, 490
Intracytoplasmic sperm injection (ICSI), 481
Intraperitoneal perforation, 444, 447
Intratubular germ cell neoplasia (IGCN), 294, 308
Intraurethral therapy, for impotence, 490
Intrauterine insemination (IUI), 481
Intravenous contrast media, 44–6
Intravenous pyelography (IVP), 6, 44–6
  films and phases, 44–6
  uses, 46
Intravenous urography (IVU). See Intravenous pyelography (IVP)
Intrinsic sphincter deficiency (ISD), 21
In vitro fertilization (IVF), 481
IPSS. See International Prostate Symptom Score (IPSS)
Isolated urinary tract infection, 134–5
Isoniazid, 258–9
Isotope renogram, 546
Ivermectin, 179

J

JJ stents, 392, 393, 594–7, 630–1, 595

K

Kaposi sarcoma, 310
Keratotic balanitis, 310–3
Kidney, enlarged characteristics and causes of, 24
Kidney stones
  characteristics of stone types, 367
  dissolution therapy, 384–5
  epidemiology, 356–7
  evaluation of stone former, 366–7
    metabolic evaluation, 366–7
    risk factors, 366
  extracorporeal lithotripsy (ESWL), 372–3
  factors predisposing to specific stone types, 362–4
    calcium oxalate, 362
    calcium phosphate, 363
    cystine, 364
    struvite, 363
    uric acid, 362–3
  flexible ureteroscopy and laser treatment, 378–9
  fragmentation, intracorporeal techniques of
    electrohydraulic lithotripsy (EHL), 374
    laser lithotripsy, 376
    pneumatic (ballistic) lithotripsy, 374
    ultrasonic lithotripsy, 374–5
  mechanisms of formation, 360
  open stone surgery, 383
  percutaneous nephrolithotomy (PCNL), 380
  presentation and diagnosis, 368
  treatment options, 370–1
  types and predisposing factors, 358–9
  watchful waiting, 370–1
Klebsiella, 542
Knife and gunshot wounds, 458
KTP laser, 87

L

Lactate dehydrogenase (LDH), 299
Laparoscopic prostatectomy, stages in, 219–20
Laparoscopic surgery, 652–3
  contraindications to, 652
  potential complications unique to, 652
  procedure specific consent forms, 653
Laser lithotripsy, 376, 646
Laser prostatectomy, 86–7
Lasers, in urological surgery, 598–600
Laser treatment, 378–9
  for intrarenal stones, 646
Leiomyoma/sarcoma, 321
Leiomyosarcoma, 188–9
Leukocyte esterase, 136
Leukoplakia, 310–3
Levofloxin, 162–3
Leydig cells, 466
LHRH agonists, 234, 235
Lidocaine, 96–7
Liposarcoma, 321
Liver, enlarged characteristics and causes of, 24
Localized prostate cancer (T1–2), 196. See also Prostate cancer
  management of, 215
    brachytherapy (BT), 228–9
    cryotherapy and high-intensity focused ultrasound (HIFU), 230–1
    external beam radiotherapy (EBRT), 226–7
    general principles, 215
    watchful waiting and active surveillance, 216–17
Locally advanced bladder cancer, 264–5
Locally advanced cancer (T3–4), 196
Locally advanced nonmetastatic prostate cancer, management, 232
  external beam radiotherapy (EBRT), 232
  hormone therapy, 232
  palliative treatment of locally advanced disease, 232
  watchful waiting/active surveillance, 232
Loin pain. See Flank pain
Long-term catheterization, 516–17
Lower urinary tract (LUT), innervation of, 500–3
  afferent innervation of bladder, 500–1

motor innervation of
  bladder, 500
  parasympathetic, 500
  sympathetic, 500
sensory innervation of
  urethra, 503
somatic motor innervation
  of urethral sphincter,
  501
Lower urinary tract
  infection, 140–1
noninfective hemorrhagic
  cystitis, 140
urethral syndrome, 141
urethritis, 140–1
Lower urinary tract
  symptoms (LUTS), 10–3,
  68, 70–1, 72–3, 242
and acute urinary
  retention, 72–3
and benign prostatic
  hyperplasia (BPH)
  clinical practice
    guidelines, 70
  digital rectal examination
    (DRE) and PSA, 70
  flow rate measurement,
    70
  post-void residual urine
    volume (PVR), 70
  pressure-flow studies, 71
  renal ultrasonography,
    71
  serum creatinine, 70
bothersome symptoms, 72
causes, 10–3
and prostate cancer, 72
uncomplicated, 74–5
Low-flow (ischemic)
  priapism, 23
Low-pressure sphincter,
  508, 518
Lumps in groin, 30–1
diagnosis, determining, 30
enlarged inguinal lymph
  nodes, 30
femoral aneurysm, 31
hydrocele of cord, 31
lipoma of cord, 31
psoas abscess, 31
saphena varix, 30
undescended testis, 31
Lumps in scrotum, 32–4
diagnosis, determining, 32–4
differential diagnosis, 32
Luteinizing hormone (LH),
  233
Luteinizing hormone–
  releasing hormone
  (LHRH), 228, 233
  side effects, 236
Lycopene, 244
Lymphadenopathy, 319

Lymphatic filariasis, 179
Lymph nodes, enlarged
  inguinal, 30
Lymphocele, 222, 634
Lymphoma management,
  309

M

Macroscopic (gross)
  hematuria, 2
MAG3 renogram, 52–3
  description, 52–3
  phases, 52
  uses, 53
Magnetic resonance imaging
  (MRI), 6, 50–1
Male posterior urethral
  injuries, 448
Male reproductive
  physiology, 466–8
  hypothalamic–pituitary–
    testicular axis, 466
  mature sperm, 466–8
  spermatogenesis, 466
  testosterone, 466
Malignant ureteral
  obstruction, 463
  bilateral ureteric
    obstruction, 463
  immediate treatment,
    463
  unilateral obstruction,
    463
Malrotation, of kidney,
  350, 351
Marshall–Marchetti–Krantz
  (MMK) procedure, 117
Mature sperm, 466–8
Maximal androgen blockade
  (MAB), 240
Meares-Stamey test, 167
Medtronic InterStim
  therapy, 105
  for nocturia, 100
Medullary cystic disease, 558
Medullary sponge kidney
  (MSK)
  definition, 336
  differential diagnosis, 336
  investigation
    biochemistry, 336
    intravenous pyelogram
      (IVP), 336
  pathology, 336
  presentation, 336
  prevalence, 336
  treatment, 337
Metabolic abnormalities, 268
Metastatic bladder cancer,
  265
Metastatic disease, 196,
  233, 319

Methotrexate, vinblastine,
  adriamycin, and cisplatin
  (MVAC), 264
Methylene-disphosphonate
  (MDP), 53
Metronidazole, 160–1
Microhematuria, 426
Microscopic/dipstick
  hematuria, 2
Micturition, physiology of,
  504–5, 660
Midstream specimen of
  urine (MSU)
  dipstick of, 140–1
  microscopy of, 140–1
Midstream urine specimen
  (MSU), 534
Mitomycin C (MMC),
  254, 258
Mitoxantrone, 240–1
Mitrofanoff procedure, 104,
  266–8
Mixed incontinence, 126
  definition, 126
  investigation and
    management, 126
  SUI component, 126
Mixed urinary incontinence
  (MUI), 20, 110–1
MR urography (MRU), 388,
  403–4
M stage of prostate cancer,
  208
MTOPS study (Medical
  Therapy of Prostatic
  Symptoms), 80–1
Multicystic dysplastic kidney
  (MCDK), 558–9
Multidetector computed
  tomography urography
  (MDCTU), 6
Multilocular cystic
  nephroma, 559
Multiple sclerosis (MS),
  bladder dysfunction
  in, 524
Multiple system atrophy
  (MSA), bladder
  dysfunction in, 524–5
Mumps orchitis, 163
Muscle-invasive bladder
  cancer. See also Bladder
  cancer
  bladder preservation,
    260–2
  locally advanced bladder
    cancer, 264–5
  metastatic bladder cancer,
    265
  palliative treatment, 263
  partial cystectomy, 260–2
  radical cystectomy,
    260–2

radical cystectomy with
    urinary diversion,
    260–2
    efficacy of, 262
    major complications, 261
    postoperative care,
        261–2
    procedure, 261
    salvage radical
        cystectomy, 261–2
radical external beam
    radiotherapy, 263

N

National Cancer Institute
    (NCI), 194
National Comprehensive
    Cancer Network
    (NCCN), 216–17
Nd:YAG laser beam, 87
Needle biopsy, 274–5
Neobladder, 266–8
Neoplasia, urological
    benign renal masses,
        276–7
    bladder cancer
        diagnosis and staging,
            254–5
        epidemiology and
            etiology, 246
        pathology and staging,
            248–51
        presentation, 252
        urinary diversion after
            cystectomy, 266–8
    localized prostate cancer
        management
        brachytherapy (BT),
            228–9
        cryotherapy and high-
            intensity focused
            ultrasound (HIFU),
            230–1
        general principles, 215
        radical external beam
            radiotherapy (EBRT),
            226–7
        radical prostatectomy,
            218–20
        watchful waiting and
            active surveillance,
            216–17
    locally advanced
        nonmetastatic prostate
        cancer, management,
            232
    muscle-invasive bladder
        cancer
        locally advanced bladder
            cancer, 264–5
        metastatic bladder
            cancer, 265

palliative treatment, 263
    radical external beam
        radiotherapy, 263
    surgical management of
        localized (pT2/3a)
        disease, 260–2
neuroblastoma, 329
    pathology and molecular
        biology, 188–9
penile neoplasia
    benign tumors and
        lesions, 310, 311
    epidemiology, risk
        factors, and
        pathology, 314–16
    premalignant cutaneous
        lesions, 310–3
    viral-related lesions, 310
prostate cancer
    clinical presentation, 196
    control, with radical
        prostatectomy, 224–5
    epidemiology and
        etiology, 190–1
    grading, 212
    incidence, prevalence,
        and mortality, 192
    palliative management
        of, 242–3
    premalignant lesions, 193
    prevention,
        complementary and
        alternative therapies,
        244–5
    risk stratification in
        management of, 214
    staging, 206–8
    transrectal
        ultrasonography and
        biopsies, 202–3
prostate cancer, advanced
    additional therapies,
        238–9
    androgen deprivation,
        mechanisms of,
        234–6
    early versus delayed
        hormone therapy,
        238
    hormone dependence of
        prostate cancer, 233
    intermittent hormone
        therapy, 238
    monitoring treatment,
        238
    prognostic factors, 233
prostate cancer screening,
    counseling before, 195
prostatic-specific antigen
    (PSA)
    density, 200
    doubling time (PSADT),
        200

free-to-total (F:T) ratio,
    200
    and prostate cancer,
        198–9
    and prostate cancer
        screening, 194
    velocity, 200
radical prostatectomy,
    218–20
    postoperative course
        after, 222–3
    prostate cancer control
        with, 224–5
    radiological assessment of
        renal masses, 274–5
renal cell carcinoma
    active surveillance, 286
    epidemiology and
        etiology, 278–9
    management of
        metastatic disease,
        292–3
    pathology, staging, and
        prognosis, 280
    presentation and
        investigations, 284
    surgical treatment,
        288–9, 290
retroperitoneal fibrosis,
    326–7
scrotum, carcinoma
    of, 320
squamous cell carcinoma
    (SCC), of penis,
    318–19
superficial UC
    management
    adjuvant intravesical
        chemotherapy and
        BCG, 258–9
    transurethral resection
        of bladder tumor
        (TURBT), 256
testicular adnexa, tumors
    of, 321
testicular cancer
    clinical presentation,
        296–8
    epidemiology and
        etiology, 294
    intratubular germ cell
        neoplasia (IGCN),
        308
    lymphoma management,
        309
    metastatic germ cell
        cancer, prognostic
        staging system for, 303
    nonseminomatous
        germ cell tumors
        (NSGCT),
        management of,
        304–7

pathology and staging, 300
seminoma, 308–9
serum markers, 299
transitional cell carcinoma (UC), of renal pelvis and ureter, 270–2
urethral cancer, 322–4
Wilms tumor, 328–9
Nephrectomy and nephroureterectomy, 632–3
anesthesia, 632
common postoperative complications and management, 632
indications, 632
postoperative care, 632
procedure-specific consent form, 633
Nephrogenic diabetes insipidus, 14–15
Nephrogenic systemic fibrosis (NSF), 274
Nephrogram phase, of IVP, 44
Nephrons, 663–4
Nephron-sparing surgery, 288–9
Nephroureterectomy, 271–2
Nesbit procedure, 622
Neuroblastoma, 329
imaging and staging, 329
presentation, 329
treatment and prognosis, 329
Neurogenic detrusor overactivity (NDO), 506–7
Neuromodulation, in lower urinary tract dysfunction, 528–9
posterior tibial nerve stimulation (PTNS), 529
sacral nerve stimulation (SNS), 528–9
Neuropathic bladder
autonomic dysreflexia, management of, 523
bladder and sphincter behavior in patient with neurological disease, 506–7
bladder dysfunction in brainstem lesions, 525
cerebrovascular accidents (CVAs), 525
frontal lobe lesions, 525
multiple sclerosis (MS), 524

multiple system atrophy (MSA), 524–5
Parkinson disease (PD), 524
peripheral neuropathies, 526
transverse myelitis, 525–6
bladder management techniques, 510–3
bladder augmentation, 512–13
deafferentation, 513
external sphincterotomy, 511
indwelling catheters, 511
intermittent self-catheterization (ISC), 511
medical therapy, 511
sacral neuromodulation, 512
urinary diversion, 513
catheters and sheaths and neuropathic patient, 516–17
condom catheter sheaths, 517
intermittent catheterization, 516
long-term catheterization, 516–17
hydronephrosis management, 522
incontinence in neuropathic patient, 518–19
causes, 518
empirical treatment, 518–19
investigations, 518
lower urinary tract (LUT), innervation of, 500–3
afferent innervation, 500–1
motor innervation, 500
sensory innervation of the urethra, 503
somatic motor innervation of urethral sphincter, 501
micturition, physiology of, 504–5
neuromodulation in lower urinary tract dysfunction, 528–9
posterior tibial nerve stimulation (PTNS), 529
sacral nerve stimulation (SNS), 528–9
recurrent urinary tract infections (UTIs), 520–1

causes, 520
history, 520
indications for treatment, 520
investigations, 520
management, 521
treatment, 520–1
storage and emptying problems, clinical consequences of, 508
high-pressure sphincter, 508
low-pressure sphincter, 508
urine storage, physiology of, 504
Neuropathic lower urinary tract, 508
high-pressure sphincter, 508
low-pressure sphincter, 508
Nifedipine, 390–1
Nitrites, 136
Nitrite testing, in urine, 36–7
Nitrofurantoin, 143–4, 145
Nocturia, 14–15
assessment of nocturic patient, 14–15
causes, 14
diagnostic approach, 14
management of, 100–1
and sleep apnea, 101
Nocturnal enuresis, 110–1, 568–9
Nocturnal penile tumescence testing, 488–9
Nocturnal polyuria, 14–15
management of, 100–1
treatment, 100–1
Non-bilharzial squamous cell carcinoma, 250
Nonexpanding retroperitoneal hematoma, 427
Nongonococcal urethritis (NGU), 141
Non-hereditary papillary RCC, 278–9
Noninfective hemorrhagic cystitis, 140
Non-neurogenic voiding dysfunction, 566–7
Nonpolyuric nocturia, 100
Nonpulsatile retroperitoneal hematoma, 427
Non-seminomatous germ cell tumors (NSGCT), 303
management of, 304–7

Nonsteroidal anti-inflammatory drug (NSAID), 390–1
Nonurological and urological flank pain, 18
N stage of prostate cancer, 207
Nück, canal of, 31
NWTSG (National Wilms Tumor Study Group), 328–9

O

Obstructive sleep apnea (OSA), 101
Ofloxacin, 162–3, 169
Oligospermia, 476
Oncocytoma, 188–9, 276
  pathology, 276
  presentation, 276
  investigations, 276
  treatment, 276
Oncogenes, 188–9
Open prostatectomy, 88–9
  complications, 89
  contraindications, 88
  indications, 88
  techniques
    suprapubic (transvesical), 88
    simple retropubic, 88–9
Open stone surgery, 383
Orchiectomy, 626–7
  anesthesia, 626
  postoperative care and common postoperative complications, 627
  procedure-specific consent form, 627
  radical, 626
  simple, 626
Orchitis, 22, 33, 163
Orthotopic neobladder, 266–8
Overactive bladder (OAB), 10–3, 20, 506–7
  definition, 122
  conventional treatment, 122
  failed conventional therapy, options for, 124–5
  intravesical pharmacotherapy, 124–5
  neuromodulation, 124
  surgery, 124
Overflow incontinence, 110–1
Oxybutynin, 82, 122, 511

P

p53, 190
Pacemakers, 602
Paclitaxel, 265
Painful bladder syndrome. See Interstitial cystitis (IC)
Palliative management of prostate cancer, 242–3
  anemia, thrombocytopenia, and coagulopathy, 243
  lower urinary tract symptoms, 242
  pain, 242
  unilateral ureteral obstruction, 242
  ureteral obstruction, 242
Palliative treatment, 263
  of locally advanced disease, 232
Papillary neoplasm of low malignant potential (PNLMP), 188–9
Papillary urothelial neoplasm of low malignant potential (PUNLMP), 250
Parapelvic cysts, 332–3
Paraphimosis, 182, 462
  definition and presentation, 462
  treatment, 462
Parasitic infections, 178–9
  genital filariasis, 179
  hydatid disease, 178
  schistosomiasis (bilharziasis), 178
Parastomal hernia formation, 641
Parenchymal transit time index (PTTI), 52–3
Parkinson disease (PD), bladder dysfunction in, 524
Partin tables, 208
PC-SPES, 244
Pediatric urology, 537–69
  abnormal sexual differentiation, 554–6
  cystic kidney disease, 558–9
  ectopic ureter, 546
  epispadias, 562
  exstrophy, 560–1
  hypospadias, 550–1
  nocturnal enuresis, 568–9
  non-neurogenic voiding dysfunction, 566–7
  normal sexual differentiation, 552–3
  posterior urethral valves, 564–5

undescended testes, 540–1
ureterocele, 548
ureteropelvic junction (UPJ) obstruction, 549
urinary tract, 538
  lower urinary tract, 538
  upper urinary tract, 538
urinary tract infection (UTI), 542–3
vesicoureteric reflux (VUR), 544–5
Pelvic floor exercises, 222–3
Pelvic fractures, 440–2
  abdominal and pelvic imaging in, 440
  and bladder injuries, 440–1
  catheterization, 440
  high-riding prostate, 442
  symptoms and signs of bladder or urethral injury in, 441–2
  urethral injuries, 441
Pelvic kidney, 348, 349
Pelvic lymphadenectomy, 261
Pelviureteric junction obstruction (PUJO), 17
Penetrating anterior urethral injuries, 452
Penetrating injuries, 420, 454
Penicillins, 534
Penis
  arteriography, 488–9
  disorders of, 182–3
    balanitis, 182
    paraphimosis, 182
    phimosis, 182
  injuries, 456–8
    amputation, 458
    fracture, 456
    knife and gunshot wounds, 458
    surgical repair of, 456–8
    treatment, 459
  neoplasia. See also Squamous cell carcinoma (SCC), of penis
    benign tumors and lesions, 310
    epidemiology, risk factors, and pathology, 314–16
    premalignant cutaneous lesions, 310–3
    viral-related lesions, 310
  prosthesis, 491
Pentosan polysulfate sodium, 174
Peptide growth factors, 188–9

Percutaneous nephrolithotomy (PCNL), 334, 380, 642–4
bleeding in, 429
complications and management, 642–4
indications, 642
outcomes, 644
postoperative management, 642
preoperative preparation, 642
procedure-specific consent form, 644
Periaqueductal gray matter (PAG), 504–5
Perinephric abscess, 150, 153
Peripheral neuropathies, 526
bladder dysfunction in, 526
Periurethral abscess, 164
Peyronie's disease, 494–5
Pfannenstiel, 628–9
pH, 36, 7
Phenoxybenzamine, 76
Phentolamine, 490
Phenylephrine, 497–8
Phimosis, 182
complications, 182
treatment, 182
Phosphatase and tensin homologue (PTEN), 188–9, 190
Phosphodiesterase type-5 (PDE) inhibitors, 490
Photoselective vaporization of the prostate (PVP), 87
Phytotherapy, 82
Plain abdominal radiography, uses of, 42
Plain CT scans, 50
Plain film, of IVP, 44
Plain-film imaging, 444–6
Plain radiography, 42
Plain tomography, 42
PLCO (Prostate Lung Colorectal and Ovarian) screening, 194
Plexopathies, 243
Pneumatic (ballistic) lithotripsy, 374
Polyruic patient, investigation of, 101
Polyuria, 14–15
Pontine micturition center (PMC), 504–5
Posterior tibial nerve stimulation (PTNS), in LUT dysfunction, 529
Posterior urethra, 106
Posterior urethral injuries in males, 448

Posterior urethral valves (PUV), 564–5
Post-micturition dribble, 110–1
Postoperative catheter displacement, 222
Post-prostatectomy incontinence, 128–9
evaluation, 128–9
incidence, 128
pathophysiology, 128
risk factors, 128
treatment, 129
Post-void residual urine volume, 58, 70
clinical usefulness of, 58
elevated residual urine volume, 58
interpretation and misinterpretation of, 58
Potassium (K$^+$) regulation, 665
Praziquantel, 178
Prazosin, 76
PREDICT study, 80–1
Prednisone, 240–1
Pregnancy, hydronephrosis of, 402
Pregnancy, urological problems in, 531–6
hydronephrosis, 536
physiological and anatomical changes, 532
biochemistry reference intervals, 533
in bladder, 532
in kidney, 532
urinary tract infection (UTI), 534
complications, 534
definition, 534
incidence, 534
pathogenesis, 534
risk factors, 534
screening tests, 534
treatment, 534
Pressure-flow studies, 60–1
Priapism, 23, 496–8
Primary testicular failure with testicular atrophy, 477–8
Primary urological neoplasms, 188–9
Pronephros, 538
Prophylactic lymphadenectomy, 319
Prophylaxis, efficacy of, 143
Proscar long-term efficacy and safety study (PLESS) study, 74–5, 78
Prostaglandin E$_1$, 490

Prostate cancer, advanced androgen-independent/castration-resistant disease, 240–1
castration-resistant prostate cancer, 241
cytotoxic chemotherapy, 240–1
second-line hormone therapy, 240
hormone therapy additional therapies, 238–9
androgen deprivation, mechanisms of, 234–6
early versus delayed hormone therapy, 238
hormone dependence of prostate cancer, 233
intermittent hormone therapy, 238
monitoring treatment, 238
prognostic factors, 233
Prostate cancer. See also Localized prostate cancer management
clinical presentation, 196
localized prostate cancer (T1–2), 196
locally advanced cancer (T3–4), 196
metastatic disease, 196
control, with radical prostatectomy, 224–5
epidemiology and etiology, 190–1
genetics, 190
hormonal influence, 190
risk factors, 190–1
grading, 212
hormone dependence of, 233
incidence, prevalence, and mortality, 192
incidence, 192
mortality, 192
prevalence, 192
and lower urinary tract symptoms (LUTS), 72
management of risk stratification in, 214
palliative management of, 242–3
premalignant lesions, 193
atypical small acinar proliferation (ASAP), 193
prostatic intraepithelial neoplasia (PIN), 193

prevention,
  complementary and
  alternative therapies,
  244–5
chemoprevention with
  antiandrogens, 245
dietary intervention, 244
and prostatic-specific
  antigen (PSA), 194
radical prostatectomy,
  218–20
staging, 206–8
  M stage, 208
  N stage, 207
  T stage, 206
transrectal ultrasonography
  (TRUS), 202–3
  with biopsy, 202
  without biopsy, 202
  biopsy protocol, 203
  prostatic biopsy,
    complications of, 203
Prostate Cancer Prevention
  Trial (PCPT), 80–1,
  198–9, 245
Prostate cancer screening
  counseling before, 195
  and prostatic-specific
    antigen (PSA), 194
Prostatic abscess, 170
Prostatic intraepithelial
  neoplasia (PIN), 193
Prostatic-specific antigen
  (PSA), 39
  derivatives
    density, 200
    doubling time (PSADT),
      200
    free-to-total (F:T) ratio,
      200
    velocity, 200
  indications for checking,
    39
  and prostate cancer,
    198–9
  and prostate cancer
    screening, 194
  and screening, 192
Prostatism, 10–3
Prostatism vs. LUTS vs.
  LUTS/BPH, 68
Prostatitis
  acute bacterial prostatitis,
    168
  asymptomatic
    inflammatory
    prostatitis, 169
  chronic bacterial
    prostatitis, 168–9
  chronic pelvic pain
    syndrome (CPPS), 169
  classification, 166
  epidemiology, 166

evaluation, 168
pathogenesis, 166
risk factors, 167
segmented urine cultures,
  167
Protein, in urine, 36
Proteus, 542
Proton beam therapy, 226–7
PSA doubling time
  (PSADT), 200
Pseudoephedrine, 492
Pseudoepitheliomatous
  micaceous, 310–3
Pseudomonas, 542
Psoas abscess, 31
Psoas hitch, 436
Pubovaginal slings, 118
  indications, 118
  outcomes, 118
  types, 118
Pulmonary embolus (PE),
  576–8
  diagnosis, 576–7
  prevention, 576
  risk factors for, 576
  treatment, 577–8
Pyelogram phase, of IVP, 44
Pyelonephritis, acute, 148–9,
  153
  differential diagnosis, 148
  investigation and
    treatment, 148–9
  pathogenesis and
    microbiology, 148
  risk factors, 148
Pyeloplasty, 650–1
  anesthesia, 650
  common postoperative
    complications and
    management, 650
  indications, 650
  postoperative care, 650
  procedure-specific
    consent form, 651
Pyonephrosis, 148–9,
  150, 153
Pyridoxine, 258–9
Pyuria, 134–5

Q

Queyrat, erythroplasia of,
  310–3
Quinolone, 520

R

Radiation Therapy
  Oncology Group
  (RTOG), 226–7
Radical and palliative
  radiotherapy, 263

Radical cystectomy, 636–8
  anesthesia, 636
  efficacy of, 262
  indications, 636
  partial cystectomy, 637
  postoperative care
    and common
    post-operative
    complications and
    management, 636–7
  procedure-specific
    consent form, 637–8
Radical external beam
  radiotherapy (EBRT),
  226–7, 263, 263
  complications, 263
  contraindications, 226
  indications, 226
  outcomes of, 227
  protocol, 226
  side effects, 226–7
  treatment of PSA relapse
    post-EBRT, 227
Radical orchiectomy, 298
Radical prostatectomy,
  218–20, 634–5
  anesthesia, 634
  common postoperative
    complications and
    management, 634–5
  complications of, 222–3
  indications, 634
  postoperative care, 634
  procedure-specific
    consent form, 635
  prostate cancer control
    with, 224–5
Radioisotope bone imaging,
  53
Radioisotope imaging, 52–3
  DMSA scanning, 53
  MAG3 renogram, 52–3
  radioisotope bone
    imaging, 53
Radiological assessment
  of renal masses. *See* Renal
    masses, radiological
    assessment
  of urinary tract, 40–1
    ultrasound, 40
    uses of, 40–1
Radiotherapy, 319
Reanastomosis, 107
Recurrent urinary tract
  infection, 134–5, 142–5
  bacterial persistence, 142
  management of, 142–5
  reinfections, 142–5
Red blood cell morphology,
  37
REDUCE trial, 80–1, 245
Referred pain, 16–19, 22
Renal adenocarcinoma, 38

Renal anatomy, 662–4
  renal blood flow (RBF), 662–3
  renal function 663–4
Renal arteriography, 274
Renal ascent and fusion, anomalies
  horseshoe kidney, 348, 349
  malrotation, 350, 351
  pelvic kidney, 348, 349
Renal blood flow (RBF), 662–3
Renal cell carcinoma
  active surveillance, 286
  epidemiology and etiology, 278–9
  histological classification, 280
  investigations, 284
  management of metastatic disease, 292–3
  pathology, 280
  presentation, 284
  prognosis, 280
  spread, 280
  staging, 280
  surgical treatment, 288–9
    immunotherapy, 292
    locally advanced RCC, 290
    local recurrence, treatment of, 290
    lymphadenectomy, 290
    metastatic RCC, 290
    molecular targeted therapies, 293
    palliative care, 293
    partial nephrectomy, 288–9
    postoperative follow-up, 289
    radical nephrectomy, 288
    surgery, 292
    tumor ablation therapy, 289
Renal duplication
  complications, 352
  definition, 352
  embryology, 352
  epidemiology, 352
  investigation, 353
  presentation, 352
  treatment, 353
Renal exploration, technique of, 427
Renal function 663–4
Renal masses, radiological assessment of, 274–5
  abdominal ultrasound, 274
  CT scan, 274
  fine needle aspiration/ needle biopsy, 274–5

Renal parenchymal disease, 4
Renal physiology
  acid–base balance, 666–7
  potassium regulation, 666
  renin–angiotensin– aldosterone system, 666
  sodium regulation, 665
  water balance, regulation of, 665
    antidiuretic hormone (ADH or vasopressin), 664
Renal trauma, 420
  classification, 420
    blunt injuries, 420
    penetrating injuries, 420
  clinical and radiological assessment, 422–4
  mechanism, 420
  staging, 423
  treatment, 426–9
    conservative (nonoperative) management, 426
    hypertension and renal injury, 429
    iatrogenic renal injury, 429
    surgical exploration, 426–9
    technique of renal exploration, 427
Renal tubular acidosis (RTA), 363, 367
Renal ultrasonography, 71, 152–3
Renin–angiotensin– aldosterone system, 666
Renogram, 52–3
Resection, 86–7
Retrograde ejaculation, 492
Retrograde pyelography, 6, 48
Retrograde urethrogram, technique of, 449, 453
Retroperitoneal fibrosis, 326–7
  benign causes, 326
  investigations, 326–7
  malignant causes, 326
  management, 327
  presentation, 326
Retroperitoneal lymph node dissection (RPLND), 306–7, 308–9
Retropubic procedure, stages in, 218–19
Retropubic suspension procedures, 117
  complications, 117
  surgery types, 117

Rhabdomyosarcoma, 321
Rifampicin, 258–9
Robinson catheter, 586, 587
Robotically assisted laparoscopic prostatectomy, stages in, 219–20

S

Sacral cord, MRI of, 93
Sacral nerve stimulation (SNS), in LUT dysfunction, 528–9
Sacral neuromodulation, 512
Salvage radical cystectomy, 261–2
Salvage radical prostatectomy, 227
Samarium-153, 242
Saphena varix, 30
Sarcomatoid, 280
Saw palmetto, 82
Schistosoma hematobium, 250
Schistosomiasis (bilharziasis), 178
Scrotal exploration for torsion and orchiopexy, 656–7
  fixation technique, 656
  indications, 656
  postoperative care and potential complications and their management, 657
  procedure-specific consent form, 657
  technique, 656
Scrotal pain, 22
Scrotal skin, carcinoma of, 34
Scrotum, carcinoma of, 320
Scrotum, lumps in. See Lumps in scrotum
Sebaceous cyst, 34
Secondary hypogonadism, 480
Secondary neoplasms, 188–9
Second-line hormone therapy, 240
SELECT Trial, 244
Self-start therapy, 145
Semen analysis, 472, 473
Seminoma, 33
  management, 308–9
Semi-rigid ureteroscopes, 646
Septicemia
  during PCNL, 642
  and urosepsis, 156–9
Serum creatinine, 70

Sexual differentiation, 552–3
abnormal, 554–6
normal, 552–3
Shy–Drager syndrome. See
Multiple system atrophy
(MSA)
Sildenafil (Viagra), 490
Silodosin, 76, 511
Simple retropubic approach,
88–9
SIOP (International Society
of Pediatric Oncology)
treatment, 328–9
Skeletal-related events
(SREs), 238–9
Sodium bicarbonate, 492
Sodium regulation, 666
Solifenacin, 122
Sorafenib, 293
South African star grass, 82
Spermatogenesis, 466, 467
Spermatozoon, 468
Sperm function tests, 472–4
Spermicides, avoidance
of, 143
Sphincter abnormalities,
112–13
Sphincter behavior in
patient with neurological
disease, 506–7
Sphincter electromyography
(EMG)
Sphincter weakness
incontinence, treatment
of
artificial urinary sphincter,
120–1
injection therapy, 116
pubovaginal slings, 118
retropubic suspension, 117
Spinal cord compression,
464
Spiral CT, 50
Spleen, enlarged
characteristics and causes
of, 24
Spongiofibrosis, excision
of, 107
Squamous cell carcinoma
(SCC), 250
of penis. See also Penis,
neoplasia
incidence and etiology,
314
investigations, 318
pathology and staging of
penile SCC, 314–16
presentation, 318
risk factors, 314
treatment, 318–19
Stab wound, 420
Staging of renal injury, 423
Staphylococcus epidermis, 542

Stenting after ureteroscopy,
646
Stents, 594–7, 595–7
indications and uses, 594
materials, 594
symptoms and
complications, 594–5
types, 594
Stereotactic body
radiotherapy (SBRT)
platforms, 226–7
Sterilization of urological
equipment, 604–5
autoclaving, 604
chemical sterilization, 604
Variant Creutzfeldt
Jacob disease (vCJD),
604–5
Stone disease, 355
bladder stones, 400
calcium oxalate stone
formation, prevention
of, 398–9
kidney stones
calcium oxalate, 362
calcium phosphate, 363
composition, 358
cystine, 364
dissolution therapy,
384–5
electrohydraulic
lithotripsy (EHL), 374
epidemiology, 356–7
evaluation, 366–7
extracorporeal
lithotripsy (ESWL),
372–3
flexible ureteroscopy
and laser treatment,
378–9
laser lithotripsy, 376
mechanisms of
formation, 360
open stone surgery, 383
percutaneous
nephrolithotomy
(PCNL), 380
pneumatic (ballistic)
lithotripsy, 374
presentation and
diagnosis, 368
struvite, 363
treatment options,
370–1
types and predisposing
factors, 358–9
ultrasonic lithotripsy,
374–5
uric acid, 362–3
watchful waiting, 370–1
ureteric stones
acute management,
390–1

diagnostic radiological
imaging, 388
indications for
intervention to
relieve obstruction
and/or remove the
stone, 392–3
management in
pregnancy, 422–4
presentation, 386–7
treatment, 394, 396–7
Storage and emptying
problems, clinical
consequences of, 508
high-pressure sphincter,
508
low-pressure sphincter,
508
Stress urinary incontinence
(SUI), 20, 110–1
significance, 20
Strontium-89, 242
Struvite, 363
Suction drains, 586, 588
Sunitinib, 293
Superficial UC management
adjuvant intravesical
chemotherapy and
BCG, 258–9
transurethral resection
of bladder tumor
(TURBT), 256
Sunitinib, 293
Superficial UC management
adjuvant intravesical
chemotherapy and
BCG, 258–9
transurethral resection
of bladder tumor
(TURBT), 256
Supra-12th rib incision, 629
Suprapubic catheterization,
88, 98–9
contraindications 98
indications, 98
suprapubic catheter (SPC),
516–17
technique, 98–9
Surveillance, active, 232
Surveillance protocol,
216–17
Systemic inflammatory
response syndrome
(SIRS), 156–9

T

Tadalafil (Cialis), 490
Tamsulosin, 76, 169, 390–1,
511
Taxanes, 265
99mTc-DMSA, 546
Telescopes and light
sources in urological
endoscopy, 606–7
Hopkins rod-lens system,
606
lighting, 606
Temsirolimus, 293
Teratoma, 33
Terazosin, 76, 169, 511

Testicular adnexa, tumors of, 321
adenomatoid tumors, 321
cystadenoma of epididymis, 321
mesothelioma, 321
paratesticular tumors, 321
Testicular appendages, 461
torsion of, 22
Testicular biopsy, 472–4, 476–7
Testicular cancer
clinical presentation, 296–8
differential diagnosis, 296
epidemiology and etiology, 294
incidence and mortality, 294
intratubular germ cell neoplasia (IGCN), 308
investigations, 296–8
lymphoma management, 309
metastatic germ cell cancer, prognostic staging system for, 303
nonseminomatous germ cell tumors (NSGCT), management of, 304–7
chemotherapy, 305–6
chemotherapy complications, 306
RPLND, 306–7
surveillance and follow-up after treatment, 306
pathology and staging, 300
seminoma, 308–9
serum markers, 299
cellular enzymes, 299
clinical use, 299
oncofetal proteins, 299
signs, 296
symptoms, 296
treatment, 298
Testicular injuries, 454
blunt trauma, testicular ultrasound in, 454
exploration in scrotal trauma, indications for, 454
history and examination, 454
mechanisms, 454
Testicular self-examination (TSE), 294
Testicular torsion, 22
definition, 460
history and examination, 460
differential diagnosis and investigations, 460

surgical management, 460–1
Testicular tumor, 22, 33
acute presentations of, 22–3
Testicular venous drainage, 478
Testis
gumma of, 33
undescended, 31
Testosterone, 64, 65, 466, 552
Tetracycline, 162–3
Third-generation cephalosporin, 520–1
Tissue transfer, 107
Tolterodine, 82, 122, 511
Transforming growth factors, 64
Transitional cell cancer/carcinoma (TCC), 6–7
of renal pelvis and ureter, 270–2
investigations, 270–1
pathology and staging, 270
presentation, 270
risk factors, 270–2
staging, 270–1
treatment and prognosis, 271–2
Transrectal ultrasonography (TRUS), 40, 70, 202–3
with biopsy, 202
without biopsy, 202
biopsy protocol, 203
prostatic biopsy, complications of, 203
Transureteroureterostomy, 434–5, 438
Transurethral electrovaporization of the prostate (TUVP), 86
Transurethral microwave thermotherapy (TUMT), 84–5
Transurethral radiofrequency needle ablation (TUNA) of the prostate, 84
Transurethral resection (TUR) syndrome, 583
Transurethral resection of bladder tumor (TURBT), 5, 254, 256, 260–2, 614–15
follow-up after, 256
indications, 614
operative and postoperative complications and their management, 614–15
postoperative care, 614

procedure-specific consent form, 615
transurethral fulguration, 256
Transurethral resection of ejaculatory ducts (TURED), 477–8
Transurethral resection of prostate (TURP), 70, 193, 203, 612–13
indications for, 88
invasive surgical alternatives to, 86–7
and open prostatectomy, 88–9
options to avoid, 94
risks and outcomes of, for retention, 94
surgical alternatives to, 84–5
Transurethral ultrasound-guided laser-induced prostatectomy (TULIP), 86
Transverse myelitis, 525–6
bladder dysfunction in, 525–6
Trial without catheter (TWOC), 94
Triamterene, 358–9
Tricyclics (amitriptyline), 122, 174
Trimethoprim, 143, 145, 520–1
Trimethoprim-sulfamethoxazole (TMP-SMZ), 169
Trospium chloride, 82, 122
T stages of prostate cancer, 206, 207
Tube drains, 586
Tuberculosis, 176–7
investigations, 177
pathogenesis, 176
presentation, 176
treatment 177
Tuberculous epididymo-orchitis, 33
Tuberous sclerosis, 558
Tumor suppressor genes, 188–9

U

UK National Institute for Clinical Excellence, 84
Ultrasonic lithotripsy, 374–5
Ultrasonography (US), 6
Ultrasound, 40
uses of, 40–1
bladder, 40
prostate, 40
renal, 40

testes, 40–1
urethra, 40
Umbilical cyst/sinus, 25
Umbilicus, 25
  causes of, 25
Uncomplicated urinary tract
  infection, 134–5, 138
Undescended testes, 540–1
Unilateral obstruction, 463
Unilateral obstruction of a
  ureter (UUO), 414
Unilateral ureteral
  obstruction, 242
Unresolved infection, 134–5
Upper tract filling, 5
Upper tract imaging study, 6
Upper tract obstruction
  ureteric strictures
    (other than UPJO),
    management of, 410–2
  ureter innervation, 417
  urinary tract obstruction,
    pathophysiology of,
    414–15
  urine flow from kidneys
    to bladder, physiology
    of, 416
Urachal abnormalities, 26
Ureteral injuries
  and bladder injuries, 440–1
  diagnosis
    of external injury, 432
    of iatrogenic injury, 432
    intraoperative diagnosis,
      432
    postoperative diagnosis,
      432
  management, 434–5
  pelvic fractures,
    association with, 441
  symptoms and signs, 433
  symptoms and signs in
    pelvic fracture, 441–2
  types, causes, and
    mechanisms, 432
Ureteral obstruction, 242
Ureteric dilatation, 646
Ureteric stones
  acute management, 390–1
  diagnostic radiological
    imaging, 388
  indications for
    intervention to relieve
    obstruction and/or
    remove the stone,
    392–3
  management in pregnancy,
    422–4
  pain, 16
  presentation, 386–7
  treatment, 394, 396–7
Ureteric strictures, 410–2
  causes, 410

definition, 410
iatrogenic, 410
investigations, 410
treatment options, 410–2
ureteroenteric strictures,
  412
Ureter innervation, 417
  afferent, 417
  autonomic, 417
Ureterocele, 548
Ureteropelvic junction
  (UPJ), 416
Ureteropelvic junction
  (UPJ) obstruction, 549.
  See also Pelviureteric
  junction obstruction
  (PUJO)
  definition, 346–7
  epidemiology, 346
  etiology, 346
  investigation, 346
  presentation, 346
  treatment
    pyeloplasty, 347
    surgery, 347
Ureteroscopes and
  ureteroscopy, 646–9
  complications, 646
  instruments, 646
  laser lithotripsy, 646
  patient position, 646
  procedure-specific
    consent form, 646
  stenting after
    ureteroscopy, 646
  technique of flexible
    ureteroscopy and
    laser treatment for
    intrarenal stones, 646
  ureteric dilatation, 646
  ureteroscopic irrigation
    system, 646
Ureteroscopic irrigation
  system, 646
Ureterosigmoidostomy,
  266, 268
Urethra, physiology of, 660
Urethra, sensory innervation
  of, 503
Urethral cancer, 322–4
  differential diagnosis, 322
  investigations, 322
  pathology and staging, 322
  presentation, 322
  risk factors, 322
  staging, 324
  treatment, 323–4
Urethral catheterization,
  94, 96–7
  indications, 96
  technique, 96–7
Urethral dilatation, 107
Urethral injuries

associated with pelvic
  fractures, 440–2
in females, 448
Urethral sphincter, somatic
  motor innervation
  of, 501
Urethral stricture disease,
  106–7
  anterior urethra, 106
  balanitis xerotica
    obliterans (BXO), 107
  management, 106
  posterior urethra, 106
  symptoms and signs, 106
  treatment options, 107
Urethral syndrome, 141
Urethritis, 140–1
Urethrography, 48
Urge urinary incontinence
  (UUI), 20, 110–1
  significance, 20
Uric acid, 362–3
Urinary diversion, 513
Urinary extravasation, 426
Urinary incontinence in
  adults, 20–1. See also
  Incontinence
  bed wetting, 21
  definitions, 20
  diagnosis and
    management, 21
  significance, 20
  total incontinence, 21
Urinary retention, acute
  causes, 91
    in men, 90
    in women, 91
  definition, 90
  definitive management
    in men, 94
    in women, 94
  initial management, 94
  pathophysiology, 90
  postoperative retention,
    risk factors for, 91
  transurethral resection of
    the prostate (TURP)
    options to avoid, 94
    risks and outcomes of,
      for retention, 94
Urinary retention, 72–3,
  242
Urinary tract, 538
  lower urinary tract, 538
  radiological imaging of,
    40–1
  upper urinary tract, 538
Urinary tract infection
  (UTI), 5
  antimicrobial drug therapy,
    146
  bacterial resistance to
    drug therapy, 146

bacterial virulence, factors increasing, 138–9
complicated, 134–5, 138
complications, 534
definition, 134–5, 534
definitive treatment, 146–7
host defenses, 139
in children, 542–3
incidence, 135, 534
in pregnancy, 534
investigations, 135–7
pathogenesis, 534
recurrent, 520–1
    causes, 520
    history, 520
    indications for treatment, 520
    investigations, 520
    management, 521
    treatment, 520–1
    risk factors, 534
route of infection, 138
screening tests, 534
treatment, 534
uncomplicated, 138
Urinary tract obstruction, pathophysiology of, 414–15
Urine culture and collection, 136–7
Urine cytology, 38
Urine dipsticks test, 2, 135–6
Urine examination, 36–7
dipstick testing, 36–7
urine microscopy, 37
Urine flow from kidneys to bladder, physiology of, 416
Urine flow rate, interpretation and misinterpretation of, 54
Urine microscopy, 37, 136
casts, 37
crystals, 37
red blood cell morphology, 37
Urine storage, physiology of, 504
Uroflowmetry, 54–6
low flow, 54–6
urine flow rate, interpretation and misinterpretation of, 54
Urolithiasis, 16
Urological and nonurological flank pain, 18
Urological contrast studies, 48
cystography, 48
ileal loopogram, 48

retrograde pyelography, 48
urethrography, 48
voiding cystourethrography (VCUG), 48
Urological eponyms, 669–72
Urological incisions, 628–9
complications, 629
lower midline, extraperitoneal, 628
midline, transperitoneal, 628
Pfannenstiel, 628–9
supra-12th rib incision, 629
Urological investigations
computed tomography (CT), 50
    uses, 50
cystometry, 60–1
intravenous pyelography (IVP), 44–6
magnetic resonance imaging (MRI), uses of, 50–1
plain abdominal radiography, uses of, 42
post-void residual urine volume measurement, 58
pressure-flow studies, 60–1
prostatic specific antigen (PSA), 39
radioisotope imaging, 52–3
radiological imaging of the urinary tract, 40–1
urine cytology, 38
urine examination, 36–7
uroflowmetry, 54–6
urological contrast studies, 48
videocystometry, 60–1
Urological surgery and equipment, 571–657
antibiotic prophylaxis, 574
catheters and drains, 584–6
circumcision, 618–19
complications, 576–8
consent, 608–9
cystoscopy, 610–11
diathermy, 601–3
endoscopic cystolitholapaxy and (open) cystolithotomy, 654
fluid balance and management of shock, 580–1
guide wires, 590–1

hydrocele and epididymal cyst removal, 620–1
ileal conduit, 640–1
irrigating fluids and techniques of bladder washout, 592
JJ stents, 594–7, 630–1
laparoscopic surgery, 652–3
lasers, 598–600
nephrectomy and nephroureterectomy, 632–3
nesbit procedure, 622
optical urethrotomy, 616
orchiectomy, 626–7
patient preparation, 572
patient safety in operating room, 582
percutaneous nephrolithotomy (PCNL), 642–4
pyeloplasty, 650–1
radical cystectomy, 636–8
radical prostatectomy, 634–5
scrotal exploration for torsion and orchiopexy, 656–7
sterilization of urological equipment, 604–5
telescopes and light sources in urological endoscopy, 606–7
transurethral resection (TUR) syndrome, 583
transurethral resection of bladder tumor (TURBT), 614–15
transurethral resection of prostate (TURP), 612–13
ureteroscopes and ureteroscopy, 646–9
urological incisions, 628–9
vasectomy and vasovasostomy, 624–5
Urological symptoms and signs
abdominal examination in urological disease, 24–5
digital rectal examination (DRE), 28–9
flank pain, 16–19
genital symptoms, 22–3
hematospermia, 8–9
hematuria I, 2
hematuria II, 4–7
lower urinary tract symptoms (LUTS), 10–3
lumps in groin, 30–1

lumps in scrotum, 32–4
nocturia, 14–15
urinary incontinence in
  adults, 20–1
Urosepsis, 156–9
  causes, 156
  empirical antibiotic
    recommendations for
    treatment of, 158–9
  investigations, 157
  management, 157
  treatment, 157–8
Urothelial carcinoma, 5,
  248–50
Uroxatral, 390–1

V

VAC (vacuum-assisted
  closure) dressing,
  160–1
Vacuum erection device,
  490–1
Vagino-obturator shelf/
  paravaginal repair, 117
Valsalva leak point pressure
  (VLPP), 21, 115
Valsalva maneuver, 266–8
Vaporization, 86–7
Vardenafil (Levitra), 490
Variant Creutzfeldt Jacob
  disease (vCJD), 604–5
Varicocele, 33, 478–80
Vascular endothelial growth
  factor (VEGF), 278–9
Vasectomy, 624–5
Vasopressin. See
  Antidiuretic hormone
  (ADH)

Vasovasostomy, 624, 625
Venous thromboembolism
  (VTE), 576–8
  prevention, 578
Vesicourachal diverticulum,
  25
Vesicoureteric reflux
  (VUR), 544–5
  in adults
    associated disorders,
      342
    classification, 342
    investigation, 343
    management, 343–4
    pathophysiology, 342
    presentation, 343
    secondary reflux, 344,
      345
Vesicovaginal fistula (VVF),
  130–1
  etiology, 130
  examination, 130
  management, 130
  surgery, 130–1
  symptoms, 130
Veterans Affairs
  Combination Therapy
  Study, 80–1
Videocystometry, 60–1
Visual laser ablation of the
  prostate (VLAP), 86
Voiding cystourethrography
  (VCUG), 48, 546
Voiding dysfunction
  major, 566
  mild, 566
  moderate, 566
Von Hippel–Lindau (VHL)
  syndrome, 278–9, 558

W

Wag artifact, 54
Warfarin, 577–8
Wasson study of watchful
  waiting vs. TURP, 74–5
Watchful waiting, 216–17,
  232, 370–1, 390–1
Water intake, 357
White blood cells, in
  urine, 36
Wilms tumor, 188–9, 328–9
  pathology and staging, 328
  presentation, 328
  investigations, 328
  treatment and prognosis,
    328–9

X

Xanthine, 358–9
Xanthogranulomatous
  pyelonephritis, 152–3
X-ray appearance of stones,
  358

Y

YAG (yttrium aluminum
  garnet) laser, 598–600
Yogurt, 144
Yolk sac tumor, 33

Z

ZD4054, 241
Zipper injuries, 459
Zoledronic acid, 238–9